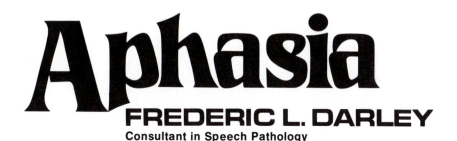

Aphasia

FREDERIC L. DARLEY
Consultant in Speech Pathology
Mayo Clinic

W. B. SAUNDERS COMPANY

Philadelphia London Toronto Mexico City
Rio de Janeiro Sydney Tokyo

W. B. Saunders Company: West Washington Square
Philadelphia, PA 19105

1 St. Anne's Road
Eastbourne, East Sussex BN21 3UN, England

1 Goldthorne Avenue
Toronto, Ontario M8Z 5T9, Canada

Apartado 26370—Cedro 512
Mexico 4, D.F., Mexico

Rua Coronel Cabrita, 8
Sao Cristovao Caixa Postal 21176
Rio de Janeiro, Brazil

9 Waltham Street
Artarmon, N.S.W. 2064, Australia

Ichibancho, Central Bldg., 22-1 Ichibancho
Chiyoda-Ku, Tokyo 102, Japan

Library of Congress Cataloging in Publication Data		
Darley, Frederic L.		
Aphasia.		
1. Aphasia. I. Title.		
RC425.D37	616.85'52	81–40739
ISBN 0-7216-2879-6	AACR2	

APHASIA   ISBN   0-7216-2879-6

Last digit is the print number: 9   8   7   6   5   4   3   2

Dedicated
to the memory of
Hildred Schuell

PREFACE

In the last act of *Love's Labour's Lost*, Berowne's courtship of Rosaline is not consummated but ends in a bargain to be fulfilled in a year and a day. Rosaline, intent on improving Berowne's character and tempering his too-sharp, victimizing wit, imposes terms—"without the which I am not to be won":

"You shall this twelvemonth term, from day to day,

Visit the *speechless sick*; and your task shall be

To enforce the pained impotent to smile."

Berowne can't believe his ears:

"To move wild laughter in the throat of death?

It cannot be; it is impossible."

But with no recourse, he agrees:

"A twelvemonth! Well, befall what will befall,

I'll jest a twelvemonth in a hospital."*

So Berowne promises that he will devote himself, his clever use of language, and his wit to make the speechless sick laugh—and in the doing of it he will learn a greater commitment to people other than himself.

His duty for a year and a day was prescribed by his lady love. The duty of speech-language pathologists treating aphasic patients is not prescribed by anyone else. It is self-prescribed—for a professional lifetime. The duty to which Berowne was committed was to make the speechless sick smile and laugh. Speech-language pathologists have an even harder task: to help them regain their power to listen and speak, to read and write—a duty requiring monumental dedication.

This book is addressed primarily to speech-language pathologists and other professionals whose responsibility it is to understand, appraise the capabilities of, and treat patients with acquired aphasia. With this intended audience, the decision about what to put in and what to leave out of a book on aphasia is simplified. Persons engaged in the rehabilitation of aphasic patients need to know the domain of aphasia and its boundaries, how to recognize it when one hears and sees it, and how to differentiate it from disorders that in some respects may resemble it but which require different treatment or warrant no

---

*William Shakespeare, *Love's Labour's Lost*, Act V, Scene II, lines 856–861, 863–864, 878–879 (emphasis in line 858 added).

treatment; how to measure the scope and the degree of a patient's language impairment; how to make a reasoned judgment about the probable outcome of the disorder—what to expect from treatment generally and from treatment of a given patient; how to develop and carry out a treatment plan tailored to individual patient needs; and how to ensure that what is done with a patient is maximally effective in getting into the patient's brain and modifying his behavior. What is less important, and is here omitted—although certainly interesting—includes a review of the history of aphasia and related disorders, a catalogue of theories about alleged typologies of aphasia, and a detailed review of anatomic-behavioral correlation in the area of language. Further, professional workers can do with fewer concepts that are essentially intuitive in their derivation; they need more empirically derived, data-oriented information about what aphasia is, the low-order laws that govern its variability, and what works in alleviating it.

This book, then, summarizes what the clinical worker needs to know so that he or she can confidently approach patients who need help, communicate empathically with them, and engage in relevant activities designed to increase the efficiency of their language processing. A great body of information is now extant on these issues. First-hand knowledge of these data can help clinicians do a professional job that goes beyond the exercise of an art to the efficient application of scientific knowledge. We all owe a debt to the hundreds of clinician-investigators who have shared with us what they have learned, and to the thousands of patients who have helped clinicians learn what aphasia is all about.

FREDERIC L. DARLEY

CONTENTS

1 • **APHASIA WITHOUT ADJECTIVES**............................... 1

How Aphasic Patients Perform................................. 3
The First Distinction: Aphasia Is Not a Speech Problem..... 8
The Second Distinction: Aphasia Is Language-Specific...... 22
The Third Distinction: Aphasia Is Not Modality-Bound....... 28
The Domain of Aphasia...................................... 41
Resolution of the Classification Problem........................ 47

2 • **APPRAISAL AND PREDICTION** 55

Purposes of Language Appraisal..................................... 55
What to Look for in the Appraisal of Aphasia 61
Tests for Evaluation of Aphasia.................................... 79
Guiding Principles in Aphasia Evaluation........................ 82
Predictions Based upon Appraisal Data 85

3 • **THE NATURAL HISTORY OF APHASIA** 110

The Period of Spontaneous Recovery............................. 110
Changing Profiles of Recovery.. 116
Prognostic Factors Related to Recovery 127

4 • **THE EFFECT OF TREATMENT** 144

Studies Without No-Treatment Control Groups................ 145
Studies Using No-Treatment Control Groups.................... 157
Individual Case Studies.. 163
Additional Testimony 175
Conclusions.. 175

5 • MAXIMIZING INPUT AND OUTPUT 186

The Arousal Power of the Stimulus 188
The Role of Cues, Context, and Redundancy.................... 197
Syntactic and Semantic Complexity............................... 204
Avoiding Information Overload.. 208
Selection of Input Modality.. 211
Variations in the Time Dimension.................................. 214
Scheduling of Stimuli Presentation 221
Situational Factors 224
The Content of Therapy 225
Other Facilitators of Output... 228
The Importance of Attitude.. 231

6 • THE TREATMENT PROGRAM 237

Where to Begin: Improving Input Processing.................... 239
Moving On: Expressive Tasks 251
Working with High-Level Patients 256
General Principles in Treatment..................................... 260
Special Management Procedures 264
The Family: Patient/Clinician 270

Index... 279

1 · APHASIA WITHOUT ADJECTIVES

Introduction
How Aphasic Patients Perform
    Auditory comprehension
    Reading
    Speaking
    Writing
    Gesture
    Effect on multiple languages
    Residual language competence
The First Distinction: Aphasia Is Not a
        Speech Problem
    Dysarthria
    Apraxia of speech
        Articulation errors not typical of
        aphasia
        Errors not attributable to impaired
        auditory perception
        Selective impairment possible
        Data from instrumental analysis of
        speech
The Second Distinction: Aphasia Is
        Language-Specific
    Dementia
    Confused language
    Emotional disturbance
    Akinetic mutism
The Third Distinction: Aphasia Is Not
        Modality-Bound
    The Wepman Model
    The Brown Model
        Central language process
        Motor speech programmer
        The speech effectors
    Clinical data supporting the models
    Non–aphasias:
        Apraxia of speech
        Word deafness
        Alexia without agraphia
The Domain of Aphasia
Resolution of the Classification Problem
References

"L'aphasie est une."

PIERRE MARIE

The concept of *aphasia* cannot readily be encompassed or its scope and its limits made explicit within a single phrase or a sentence. Dictionaries try to do it. *Dorland's Illustrated Medical Dictionary* (1981) defines aphasia as "Defect or loss of the power of expression by speech, writing, or signs, or of comprehending spoken or written language, due to injury or disease of the brain centers." This definition suggests a spectrum of disorders of both input and output attributable

1

to cerebral dysfunction. For *dysphasia,* commonly used to refer to a lesser degree of severity of the same problem, this dictionary supplies a quite different definition: "Impairment of speech, consisting in lack of coordination and failure to arrange words in the proper order, due to a central lesion" implicating only the speaking modality and seeming to suggest some type of motor dysfunction in the term "lack of coordination."

Stedman's Medical Dictionary (1976) defines aphasia as follows: "Logagnosia; logamnesia, logasthenia; impaired or absent communication by speech, writing, or signs, due to dysfunction of brain centers in the dominant hemisphere." This definition appears to implicate primarily expressive modalities, an emphasis also found in the definition of *dysphasia:* "Lack of coordination in speech, and failure to arrange words in an understandable way; related to cortical damage."

Such definitions suggest no clear basis for differentiating aphasia from other kinds of communication disorders and supply no practical limits for the person interested in appropriate management of the disorder. Aphasia does not designate some general dysfunction in communication. Not all disordered communication is aphasia. The term "aphasia" should refer to a specific, definable entity (1) with recognized features differentiable from the features of other communication disorders, (2) with agreed upon limits, and (3) approachable in rehabilitation in a coherent manner with a rationale of demonstrable validity. In our consideration of aphasia we are concerned in part with nomenclatural problems, for the domain of aphasiology is littered with an incredibly diverse terminology, which often obscures communication among those involved in the management of patients. But we are also importantly concerned with daily clinical challenges of differential diagnosis and clarification of boundaries between communication disorders, which are not always clear-cut.

The problem does not relate to etiology. The cause of the problem may be vascular (impaired blood flow because of embolus, thrombosis, or hemorrhage), traumatic (contusions or lacerations of variable origin), neoplastic (space-occupying growths that impinge on cortical tissue, destroy it, or interrupt blood flow to it), infectious or inflammatory (abscess, meningitis, encephalitis), or surgical (harm to brain tissue incidental to some surgical procedure). Whatever the etiology, the symptoms are the same and result from interference with the function of the circuitry crucial to communication. Our concern is with the specific changes in communication that resulted from the insult to the brain.

Our goal is to develop a description of the domain that is reasonably embraced by the term aphasia and to sift through the terminology in order to arrive at a group of words that can designate entities precisely. We need nomenclature that clarifies boundaries between disorders, suggests the differential dynamics for the disorders, and can be used without the necessity for some intervening step of explanation.

HOW APHASIC PATIENTS PERFORM

As a first step we will consider the scope of aphasic patients' language difficulties.

Auditory Comprehension. The inefficiency of aphasic patients in listening may make them seem at times as if they were hard of hearing. Severely aphasic patients may not be able to recognize single spoken words; they cannot select the appropriate object or picture when told the name of it, a difficulty variably designated "word deafness," "auditory imperception," and "auditory verbal agnosia" (Schuell, 1953). Even if they can recognize a single word, they may in the absence of that stimulus be unable to evoke the auditory image of it and need to have it repeated before they can again respond meaningfully, a problem that Schuell called "impairment of reauditorization" (Schuell, 1954). They may confuse words that are closely associated in meaning or similar in sound, or their difficulties may be random and they indicate that they "don't know" the word (Schuell and Jenkins, 1961b). Problems of word recognition are evidenced in conversational difficulties and confirmed in performance on vocabulary tests (Schuell et al., 1961). Difficulties not only are evidenced in appreciating the denotation of words (the relationship between the word and its referent) but also extend to reduced appreciation of the connotations of words (Gardner and Denes, 1973). Less severely aphasic patients may display less difficulty in recognizing and appreciating the meaning of single words but will likely have difficulty in comprehending sentences (DeRenzi and Vignolo, 1962; Parisi and Pizzamiglio, 1970; Shewan and Canter, 1971; Waller and Darley, 1979). The longer the sentences and the greater their complexity in terms of vocabulary level and syntactic structure, the greater the difficulty. Listening to paragraph-length material, aphasic patients lose details, and in retelling such narratives, they omit mention of salient points (Waller and Darley, 1978). Comprehension is limited by the unfailing presence of a restriction of auditory retention span. Whether asked to repeat series of syllables, words, digits, letters, or sentences or point to a series of objects or pictures in response to spoken instructions, aphasic patients show that they cannot retain, order, and recall sequences as long as they used to be able to (Schuell, 1953; Albert, 1972; Brookshire, 1972, 1975; Flowers, 1975). They sometimes say that they cannot "listen fast enough." They only partially execute two- or three-step commands and make more errors when required to process increasing numbers of bits of information (DeRenzi and Vignolo, 1962). They invariably need more processing time. Patterns of auditory impairment vary from patient to patient (Brookshire, 1978), although patients may display more than one pattern. Some show primarily a *retention deficit*, performing more poorly as messages increase in length. Some show an *information capacity deficit*, being unable simultaneously to receive and process input, therefore missing parts of messages. Some are hindered by *noise buildup*, performing more poorly from the beginning to the end of the input, while others show *slow rise time*, missing initial parts but comprehending later parts of the input. Some seem to fade in and out in understanding input because of *intermittent auditory imperception*.

Reading. Visual recognition of printed words is impaired in severe cases, aphasic patients making errors in matching words to pictures or objects (Schuell and Jenkins, 1961b). The single word in isolation may look unfamiliar and somehow "wrong." Confronted with sentences, patients may struggle through a sentence word by word, misreading words and not appreciating their errors, failing to recognize the identity of certain words, and failing also to derive the meaning from the syntactic structure of the sentence. When they have finished their word-by-word struggle, their grasp of the meaning may have evaporated and they must struggle through it again. When they try to cope with material of greater length and complexity, problems parallel to those experienced in listening appear; they overlook or fail to retain details when they answer questions about the material or try to recount it.

Speaking. When aphasic patients attempt to speak, words elude them. Problems in retrieving specific words from the lexicon are evident in many ways. When they try to name familiar objects or pictures their responses may be slowed, they may fail to evoke the correct word, they may substitute a word related to the target word in any of several ways, they may produce an unrelated word, or they may be unable to produce any word (Schuell and Jenkins, 1961b; Geschwind, 1967; Ettlinger and Moffett, 1970; Rochford, 1971). Regardless of the sensory modality through which the stimulus object is presented — visual, olfactory, tactile, or auditory presentation of its characteristic sounds — the naming difficulty persists (Goodglass et al., 1968), and "noise" and distraction in the environment increase the difficulty (Winchester and Hartman, 1955). Not only do aphasic patients have trouble with such *convergent* semantic behavior (selecting and producing a specific word linked to the stimulus), but they demonstrate as well impairment of *divergent* semantic behavior. That is, when they engage in a broad search of memory storage in order to proliferate ideas and produce a flow of related words — for example, all the words they can think of beginning with a given letter or lists of categorical items like animals or things people eat — they demonstrate restriction of flow and flexibility in word retrieval, quickly depleting their "reservoir of associations" (Chapey et al., 1976, 1977; Birbaumer et al., 1972). They may use various strategies to help themselves in word retrieval: delay (taking or asking for additional time), semantic association (producing opposites, in-class associations, part-whole associations, or serially related items), phonetic association (producing some other phonetically related word), description (explaining what they are trying to say), or generalization (using some general "empty" word in place of the desired word) (Marshall, 1976).

Even if they display little difficulty in retrieving specific words (so-called anomia), the speech they produce in conversation is characterized by a reduced variety of vocabulary; they use fewer different words than normal subjects do in a sample of any given size (Howes, 1964). Not only do nouns occur less frequently, as might be suggested by the misnomer anomia, but also words of other grammatical classes show decreased use, aphasic patients retaining the more frequently occurring words of the language and failing to employ those used less frequently (Wepman et al., 1956).

They have difficulty repeating what they hear, particularly as the input becomes longer and more complex (Brown, 1975). They can no longer spell words aloud as well as they used to (Thurston, 1954; Noll and Hoops, 1967).

When they try to formulate and express ideas orally, aphasic patients may verbally beat around the bush without coming to the point satisfactorily, they may settle for an abbreviated, disjointed statement that lacks details and precision, or they may produce overly long, redundant responses. Their problem in retrieving specific words and organizing them into precise sentences is obvious. They produce their sentences more slowly, and they produce fewer content units per minute than they used to or than normal subjects do (Yorkston and Beukelman, 1980). Their sentences show not only restricted use of vocabulary but also restricted use of various grammatical sentence types; they use fewer optional transformations than normals and do not use syntactic transformations that add words to the sentence; their syntactically correct sentences still show reduced semantic specificity (Schuell et al., 1969). Their arrangement of words into sentences may be defective, and their use of inflectional morphemes may also be limited, these features of syntax and morphology sometimes appearing to be impaired independently (Goodglass and Berko, 1960).

Some patients manage no more than a telegraphic kind of speech, producing primarily substantive words with omission of function words, whereas other patients are relatively unable to produce the substantive words. Still other patients with severe impairment of auditory comprehension may produce a continuous flow of meaningless jargon or fluent speech full of neologisms, seemingly unaware that they are not communicating and even denying that they have a communication difficulty. This copious flow of speech may be largely unintelligible but it resembles the mother tongue by retaining its typical prosodic and some syntactic aspects. Associated euphoria, denial of illness, and other aspects of personality and adjustment suggest a possible anosognosic aspect to this specific language behavior (Kinsbourne and Warrington, 1963; Weinstein et al., 1966; Kertesz and Benson, 1970; Weinstein and Lyerly, 1976).

Writing. When they try to write, aphasic patients may forget how words should look and may be confused as to how to form certain letters. In writing words to dictation, they may produce association errors ("home" for "house"), distort or reverse letter forms, confuse letters with similar visual configurations, substitute words that sound like the given word, or omit or substitute letters (Schuell and Jenkins, 1961b; Boone and Friedman, 1976). They may make numerous efforts at self-correction, often unsuccessfully. Spelling performance in writing demonstrates a predictable and orderly breakdown, patients having increased difficulty as words increase in length and decrease in frequency of usage (Bricker et al., 1964).

In writing sentences spontaneously or to dictation, in addition to the misspelling or distortion of words, the intended meaning may be altered by wrong word choice or word omission, or the resulting group of words may be only nonsense, conveying no message (Keenan, 1971; Keenan and Brassell, 1972). Less impaired patients' spontaneous writing may be sparse and produced more slowly than average, with evidence of self-corrected errors.

Gesture. Aphasic patients show reduced appreciation of the meaning of gesture and pantomime (Duffy et al., 1975; Gainotti and Lemmo, 1976). They are likewise impaired in ability to communicate meaning through pantomime and gesture (Goodglass and Kaplan, 1963; Schlanger et al., 1974).

Effect on Multiple Languages. When aphasic patients are bilingual or proficient in several languages, they demonstrate the same impairments in all languages they speak, although perhaps to different degrees (Lambert and Fillenbaum, 1959; Charlton, 1964; Watamori and Sasanuma, 1976, 1978; Voinescu et al., 1977).

Residual Language Competence. When globally aphasic patients demonstrate very severe impairment in all modalities, one might conclude that they have lost all language competence. Studies have demonstrated, however, that despite severe language handicap, aphasic patients retain some language capacities to an unexpected degree. For example, they show recognition that a foreign language they hear is not their native language; they can discriminate between nonsense (jabberwocky) and meaningful language (Boller and Green, 1972). They retain an appreciation of the relationship of stress to meaning, for they can differentiate nouns from verbs (con'vict versus convict') where the differentiating characteristic is stress (Blumstein and Goodglass, 1972).

When presented with an assortment of grammatical sentences and ungrammatical sentences containing violations of syntax or semantic structure or both, they make few errors in sentence evaluation, rarely evaluating grammatical sentences as being ungrammatical. "Aphasics' knowledge of the grammatical form of function words and morphological endings does not appear to have been significantly altered. . . . Some aspects of linguistic competence may still be functioning adequately in aphasia" (Bliss et al., 1976a). Although sometimes they are unable to evoke the name of something, they demonstrate the "tip-of-the-tongue" effect noted in normal subjects (Goodglass et al., 1976). A high percentage of the time they can guess the correct initial letter of the intended word, the number of syllables it has, and the relative size of the word (big, medium, small): "For many of these aphasics, the unnamed target word is present in some 'schematic' form somewhere in the linguistic system. . . . Some representation of that word must be resonating in the internal dictionary in order to allow these generic properties to be 'read off.' . . . An aphasic's inability to name an object may only reflect an inability to bring these generic properties into a linguistic 'gestalt' " (Barton, 1971). Asked to repeat grammatical and ungrammatical sentences, they repeat correctly more grammatical than ungrammatical sentences; these results suggest that "aphasics are to some extent guided by greater residual linguistic knowledge or competence than might be inferred from their spontaneous production" (Bliss et al., 1976b). Globally aphasic patients have been taught alternative modes of communication, suggesting that central language processing is still possible at some level. Glass and co-workers (1973) reported that seven globally aphasic patients despite gross deficits in natural language learned an artificial language system using cut-out paper symbols for words. "Despite massive language loss, globally aphasic patients retain a rich contextual system and at least some capacity for symbolization and primitive linguistic functions. . . . Aphasia may impair symbolization but even in global aphasia the capacity for using symbols is not totally abolished." Gardner and co-workers (1976) taught a visual communication system to eight aphasic patients with little or no ability to communicate using natural language. The system involved the use of cards carrying simple geometric or ideographic forms denoting meaningful units. Patients learned to use this system with various levels of achievement; some were able to carry out commands, answer questions, and describe actions; others went further in using the system to express desires and feelings. "Evidence suggests that some severely aphasic patients can master the basics of an alternate symbol system. Moreover, several indices suggest that the communication consequences of the system are appreciated, and that at least some of the cognitive operations entailed in natural language persist despite severe aphasia."

Now that we have described the scope of aphasic patients' language dysfunction, we can proceed to determine how this cluster of behaviors can be differentiated from other neuropathologic disorders of communication. We will make three distinctions, which collectively supply us with necessary concepts and nomenclature.

THE FIRST DISTINCTION: APHASIA IS NOT A SPEECH PROBLEM

Aphasia is a language problem, not a speech problem. It is not the result of difficulties in either the programming or the execution of certain muscular movements. It does not relate to any dysfunction in the basic motor speech processes, the mechanics of exteriorizing ideas through speech. Rather, it has to do with how efficiently one processes the symbolic code that constitutes language. The term aphasia designates an impairment of one's ability to decode (interpret) and encode (formulate) conventional meaningful linguistic units, that is, morphemes and larger syntactic units — phrases, clauses, sentences. The aphasic patient has some degree of difficulty interpreting the language he or she receives (hears or reads) and formulating and expressing coded language (speaking, writing, gesturing) despite normal sensation and normal functioning of the musculature of the oral mechanism and the limbs.

The first distinction leads us to segregate aphasia from two kinds of motor speech disorders: the dysarthrias and apraxia of speech.

Dysarthria. Patients who display dysarthria alone have no trouble dealing with the symbolic code. They read and understand words, can answer questions about what they have read, write appropriate answers, and speak appropriate words — but they do not speak them efficiently, for they have incurred a lesion of the central or peripheral nervous system that causes slowness, weakness, incoordination, or alteration of tone of the muscles used in speech. The result is some impairment in any or all of the following basic motor speech processes:

1. Respiration, which provides the raw material for speech. The patient may have inadequate breath support for speech, may "run out of breath." He or she may try to speak with insufficient lung volume and make effortful grunts at the ends of phrases. Inhalation may be audible (stridor), or there may be episodes of forced inhalation and exhalation.

2. Phonation, the breath stream setting into vibration the adducted vocal folds. Phonation may be interrupted by unwarranted stoppages. The pitch of the voice may be inappropriately high or more usually inappropriately low, and there may be pitch breaks. There may be monotony in pitch usage, or sometimes an evident vocal tremor. The overall loudness level of the voice may be inadequate, or there may be a

progressive deterioration of loudness as speech proceeds. In some cases there may be marked monotony of loudness, in other cases excessive variations in loudness level. The quality of the voice may be impaired, sometimes being harsh, at other times breathy, sometimes hoarse (a combination of both harshness and breathiness), sometimes characterized by a distinctive strained-strangled sound.

3. Resonance, the selective amplification of the vocal tone by the pharynx, oral cavity, and nasal cavities. The voice may be characterized by an excessive degree of nasal resonance (hypernasality), and there may be nasal emission of air, which is audible or noted when a mirror is held beneath the nares and becomes clouded. Both conditions result from palatopharyngeal incompetence.

4. Articulation, the breath stream being shaped into phonemes (speech sounds) through impedances produced by the tongue, teeth, and lips. Articulation may be imprecise, with breakdowns sometimes occurring irregularly, but oftentimes consistently. Speech sounds may be slighted, elided, or omitted; there may be voicing errors. Phonemes may be prolonged or they may be repeated. Not only consonants but also vowels may be imperfectly produced. The greater the impairment of articulation, the more likely will intelligibility be impaired.

5. Prosody, the grouping of rapidly sequenced sounds into words strung together into phrases at different rates, with variations in time, pitch, and loudness that accomplish emphasis, lend interest to speech, and characterize individual and dialectal modes of expression. Rate may be slowed overall, or there may be acceleration of rate during contextual speech, or rates may be variable; sometimes speech is produced in short rushes. Phrases may be unusually short because of air wastage due to inefficient valving of the breath stream at the glottis or the palatopharyngeal sphincter, or both. Syllable and word stress may be reduced overall or may be equalized, with excess stress on usually unstressed words and syllables.

These aberrations of speech typically occur in certain clusters resulting from impairment of given portions of the total motor system. It is possible to recognize distinctive patterns of dysarthria. These have been identified as flaccid (lower motor neuron impairment), spastic (bilateral upper motor neuron impairment), ataxic (cerebellar dysfunction), hypokinetic (extrapyramidal problems seen in parkinsonism), hyperkinetic (resulting from a variety of extrapyramidal movement disorders), and mixed (Darley et al., 1969a, 1969b, 1975).

In dysarthria, the patient's *speech* is disturbed because there is impaired innervation of muscles responsible for speech execution. As a result, the breath stream is not properly shaped by the series of musculoskeletal valves that constitute the speech apparatus. But all these problems occur later in the process of language formulation and relate strictly to the exteriorization of language through the modality of speech. The patient with dysarthria is not aphasic.

Apraxia of Speech. Another type of patient with impaired speech is like the dysarthric patient in that he or she demonstrates good command of the symbol system. But this type of patient has trouble speaking because of a cerebral lesion that prevents his executing voluntarily and on command the complex motor activities involved in speaking, despite the fact that muscle strength is undiminished. The disorder in this case is designated an apraxia of speech. As he speaks, the patient appears uncertain as to how to position his articulators correctly. He visibly and perhaps audibly gropes to produce correct articulatory postures and to accomplish sequences of these postures in forming words. His articulation is frequently off-target. He often, indeed usually, recognizes that he is off-target, and he tries to correct the error, often effortfully. His errors recur nonetheless, but they are not always the same; the errors on a series of trials may be highly variable. As the speaker tries to avoid error by carefully and deliberately programming his muscle movements, he may slow down, space his words and syllables evenly, and stress them evenly; as a result, the prosody of his speech as well as his articulation is altered to some degree.

The orderliness and predictability of certain aspects of apraxic speech have been demonstrated in a series of studies:

1. Articulatory errors increase as the complexity of motor adjustment required of the articulators increases. Vowels evoke fewer errors than singleton consonants. Of the singleton consonants, affricative and fricative phonemes evoke the most errors. Most difficult of all are consonant clusters (Shankweiler and Harris, 1966; Johns and Darley, 1970; Deal and Darley, 1972; Trost and Canter, 1974; LaPointe and Johns, 1975; Dunlop and Marquardt, 1977; Burns and Canter, 1977). Palatal and dental phonemes are significantly more susceptible to error than other phonemes classified according to place of production (LaPointe and Johns, 1975). Repetition of a single consonant such as /puh/, /tuh/, or /kuh/ is ordinarily accomplished more easily than repetition of the sequence /puh-tuh-kuh/ (Rosenbek et al., 1973); on the latter task the patient is typically unable to maintain the correct sequence, even when he is repeatedly given a model to imitate.

2. There is some evidence that initial consonants tend to be misarticulated more often than consonant phonemes in other positions (Shankweiler and Harris, 1966; Hecaen, 1972; Trost and Canter, 1974). Burns and Canter (1977) found that five patients with conduction aphasia and five with Wernicke's aphasia (mostly with posterior lesions) made what they called phonemic paraphasic errors more frequently in the final than in the initial position of words. However, Johns and Darley (1970) reported that in patients with apraxia of speech "no single position in the word emerged as characteristically more difficult"; LaPointe and Johns (1975) found error percentages for initial, medial, and final positions to be nearly equal; and Dunlop and Marquardt (1977) found phoneme position unrelated to occurrence of error.

3. On repeated readings of the same material, patients with apraxia of speech demonstate a consistency effect, tending to make errors at the same loci from trial to trial; they also demonstrate some adaptation effect, tending to make fewer errors on successive readings (Deal, 1974). The amount of reduction of errors is not great, and it is variable from subject to subject.

4. Phonemes occurring with relatively high frequency in the language tend to be more accurately articulated than phonemes which occur less frequently (Trost and Canter, 1974).

5. Analysis of substitution errors made by apraxic patients according to the system of distinctive features indicates that the errors are variably related to the target sounds. Trost and Canter (1974), using a four-factor system, found that approximately 88 per cent of the errors were one- or two-feature errors, most of the rest being three-feature errors. Slightly over half of the place errors observed were off-target by one place, but about one third were off by two places. Errors according to manner of production (degree of oral articulatory constriction) tended to be off to a greater extent: 46 per cent of the errors were two degrees off, 31 per cent were one degree off, 11 per cent were three degrees off, and 12 per cent were four degrees off. Martin and Rigrodsky (1974) found that more than 60 per cent of the errors were either one or two features away from target; they believed that "the high degree of similarity between the error and the desired phoneme . . . is not a haphazard occurrence of errors. . . . They are related to the stimuli . . . and may be reflective of either perceptual problems or memory decay." LaPointe and Johns (1975) determined whether the substitutions made by their 13 apraxic patients were errors of placement, manner, or voicing, or combinations of these; they found that 38 per cent of the errors were defective in two or more features and "bore little acoustic resemblance to the target sound."

6. When errors made by apraxic patients are analyzed with regard to sequential aspects, three types of error are observed: anticipatory (prepositioning), reiterative (postpositioning), and metathesis (the order of two phonemes being reversed) (LaPointe and Johns, 1975). All 13 subjects in LaPointe and Johns' study produced some sequential errors, but the percentage of such errors relative to the total number of substitution and initiation errors was small (7 per cent). Anticipatory errors outnumbered reiterative errors by a ratio of 6:1; metathesis of phonemes occurred rarely. Burns and Canter (1977) found more errors of phoneme sequencing among their "posterior" conduction aphasic patients and Wernicke's aphasic patients than Trost and Canter (1974) did among their "anterior" Broca's aphasic patients.

7. Apraxic patients display a marked discrepancy between their relatively good performance on automatic and reactive speech productions and their relatively poor volitional-purposive speech performance. "Words and phrases highly organized by practice and usage tend to sound normal" (Schuell et al., 1964). Such islands of fluent,

well-articulated speech appear in conversation, punctuated by episodes of effortful, off-target groping.

8. Imitative responses tend to be characterized by more articulatory errors than does spontaneous speech production. This holds true for single monosyllabic words as well as for material of greater length and complexity. Some patients display remarkably long latencies between the presentation of a stimulus word and their repetition of it (Schuell et al., 1964; Johns and Darley, 1970; Trost, 1970).

9. Articulation errors increase as length of word increases. As the patient produces a series of words with increasing number of syllables (door, doorknob, doorkeeper, dormitory), more errors are noted in the longer words. Such errors typically occur in the syllable common to all of the words, not just in the added syllables (Johns and Darley, 1970).

10. In oral reading of contextual material, articulatory errors do not occur at random; they are more frequent on words that carry linguistic or psychologic "weight" and that are more essential for communication (Deal and Darley, 1972). Words have been assigned weights on the basis of four characteristics: grammatical class (noun, adjective, adverb, verb); difficulty of initial phoneme (affricative, fricative, or consonant cluster); position in the sentence (one of the first three words); and word length (more than five letters long). Thus, a word weighted 4 would be a noun, adjective, adverb, or verb more than five letters long, beginning with an affricative, fricative, or consonant cluster, occurring as one of the first three words of the sentence. The combination of word length and grammatical class has been found to be an especially important determinant of the loci of errors. The difficulty level of initial phonemes also has a particularly negative effect on articulatory accuracy when combined with grammatical class. Grammatical class alone has not been found to be significantly related to occurrence of error (Deal and Darley, 1972; Dunlop and Marquardt, 1977). In general, when the complexity of a required response is increased, more errors occur. Any single characteristic may be insufficient to elicit error, but if characteristics are combined, their joint effect may be powerful enough to induce inaccuracies.

11. Correctness of articulation is influenced by mode of stimulus presentation (Johns and Darley, 1970; Trost and Canter, 1974). Patients tend to articulate more accurately when speech stimuli are presented by a visible examiner (auditory-visual mode) than when they imitate a stimulus presented by tape recorder (auditory mode) or spontaneously produce a word printed on a card (visual mode).

12. Attainment of the correct articulatory target is facilitated more by repeated trials of a word than by increase in the number of stimulus presentations (Johns and Darley, 1970). Patients are more likely to be on-target if they are given a model once and have three opportunities to imitate it than if they are permitted a single trial or are given three presentations of a model but only one trial to imitate it.

13. Accuracy of articulation in apraxic patients is not significantly influenced by a number of auditory, visual, and psychologic variables:

a. When patients perform a task under two conditions, one while observing themselves in the mirror and the other without such visual monitoring, the difference in the number of errors they produce is not statistically significant (Deal and Darley, 1972). Apparently patients with apraxia of speech cannot use the information derived from visual monitoring, at least without specific instructions as to how and why this information should be used.

b. Introduction of masking noise that prevents patients from hearing their own speech does not significantly alter the number of articulation errors they make (Deal and Darley, 1972).

c. Articulatory performance is not improved when the patient is given an opportunity to delay an imitative response (Deal and Darley, 1972). In three conditions of enforced latency (no delay in repetition after presentation of stimulus, 3-second delay, and 6-second delay), apraxic speakers displayed no significant differences in articulatory accuracy.

d. Articulatory accuracy is not influenced by the instructional set created in the speaker (Deal and Darley, 1972). Patients do equally well (or poorly) in reading passages whether told that the passage is extremely easy, that it is loaded with hard words and phonemes and is extremely difficult, or that the degree of difficulty is unknown.

e. Incidence of errors is not significantly influenced by imposing upon the patient's speech an external auditory rhythm (Shane and Darley, 1978). When rhythmic auditory stimulation provided by a metronome was imposed at each subject's own oral reading rate as well as at 75 per cent and 125 per cent of this rate, articulatory accuracy did not significantly improve.

The apraxic patient's problem is not dysarthria, for on neurologic examination one finds no significant evidence of slowness, weakness, incoordination, or alteration of tone of the speech musculature; furthermore, whereas in dysarthria all of the basic motor processes are variably involved, in apraxia of speech the continuing impairment is specifically articulatory, with prosodic alterations at times following as probably compensatory phenomena. At the onset of the problem, the patient may experience difficulty initiating phonation at will, but once this difficulty passes, as it usually does in a few days, phonation and resonance are normal and articulation stands out as primarily deviant, with some involvement of prosody. Furthermore, whereas in dysarthria the articulatory errors are characteristically errors of simplification (distortions and omissions), in apraxia of speech these errors are supplemented by a preponderance of errors that must be considered complications of speech (substitutions of other phonemes, additions of phonemes, substitutions of a consonant cluster for a single consonant, repetitions of phonemes, and prolongations of phonemes).

The apraxic speaker also shows that the difficulty in articulation is not a problem in the processing of meaningful linguistic units. When he has trouble articulating a given word, he gives clear evidence that his trouble is not in word finding. He demonstrates by his repeated trials that he has the word clearly in mind. He may be able to write it, and he answers correctly when asked to choose from among a group of words the word he is trying to say. His problem involves the processing not of the meaning-bearing elements of language but rather of non-meaningful elements, the programming of the elemental speech postures and their sequences.

Apraxia of speech can occur in relatively pure form. The pattern of apraxic patients' performance in the various language modalities on a test battery reveals that speaking performance is significantly worse than performance in listening, reading, and writing. This disproportionate difficulty is commonly observed in clinical testing and has been documented in a group investigation summarized here.

In order to discern what patterns of communication impairment differentiate groups of patients having different neurogenic disorders of communication, Halpern and co-workers (1973) and DiSimoni and associates (1977) administered a standard language examination to five groups of patients. The groups studied by Halpern and collaborators represented aphasia, generalized intellectual impairment (dementia), confused language, and apraxia of speech. DiSimoni and his co-workers studied chronic schizophrenic patients.

The 10 patients assigned to each of the four groups studied by the Halpern group met criteria for these designations following complete neurologic examination, including tests of mental status and language performance. The language examination contained 21 subtests, which yielded scores on the following six functional categories: auditory retention span (three subtests), auditory comprehension (five), reading comprehension (six), naming (one), writing words to dictation (one), and arithmetic (two). Three subtests (defining seven words, explaining three proverbs, and telling three things every good citizen should do) required oral expression of ideas; error criteria were established to permit quantitative scoring of the responses in terms of four categories: syntax (errors included use of improper grammatical inflection and addition of, deletion of, or substitution for syntactic words); adequacy (erroneous responses included substitution, deletion, and addition of substantive words; the degree of elaboration of the response also entered into the judgment of adequacy); relevance (errors were bizarre responses that appeared unrelated to the stimulus without apparent awareness of error or attempt to self-correct); and fluency (errors included excessive hesitation and sparseness in responses).

In all 10 categories, responses were evaluated on a percentage-of-error basis so that comparison could be made of performances tested by different numbers of items. Descriptive terms were then applied to ranges of percentages according to the Sklar Aphasia Scale (Sklar, 1966): 0 to 10 per cent was considered no impairment; 11 to 30 per cent, mild impairment; 31 to 60 per cent, moderate impairment; 61 to 90 per cent, severe impairment; and 91 to 100 per cent, total or global impairment.

Table 1–1 presents the rank order of the percentages of impairment of the 10 language categories for all five groups studied. Five categories, given in italics, tended to differentiate the groups (reading comprehension, auditory retention span, fluency, writing to dictation, and relevance). Impairments in the other five categories (auditory comprehension, adequacy, arithmetic, naming, and syntax) did not differentiate the groups. Auditory comprehension occupied a central position in the rank order of each of the groups and in every group fell near the mean; therefore, it served as a kind of standard reference point.

Considering the group of patients with aphasia, it can be seen that they showed impairment in all 10 language categories — moderate in six of them, mild in four. Even the mild impairments, however, tended toward the moderate range, and the overall rating (mean, 31) was in that range. The aphasic group showed moderate impairment with regard to adequacy, auditory retention, arithmetic, auditory comprehension, fluency, and naming. Relevance and writing to dictation were least impaired, adequacy and auditory retention span most impaired. Auditory retention span stood out as particularly impaired in aphasia, less so in the other disorders.

Considering the group with apraxia of speech, these subjects showed mild impairment in seven categories, normal performance in three. The overall rating (mean, 14) fell in the lower portion of the mild range. This finding of only mild impairment of overall language functions indicates that apraxia of speech is a disorder of something other than language. Except for arithmetic, only aspects of oral expression of ideas (adequacy, fluency, and syntax) were more than slightly impaired. The prominence of impairment of fluency is a characteristic that distinguishes the apraxia of speech group from the other groups. Most of their errors in fluency were in pausing and hesitating. The groping for articulatory placement and the patient's repeated efforts to produce words correctly appeared to cause lack of fluency.

It was precisely this observation of disproportionate impairment of speaking in two patients that led Broca (1861) to posit the impairment of a separate "faculty." He recognized that some patients suffer impairment of the "general faculty of language," which he called *verbal amnesia*; but to account for the behavior of his patients, he suggested impairment of an additional faculty, the "faculty of articulated language," which he called *aphemia*. "What they have lost, then, is not the faculty of language, it is not memory for words, nor is it the activity of nerves and muscles of phonation in articulation; it is

Table 1-1 Rank Order of Percentages of Impairment of 10 Language Categories for Five Groups of Patients Studied by Halpern and Associates (1973) and DiSimoni and Co-workers (1977) (Categories Listed in Italics Best Differentiate the Five Groups)

Rank Order	Aphasia (%)	General Intellectual Impairment (%)	Apraxia of Speech (%)	Confused Language (%)	Schizophrenia (%)
1	Adequacy, 43	Adequacy, 45	Adequacy, 30	Arithmetic, 54	Relevance, 45
2	*Auditory Retention,* 42	*Reading Comprehension,* 41	Fluency, 22	*Reading Comprehension,* 47	Arithmetic, 42
3	Arithmetic, 36	Arithmetic, 40	Arithmetic, 21	*Writing to Dictation,* 44	*Reading Comprehension,* 22
4		Auditory Comprehension, 29	Syntax, 20	Relevance, 40	*Fluency,* 17
4½	Auditory Comprehension, 33 / *Fluency,* 33				
5		*Auditory Retention,* 18		Adequacy, 28	Auditory Comprehension, 13
5½			Auditory Comprehension, 13 / *Writing to Dictation,* 13		
6	Naming, 31	Naming, 16		Auditory Comprehension, 24	*Auditory Retention,* 10
7	Syntax, 27	Syntax, 11	*Auditory Retention,* 11	Syntax, 21	*Writing to Dictation,* 9
8	*Reading Comprehension,* 24		Naming, 7	Naming, 19	*Adequacy,* 6
8½		*Relevance,* 10 / *Writing to Dictation,* 10			
9	*Writing to Dictation,* 21		*Reading Comprehension,* 6	*Auditory Retention,* 17	Naming, 3
10	*Relevance,* 18	*Fluency,* 9	*Relevance,* 2	*Fluency,* 14	Syntax, 2
Mean	31	22	14	28	17

*Adequacy is italicized in this group as it differentiates schizophrenia from the other four disorders.

From DiSimoni, F. G., Darley, F. L., and Aronson, A. E.: Patterns of dysfunction in schizophrenic patients on an aphasia test battery. J. Speech Hearing Disord., 42:498–513, 1977.

something else, it is a particular faculty . . . for coordinating the proper movements of articulated language, or more simply the faculty of articulated language since without it articulation is not possible."

The notion continues to be advanced, nevertheless, that these articulatory phenomena, which we consider to constitute an independent problem and which we designate apraxia of speech, are a manifestation of impairment of *language* processing, therefore a form of aphasia. The hypothesis is that this language impairment is at the phonologic level (Martin and Rigrodsky, 1974). This point of view is also reflected in the terminology often applied to the articulatory errors — *phonemic* or *literal paraphasias*. It is suggested that the patient who makes these errors is making faulty selection of intended phonemes rather than incorrectly programming the production of correctly selected phonemes. It is posited that his articulatory behavior is simply "part of the disruption of an entire system" (Martin, 1974). Several lines of evidence discount this notion.

Articulation Errors Not Typical of Aphasia. If there were indeed a "hierarchical interdependence of all speech events on virtually all levels of analysis, from muscle ordering to word and phrase ordering" (Lenneberg, 1967), we would expect that all patients who show some impairment of internalized linguistic rule structure (aphasic patients) would display it with regard to phoneme selection and combination. But the obvious fact that faces anyone who works with a spectrum of patients with cerebral damage is that *not all* aphasic patients display phonologic impairment. Halpern and co-workers (1976) studied 30 adult aphasic patients, none of whom demonstrated dysarthria, and none of whom displayed the kind of inconsistently off-target articulatory errors described in the preceding paragraphs. These patients were presented with a test of phoneme production in one- and two-syllable words, the words to be repeated after an auditory stimulus and spoken spontaneously in response to printed stimuli; a sample of conversational speech lasting from 3 to 5 minutes was also elicited. Phonemic errors occurred on only 2 per cent of the target phonemes in the articulation test, and 28 of the 30 subjects made no articulation errors during the sample of spontaneous speech obtained.

It is only *some* aphasic patients who display articulatory impairment, and the separateness of this disorder from their aphasia has been remarked by several investigators. Bay (1964) in a study of what he called "80 unselected aphasic patients" reported a distinct subgroup: "A well-defined and frequent group of speech disorders is marked by a distinct apraxia of the articulatory muscles and impaired tongue movements. . . . These patients show practically no receptive disorders but a uniform disturbance of the expressive speech performances." In various publications, Bay has reiterated his conviction that it is "a motor disorder independent of language, and we must distinguish this motor disorder from the linguistic disorders which we call aphasia."

Similarly, Wepman and associates (1960) reported encountering in clinical practice "patients who had little or no difficulty formulating concepts into words, despite apraxic and dysarthric language efforts." They recognized a modality-bound, nonsymbolic problem requiring differentiation from aphasic problems of symbolic formulation. Similarly, Schuell and co-workers (1964) found a group of aphasic patients with a condition designated minor syndrome B, whose speech was hesitant and labored, with many articulatory errors, usually without auditory problems except mild reduction of auditory retention span. "Phoneme discrimination appeared adequate, but this did not prevent articulatory errors. Intensive auditory stimulation increased vocabulary and retention span but did not improve articulation." They further stated that what helped patients with minor syndrome B was not intensive auditory stimulation but "facilitation by means of strong rhythmic drill on consonants and consonant blends, first in nonsense syllables, then in various positions and combinations in words, phrases, and sentences."

Errors Not Attributable to Impaired Auditory Perception. There is no support in the literature for the idea that the errors made by apraxic patients are attributable to impairment of auditory perception of phonemes, conceivably causing phonemic selection errors. Shankweiler and Harris (1966), who studied the phonemic production of five apraxic patients, reported the performance of four of these patients on a test of speech perception. Each patient listened to a tape recording of three 75-word lists of real word monosyllables; he encircled each word he heard in a set of five possible matches for that word, all foils being closely related to the target word. Two patients performed as well on this test as normal controls; one of these showed the greatest impairment of articulation of all five members of the group. "This dissociation strongly confirms the impression that severe phonetic disintegration can occur independently of impaired recognition of speech sounds." The two other patients performed less well for reasons that were not clear, possibly because of reading impairment, but the errors they made in perception were unrelated to the errors they made in production.

Johns and Darley (1970) also tested the auditory perception of their 10 apraxic patients. The patients listened to a recording of 60 monosyllabic words (30 nonsense, 30 real) and circled each as found in a closed-response set of acoustically and orthographically similar words printed on an answer sheet. The apraxic group attained a mean of 92 per cent correct identification on the total list of words, 98 per cent correct on the real words.

Aten and co-workers (1971) explored the auditory perceptual skills of this same group of patients further. Meaningful two- and three-word minimally varied auditory sequences were presented to the subjects, who responded by pointing to appropriate pictures sequentially on a sheet containing up to six foils, ruling out correct response by chance.

Four apraxic subjects made inferior scores, three made intermediate scores, and three scored within the range established by matched normal subjects.

Square (1981) contrasted the performances of 4 "pure" apraxic patients, 10 aphasic patients without apraxia of speech, 10 aphasic patients who were also apraxic, and 10 normal control subjects on a comprehensive battery of perceptual tests. Seven tests measured speech discrimination, four tested temporal ordering of auditory stimuli, and three tested internal or self-initiated speech discrimination. She found that her "pure" apraxic subjects performed most like the normal control subjects on all tasks, whereas patients who were aphasic (whether demonstrating an associated apraxia of speech or not) performed significantly less well on the tasks. The data clearly point to a motor programming disability on the part of the apraxic patients rather than a phonemic selection disorder as an explanation for their articulatory production difficulties.

Data are in agreement that severe articulatory impairment can occur independently of and in the absence of impaired perception of speech sounds measured in a variety of ways.

Selective Impairment Possible. The reasonableness of the idea of isolated, selective impairment of the mechanism for programming articulatory movements independently of other aspects of communication is supported by both neurophysiologic theory and clinical data. Darley and associates (1975) have proposed a neurophysiologic model of communication that presents an interconnected, interrelated, and interdependent system divisible into successive levels of complexity: the lower motor neuron level, the vestibular-reticular level, the upper motor neuron level, the cerebellar level, the conceptual-programming level, and the integrative-formulation level. It is well known that the various dysarthrias result from selective impairment of the lower motor neuron level, the vestibular-reticular level, the upper motor neuron level, and the cerebellar level. The existence of oral encoding difficulties in the absence of significant phonologic decoding problems, aphasia, or dysarthria strongly suggests that a separate system subserving motor programming exists — the conceptual-programming level. Such a system may be interrelated with language and muscle movements but retains a function independent of them. Breakdown is conceivable at this as well as at any of the other levels.

Moving from theory to clinical data, the independence of apraxia of speech from aphasia has been confirmed by the work of Mohr and colleagues (1978). They studied the lesions in 20 cases observed since 1972, documented by autopsy, computed tomography, or arteriogram, and reviewed autopsy records from Massachusetts General Hospital for a 20 year period as well as published cases since 1820. They concluded that infarction of Broca's area, long thought to be the critical area related to motor or Broca's aphasia, does not cause Broca's aphasia:

The infarction affecting the Broca area and its immediate environs, even deep into the brain, causes a mutism that is replaced by a rapidly improving dyspraxic and effortful articulation, but ... no significant disturbance in language function persists. The more complex syndrome traditionally referred to as Broca aphasia ... is characterized by protracted mutism, verbal stereotypes, and agrammatism. . . . [It] results from a large infarct in the sylvian region, encompassing much of the operculum, insula, and subjacent white matter in the territory of the upper division of the middle cerebral artery serving the dominant ... cerebral hemisphere. Clinically, the syndrome is the late development of an initially more profound total aphasia.

Data from Instrumental Analysis of Speech.   Several laboratory studies using a variety of instrumental techniques are in agreement in supporting a motor programming as opposed to a phonemic selection basis for apraxia of speech. Shankweiler and co-workers (1968) reported on the articulatory performance of two apraxic patients and used electromyographic recordings to study the activity of their lips, tongue, and mandible during speech. They report that even though certain articulations were wrong, they could be identified as the intended sound. Electromyographic data from one of the patients, the less severely affected one, indicated that he had the correct labial phoneme targets in mind in articulating certain words, although his productions were defective, more so in the initial position than in the terminal position.

Itoh and co-workers (1979) reported on fiberscopic observations of velar movements during speech of a patient diagnosed as having "a relatively 'isolated' form of apraxia of speech." Repeated utterances of the same word showed a marked variability in the patterns of velar movements; despite such variability, the general successional pattern of velar gestures for a given phonetic context approximated the normal pattern. "This result seems to indicate that the observed variation in the pattern of velar movements and the resultant phonetic change do not stem from a selection or retrieval error of a target phoneme in the process of speech production, namely, an error of phonological processing. . . . We assume that this type of behavior in the apraxic patient is indicative of a 'motor' impairment or of difficulty in the process of programming 'the positioning of speech musculature.'. . . Although it is hazardous to generalize on the basis of a single case, these observations seem to indicate that an articulatory disorder distinct from dysarthria can occur as a discrete motor impairment, which seems to be a reflection of faulty programming of the speech musculature and thus fits well within the generic term 'apraxia of speech.'. . . It is concluded that the mechanism responsible for the organization (or reorganization) of neural commands and for the time programming of articulators in this patient is not functioning appropriately, resulting in an articulatory disorder, for which the term or concept of apraxia of speech is appropriate and that this type of disorder can occur independently of a phonological impairment."

Itoh and associates (1980) studied the temporal organization of articulatory movements in a patient diagnosed as having an "isolated" apraxia of speech using pellet tracking techniques with an x-ray microbeam system. Whereas the movement patterns of the apraxic patient in the repetition of the monosyllable /pa/ were as regular as those of a normal subject, the temporal organization among different articulators was sometimes disturbed in the production of a meaningful Japanese word. "This finding seems to indicate that the motor programming for the temporal organization of different articulators becomes difficult in apraxia of speech under certain conditions, resulting in inconsistent articulation errors. . . . These results seem to offer additional support for our view (1) that an articulatory disorder due to brain damage, which is distinct from both aphasia and dysarthria, can occur as a discrete motor impairment reflecting faulty programming of the speech musculature and (2) that the term apraxia of speech is appropriate for describing such a disorder."

Itoh and associates (1979) analyzed wide-band spectrograms made from recordings of four young normal subjects, four aged normal subjects, and four subjects with apraxia of speech, reading a list of 100 Japanese monosyllables. Their focus of attention was voice-onset time (VOT) as related to supraglottal articulatory adjustments. They found that the patterns of VOT in the apraxic subjects were markedly different from those displayed by the normal subjects, a difference also reported by Freeman and co-workers (1978) in one apraxic subject; by Blumstein and colleagues (1977) in a group of "anterior aphasics"; and by Blumstein and collaborators (1980) in four patients with Broca's aphasia and four with conduction aphasia. "This result can be interpreted to indicate that the control over the timing of laryngeal and supralaryngeal articulatory events is disturbed in this subject group. . . . The findings of our previous studies examining the movements of the articulators during speech in an apraxic patient allow us to conclude that inconsistent articulatory errors, which were the major characteristics of apraxic speech, could be attributable to an impairment of time programming for the appropriate phoneme rather than to a defect in selecting an appropriate phoneme. The present results seem to offer additional support for such a view."

We conclude this discussion of the first distinction to be made by reiterating that both dysarthria and apraxia of speech can occur in association with a true language disorder. Apraxia of speech is often, indeed usually, observed to coexist with aphasia. When they occur together, the combination is often called motor aphasia or Broca's aphasia, but our contention is that the articulatory disorder is not an integral part of the aphasia. The aphasic patient who displays apraxic speech errors has two disorders, each of which requires independent treatment with different rationales and procedures.

THE SECOND DISTINCTION: APHASIA IS
LANGUAGE-SPECIFIC

The aphasic patient's difficulty is in the processing of the language code, however received or expressed, whether by listening, reading, speaking, writing, or gesturing, and this dysfunction is disproportionate to dysfunction in other cognitive areas.

That is not to say that aphasic patients show no cognitive dysfunction. Neuropsychologic studies reveal various perceptual and cognitive impairments. Investigators have shown, for example, that their abstract thinking, as tested by the Weigl Sorting Test, is impaired (DeRenzi et al., 1966). More than other brain-damaged individuals they show impaired recognition of meaningful environmental sounds and noises (Spinnler and Vignolo, 1966). They show deficits in knowledge of the body schema, ability to locate embedded geometric figures, solving of complex visual problems, and map-reading and pathfinding (Weinstein, 1964). They are slower and make more errors than nonaphasic subjects in other visual discrimination tasks (Rosenberg and Edwards, 1964). They perform less well than nonaphasic brain-damaged subjects on various tests of cognitive function, including the Raven's Coloured Progressive Matrices, sorting tests, and block design tests (Archibald et al., 1967).

Scattered reports suggest that aphasic patients do no more poorly than nonaphasic subjects on tasks involving "thinking" and problem solving (Meyers, 1952–53) and that patients tested psychometrically prior to neurosurgery (with normal language) and again following neurosurgery (now severely aphasic) show no loss of intellectual performance (Lebrun and Hoops, 1976). But a number of investigations have indicated that on standard intelligence tests aphasic patients earn IQ scores that are depressed in comparison with their expected premorbid intelligence or with the performance of subjects with comparable school achievement (Wepman, 1951; Welman, 1964; Caceres and Maurtua, 1968; Van Dongen et al., 1972; Orgass et al., 1972). Since intelligence and language are so interwoven, it is not appropriate to conclude that aphasic patients with depressed IQs have suffered a loss of intelligence. Members of a conference devoted to the subject of intelligence and aphasia (Lebrun and Hoops, 1976), after a comprehensive discussion of the cognitive performance of aphasic patients and ways to assess it, concluded:

> There is no overall estimation of intelligence which is applicable to aphasics. Specific aphasic patients suffer to different degrees on different tasks which comprise a typical and traditional intelligence test. Some of these tasks necessitate some type of verbal mediation, even if that mediation be internal. Aphasics find their greatest difficulties in attempting to complete any task requiring any variety of verbal mediation. Hence, performance of aphasics varies from subtest to subtest depending upon the degree to

which verbal mediation is necessary. . . . Intelligence is a competence which can only be tapped indirectly. This competence underlies a large variety of activities. Language is but a tool at the disposal of intelligence. It enables some aspects of intelligence to manifest. Aphasia impairs the display of intelligence by means of language.

An important point follows: although most studies indicate that aphasic patients show some "loss" of intelligence (as measured by IQ), as they recover language function they demonstrate gains in IQ (Wepman, 1951; Welman, 1964; Culton, 1969; Wertz et al., 1978). Their apparent intellectual decline is reversible. This factor distinguishes them from other groups of patients who demonstrate progressive loss of intellectual ability and other extensive impairments of problem solving and social interaction. Aphasic patients present a much more focal deficit, implicating language functions disproportionately, than do patients identified as having various cognitive and interactional disorders. Four of these groups, which can be differentiated from aphasia, will be discussed.

Dementia. Patients suffering from a progressive degeneration of the brain, sometimes called organic brain syndrome, display insidious onset and gradual progression of generalized intellectual impairment. These patients are identified as demented (senile or presenile dementia). One feature of their dementia is at least mild across-the-board language difficulty.

Ordinarily demented patients have little or no difficulty recognizing single words that they hear or read, matching words and pictures, and naming pictures and objects. They usually display some difficulty in auditory retention, but it is usually not severe, at least in the early stages of the disease; for example, they can repeat sentences unless they are quite long, and they can repeat several digits forward and backward although not as many as normal adults. When they talk, their sentences are well constructed; their vocabulary is not unusual. However, the more abstract the verbal task, the more trouble they have. They usually have difficulty explaining proverbs, sometimes failing to see how two proverbs are different (" 'Don't count your chickens before they're hatched.' Well, that's the same as 'Don't put all your eggs in one basket' "). They may explain proverbs in concrete terms rather than abstract generalizations from them ("You might break all your eggs"). Paucity of ideas was demonstrated by one demented patient when asked what every good citizen should do: "He should be neighborly. He should help his neighbor — but that goes back into the same idea. He should be kind to his neighbor; say hello to his neighbor — things like that." Although he recognized that he was not succeeding in listing separate items, he was unable to improve his performance.

Demented patients tend to be slow in responding to all stimuli, ramble in their answers, forget what they are doing or talking about, become easily mixed up on how to mark written responses, wander in their attention, give up on tasks easily, be unsure of their answers, and repeatedly offer expressions of inadequacy and bewilderment. They do not typically make significant syntactic errors in their responses, nor in word retrieval do they come up with bizarre choices. Their speech is generally free of phonetic errors. They do not confabulate. (According to one dictionary, to confabulate is to "give answers and recite experiences without regard to truth.") Whereas aphasic patients display a language disorder disproportionate to their overall level of cognitive function, demented patients demonstrate comparable degrees of impairment on a wide range of mental tasks. They demonstrate difficulty in new learning; they are poor in recall of general information; they often seem to have forgotten the basic operations involved in arithmetic.

For a comparison of demented and aphasic patients, we return to the study by Halpern and co-workers (1973). One of their groups was composed of 10 patients with generalized intellectual impairment; they demonstrated a broad depression of their mental faculties on neurologic and psychometric testing. On the language battery administered, this group was deficient in seven of the 10 language categories (Table 1–1). The overall rating (mean, 22) was in the middle of the mild range. In three categories the demented patients were moderately impaired (adequacy, reading comprehension, and arithmetic), and in a fourth (auditory comprehension) they were nearly in that range. Their syntax (at 11 per cent) was almost unimpaired, and in three categories (relevance, writing words to dictation, and fluency, at 9 and 10 per cent) they were just within the range of no impairment. These findings indicate that demented patients demonstrate a mild general reduction in capacity; they have some impairment of most language functions and greater disability in the same functions (adequacy, arithmetic) that are generally most difficult for the other groups.

It is often difficult to determine whether a patient with mild language dysfunction has a language-specific problem (aphasia) or whether his language difficulty is part of a more comprehensive "thinking" problem. Ultimately the differentiation depends upon the total pattern of results obtained in language and psychometric testing. This differentiation is an important one to the neurologist, since aphasia connotes a focal lesion, whereas dementia suggests a more diffuse, probably degenerative process.

Confused Language. Neurologists identify a specific impairment of mental function as a "confused state" or "confusion." "In confusion the patient's responses demonstrate that he fails to comprehend his surroundings. He may think he is at home rather than in the hospital and he may misidentify people. He is likely to be disoriented in time. He tends to misinterpret events. His clarity of thinking and his memory of recent events are impaired" (Mayo Clinic, 1976).

Several features characterize the altered communication of confused patients. They typically have some difficulty tracking a conversation. They may respond well to specific commands and questions, giving accurate answers when asked to name objects, read words and sentences, and do simple arithmetic. But on less structured tasks, given more freedom in response, as when asked open-ended questions or required to explain proverbs or the functions of objects, they may "wander away," produce irrelevant and peculiar responses, and confabulate. For example, a patient asked to list three things that he had done that day replied, "I stayed away above time, and I tried to grasp things that were unheralded before me, and I tried to reminisce, which was impossible." Another patient answered, "I don't know if I tried any desserts; I suppose I did. You would have to figure them out. I gave friends new models of things to go by, I suppose." A patient who was asked what every good citizen should do responded, "You should go to the store and enter inside, and then you should get shoes started; and you should help to have the Volkswagen go and you should help the Volkswagens with your store."

Confused patients are usually unaware of the inappropriateness and bizarreness of their responses, ordinarily less aware of their errors than aphasic patients are of theirs. They think they are making sense even when their responses are inadequate and irrelevant. A hospitalized patient who was asked to list three things he had done that day replied, "First I drove the car. Two, I made somebody happy that wasn't. And I made the United Press paper real happy." When the accuracy of his statement was challenged, he defended it. The syntactic structure of responses made by confused patients is typically more correct than the structure of responses made by aphasic patients. Confused patients usually demonstrate normal syntactic structure even when the word choice and content of the sentence are inappropriate. Speech is typically fluent and without articulatory or phonatory distortion. For example, the voice, articulation, prosody, and syntax of a confused college student who had incurred a closed head injury in an automobile accident were all within normal limits when he listed three things that every good citizen should do: "He should watch out for mailboxes. He should watch out for people. He should watch out for papers." Another confused patient with fluent speech and good syntax replied, "He should build on the right side. He should build on the left side. And he should build on the west side."

It is this pattern of a high degree of irrelevance of content coupled with paradoxically adequate syntax and fluency that differentiates the language performance of confused patients from that of aphasic patients. Halpern and co-workers (1973) found that the 10 confused patients in their study showed impairment of all 10 language categories measured (Table 1–1). The overall rating (mean, 28) fell near the upper border of the mild range, and four of the group scores were within the moderate range. These patients showed impairment of arithmetic, reading comprehension, and writing to dictation. Relevance had fourth rank among this group and differentiated them from the other groups. They gave bizarre responses to various stimuli, indicating reduced clarity of thinking and accuracy of remembering, and, unaware of the irrelevance of their responses, they made no attempt at correction. Writing words to dictation, which ranked third in impairment in this group, was less impaired in the other groups. The functions involved in writing words after hearing them spoken and the concentration required to do it apparently were beyond the capacity of the confused patients. Most of their writing errors were misspellings, but some were bizarre responses unrelated to the stimulus. The finding that confused patients failed more often to comprehend what they read than what they heard may be attributable to their inability to keep their attention on a silent stimulus (reading) as closely as on the auditory stimuli presented actively by the examiner.

Confusion is often but not necessarily traumatically induced. Unlike most other acquired language disorders, it is often, but not always, transient. Brain lesions in these cases have usually been found to be disseminated, either multiple focal lesions or a combination of focal and diffuse (Halpern et al., 1973).

Emotional Disturbance.   Some individuals, in response to life's problems and interpersonal conflicts, develop psychogenic disorders of communication including muteness. Such conversion reactions are defined as "specific, relatively persistent physical symptoms or syndromes which exist in the absence of sufficient causative, physiological pathology. They constitute an unconscious simulation of illness by the patient, who is convinced of their somatic origins; and they enable the patient to remain relatively unaware of conflict, stress, or inadequacies which would otherwise be emotionally disturbing" (Ziegler et al., 1963). Such patients who have gone beyond psychogenic aphonia (resorting to whispering) and have become totally mute may because of their restricted expressive performance appear to be aphasic or anarthric. However, they make no pretense of not understanding what they hear or read. They demonstrate a marked discrepancy between receptive and expressive abilities. Furthermore, they do not appear to be worried about their silence; they seem blandly to accept their inability to express themselves and they display no drive to communicate vocally. Such patients are thus quite different from patients in other categories described here. Aphasic patients, in contrast, demonstrate impairment of both reception and expression. Aphasic and demented patients typically indicate that they want to communicate even though communication may be a struggle and what they produce is fragmentary at best. Patients have been seen who in their apparent effort to protect themselves have retreated from psychogenic aphonia, when they are at least willing to whisper, to a mute state, in which they neither phonate nor whisper but resort to writing, to a condition in which they seemingly are unwilling even to write.

Another type of psychiatric patient is the chronic schizophrenic. The behavior of these patients is characterized by disturbance in reality relationships and concept formation, with associated affective, behavioral, and intellectual disturbances in varying degrees and mixtures. They show tendencies to withdraw from reality, inappropriate moods, unpredictable disturbances in stream of thought, regressive tendencies, and sometimes hallucinations.

Investigators have detailed various aspects of the language performance of schizophrenic patients (see DiSimoni et al., 1977, for a review of these observations). Reports indicate that their language does not consistently fulfill normal communicative function because it is often not used primarily for informational purposes. There may be perseveration of ideas and preoccupation with certain themes. Speech may be abnormal in prosody. Patients reportedly sometimes demonstrate syntactically disordered language or stylized constructions, and they may telescope their ideas. They may exhibit disorientation with regard to time, place, or person and may confabulate and present fictitious versions of past events. They may make errors in word choice or pronunciation that sound paraphasic, and they may produce neologisms.

DiSimoni and co-workers (1977) administered a 26 subtest language battery to 27 state hospital patients diagnosed as chronic schizophrenics. Their profile of performance was different from that of the aphasic, demented, and confused patients studied by Halpern and associates (Table 1–1). They usually communicated readily and had no difficulty making their wishes known, but they often introduced extraneous conversation reflecting their preoccupations. Their responses were typically well worded and grammatically complete. The features that most clearly distinguished them from aphasic patients were a high degree of general communicative adequacy, in contrast to aphasic patients' general inadequacy of expression, and a high incidence of irrelevance in their comments, in contrast to the high degree of relevance found in the remarks of aphasic patients. In addition, listening, reading, and writing functions were relatively unimpaired in the schizophrenic patients, whereas they are typically impaired to a degree comparable to speaking impairment in aphasic patients. Auditory retention span was only mildly disrupted in schizophrenic patients, whereas it was severely impaired in the aphasic patients.

Duration of illness was found to be negatively correlated with performance on most of the language subtests, indicating that the longer the subjects had been schizophrenic, the poorer their performance was in virtually every dimension tested. It appears that as the duration of their illness increases, schizophrenic patients deteriorate in language performance first in the direction of the profile shown by confused patients and ultimately toward the profile characteristic of demented patients.

Akinetic Mutism. Some patients with neurologic lesions present what has been called an akinetic or trance-like mutism. The clinical picture is one of the patient lying in bed motionless and atonic, sleeping more than normally but easily aroused, and making no spontaneous movement and no sound. In extreme forms of the disorder, the patient lies inert, mute, and immobile except that his open eyes follow events in the environment, indicating consciousness and seeming to "give promise of speech." Some observers have described lesser degrees of the disorder; in less complete manifestations the patient responds imperfectly after a long latent period with monosyllabic words or brief sentences, sometimes in a whisper, often in a monotone.

This disorder has been related to the existence of tumors in the region of the third ventricle, metastatic tumors in the midline of the midbrain, ischemia in the area of supply of the basilar artery, encephalitis, and traumatic lesions of the frontal lobes. Through some mechanism, these patients are inhibited in their cortical motor functions even though the lesions may be in the brainstem. Follow-up studies indicate that patients improve but display residual mental and speech defects (Klee, 1961).

THE THIRD DISTINCTION: APHASIA IS NOT MODALITY-BOUND

Analysis of the performance of patients with a broad spectrum of communication problems reveals that some patients with apparent language disorders demonstrate trouble with only a single input or output modality, adequately processing the symbol system in other modalities. Patients can be differentiated with regard to whether (1) their impairment is related to some central mechanism for processing language input and output or (2) they present modality-bound problems of transmission, along either sensory or motor channels. The concept most in accord with the facts is that aphasia is a multimodality

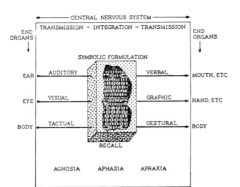

Figure 1-1. The Wepman model: An operational diagram of language functions in man. (From Wepman, J. M., and Van Pelt, D.: A theory of cerebral language disorders based on therapy. Folia Phoniatr., 7:223–235, 1955.)

symbolic disorder resulting from malfunction of a central integrative mechanism not bound to any particular transmission channel — of ingress or egress — but making use of and relating to all of them. The importance of the distinction is highlighted by consideration of two models of language behavior that have been proposed.

The Wepman Model. Wepman and VanPelt, drawing upon their experience with a range of communication problems related to brain dysfunction, elaborated "a theory of cerebral language disorders based on therapy" (1955). Their diagram of human language functions presents graphically a concept of a differentiated symbolic and non-symbolic language schema (Fig. 1–1).

> It should be recognized at the outset that no specific neurophysiological substrate is suggested for it. The same neural structure responsible for symbolic function and recall is predicated as being responsible for the transmission of neural impulses through the central nervous system. The present conception stresses that the two functions can be differentiated by the language defects observed subsequent to their unique disruption. Thus, two basic types of language defects are held to occur as the result of central nervous system disorders: (1) disorders of symbolization (aphasia); (2) nonsymbolic disorders (agnosia, apraxia).
>
> The very specific receptive nature of the agnosias and the equally specific expressive nature of the apraxias are shown. From this it follows that damage to the cortex can uniquely affect the modalities of reception and expression. Likewise, quite separate from these defects of a specific kind are shown the integrative losses that can exist due to cortical disruption where no particular modality is affected but only the absolute power to formulate symbols. . . . It is suggested here that an experienced examiner can differentiate between breakdowns in the transmission system which deny new stimuli reception to the integrative mechanism and those breakdowns which reduce the ability to recall old specific imagery. . . . The agnosias and the apraxias are presented here as the language problems of transmission. As such, of course, they are considered to be nonsymbolic in nature. Any disruption of the purely transmissive function of the cortex, whether it be along the lines of ingress or egress, whether it be along the paths of auditory reception or verbal expression, will affect the particular modality in question without affecting other modalities. From this it follows that the agnosias and the apraxias may appear quite uniquely. This is a state that is commonly seen in therapy.
>
> The classic definition of aphasia is that of difficulty with the basic function of language in relation to cortical activity, the inability to form symbols. In the present context it is held that only certain language problems consequent to cerebral damage fall into this category. Integration of the cortex for symbolic formulation implies the accessibility of previous learning. Underlying the cortical language process is the ability to integrate present stimuli with available symbols formed from past stimuli. . . . Defects of integration due to cortical disruption are felt to affect the accessibility of recall of previously available language symbols. By this reasoning, then, aphasia becomes a problem of recall and associa-

tion of old learning with new stimuli. From innumerable cases in therapy it seems to the present writer that the aphasic patient actually loses nothing of his past learning; rather, he loses the ability to recall from his past to the present. It appears as though the mechanism of integration were affected; not the storage of previous learning, but the means of making available the symbols stored. From this it would follow that when previous learning is actually lost the problem is not one of aphasia, but of intellectual deterioration.

In disorders of symbolic formulation, it is here held that modalities of reception and expression may be intact. When this is so, the patient will be able to function within each part of the complex language act, but will be limited in his function due to the generalized problem of recall.

Patients with integrative defects appear to have a generalized language disorder. They appear to be unresponsive to direct therapy for the defect in symbolization lowers their level of comprehension. They do respond to stimulation therapy. They always have an element of recall difficulty because of the inextricable relation between recall and symbolization.

Subsequently, Wepman and co-workers (1960) developed their model further and presented a revised diagram (Fig. 1–2), which more clearly demonstrates the effect of feedback, both internal and external, upon the language process and which emphasizes levels of function — the reflex level, the perceptual level, and the conceptual level. At the

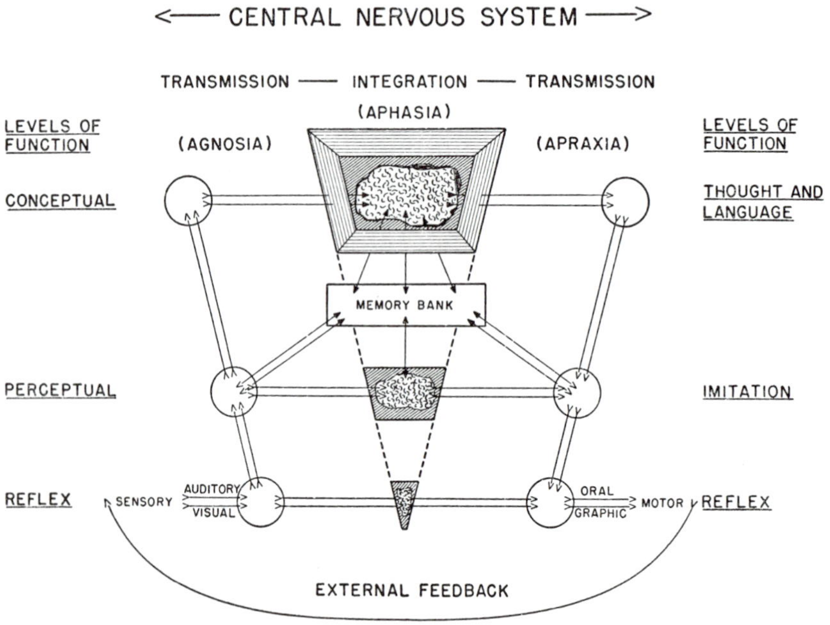

Figure 1–2. Wepman's revised model: An operational diagram of the levels of function in the CNS. (From Wepman, J. M., et al.: Studies in aphasia: background and theoretical formulations. J. Speech Hearing Disord, 25:323–332, 1960.)

lowest level of function, when a stimulus is received, reflex behavior ensues with recall playing no role in the system, "since reflex action is thought to leave no apparent trace within the system. . . . When the stimulus is shunted to the next higher level (the perceptual level), it is seen to be bound to the original receptive modality. Transmission across the system here is seen as the capacity of the organism to transmit percepts which may leave their trace on the memory bank but have no meaning to the individual. Across this bridge flows the echoic language of the infant, the parrot, or of any speaking organism."

At the concept-formation level, "the modality-bound stimulus is seen to have its effect both upon the memory bank for the arousal of associations and upon the integrative process where incoming stimuli are thought to combine with the associations from the past to form a state of meaningfulness. . . . Meaning invested in diverse symbols and associations becomes transformed into the symbols and symbol sequences of language — the conventional word patterns and grammatical forms which are part of the individual's repertoire of highly overlearned habits. Selection of language symbols may be called the semantic process; articulation of language symbols in discursive expression, the syntactic process. The specific form of expression follows the specific modality selected — speech, writing, or gesture." This higher level symbolic activity, then, transcends modality. Wepman and associates conclude:

> Aphasia is seen as a disruption of the integrative process after the stimulus is free of its input modality. The defect in language may fall at any point in the process: in the arousal of a meaningful state, in the semantic process of word selection, or in the syntactic process. . . . The present concept shows a triad of events in which modality-bound input leads to integration and symbol formulation which in turn lead to modality-bound motor output. The model shows the agnosias and apraxias as transmissive disorders, nonsymbolic in nature, bound by the pathways of reception and expression. The aphasias are shown as disruptions in the symbolic language process.

These authors point out that their model has direct clinical implications for diagnosis and the planning of therapy. They contrast the direct training procedures effective for the agnosias and apraxias with the indirect stimulative approaches found useful for aphasia.

The Brown Model.   Another model has been proposed by Brown (1968). His model posits a unitary three-level language- and speech-processing mechanism, designated the central language processor, the levels of which are correlated with certain geographic areas of the brain.

Central Language Process.   The normal language modalities of listening, reading, speaking, and writing as well as the subsidiary modalities of somatosensory-spatial perceptions and gestures are integrated with other conscious experiences in the central language process (designated variably by others as inner speech, language formulation, and symbolic formulation). Its efficient performance requires the integrity of the posterior portion of the dominant (for language) temporal lobe and poorly defined portions of adjacent midtemporal, inferior parietal, and anterior occipital lobes. The chief functions of the central language process are the transformation of language received into meaningful content and the conversion of meaningful internal content into language for exteriorization. In order to accomplish these functions, the central language process must:

1. have access to the lexicon (vocabulary) of stored words that the individual has developed throughout his life experience;

2. have access to the body of grammatical rules (morphology, syntax) for modifying, combining, and ordering words, rules abstracted over the years from heard language models;

3. have the ability to retain ongoing language events long enough to process them and the ability to evoke them spontaneously when they are not present (re-auditorize);

4. have the capacity to exercise a selection from among various inputs and outputs. A variety of input material is experienced continuously — auditory, visual, somatosensory — as are internal events, such as feelings, thoughts, perceptions, and concepts. A selection from all these inputs must be made, with attention focused on the most important input for the situation. On the output side, since many responses are possible to any given stimulus, a search must be made of these alternatives, an appropriate selection made, and action taken to respond.

The central language process has direct access to both input modalities — listening (auditory speech) and reading (visual-verbal) input — as well as to all output modalities — spoken (motor speech), written, and gestural output. It receives input from certain analyzers. Analysis of the occurrence and sequence of phonemes that make up spoken words is the function of the auditory speech analyzer; it requires the integrity of the midtemporal lobe of the dominant (for language) hemisphere. The visual language analyzer analyzes the input of words that are read; the integrity of the dominant hemisphere's supramarginal and angular gyri appears to be essential for its ongoing function. The central language process integrates and transforms these language inputs into meaningful content and then converts portions of this content into a form for exteriorization. It selects words and word sequences and converts them into a neural code of directions transmitted to the second level of the mechanism, the motor speech programmer.

Impairment of the central language process results in aphasia with consequent dysfunction in all language modalities. Retrieval of vocabulary from the lexicon is slowed or otherwise defective; use of grammatical rules is impaired and comprehension of the meaning in syntax is defective; there is restriction of auditory retention span and impairment of capacity to re-auditorize; flaws appear in the capacity to select from the hierarchy of input and output. The various problems are manifested in all modalities, not just one or two, because a central mechanism has been damaged, not simply a transmission channel.

Motor Speech Programmer. The second level of the mechanism, driven by the central language process, performs the task of motor programming. This task requires the selective application of some 100 speech muscles at the proper time, in the proper order, and for the correct duration to produce the desired speech sounds in the desired sequence. The average speech muscle is composed of 100 motor units, and the 100 speech muscles during conversational speech produce speech sounds at the rate of about 14 per second; the production of speech, then, requires something like 140,000 neuromuscular events per second. Such activation and control is beyond our volitional capacity; it follows that the sequential production of speech sounds in conversation is a result of activation of preprogrammed chains of neural output. Perhaps such preprogramming takes place during infancy and early childhood through babbling and articulatory practice. The trained motor speech programmer ends up able to activate the preprogrammed chains in the appropriate order.

Function of the motor speech programmer depends upon the integrity of the posterior part of the third frontal gyrus, commonly known as Broca's area, of the language-dominant hemisphere, and of tracts by which it is connected to the more posterior zone housing the central language process. Damage to the programmer and its connecting tracts results in apraxia of speech.

For most language operations, it would have to be assumed that the motor speech programmer is driven and directed by the central language process. There is evidence, however, that it can be driven by the auditory speech analyzer without the intervention of the central language process. Such would be the situation when we parrot or echo what we hear without true comprehension of the material; we may repeat foreign words and phrases without understanding them, and we may echo nonsense syllables. Patients have been described who echo what they hear without evidence of comprehending it (echolalia). This has been noted when a lesion involves the posterior part of the temporal cortex but spares the midtemporal gyrus, the inferior frontal speech area, and the arcuate fasciculus connecting the two (Denny-Brown, 1965). Thus, the auditory speech analyzer, the motor speech programmer, and their subcortical connections are intact, but the central language process has been either destroyed or isolated (disconnected) from the auditory speech analyzer.

It is also possible for the motor speech programmer to be driven directly by the visual speech analyzer, since normal persons have the experience of being able to read foreign words or nonsense syllables that convey no meaning. It is also possible that the motor speech programmer may perform autonomously without adequate direction or control, perhaps activated by structures within the frontal lobe or thalamic nuclei; this mechanism could account for the phenomenon of jargon that occurs when the central language process is severely damaged.

The Speech Effectors.   The third stage in this model is constituted by the effectors of the speech act. These include neurons in the motor strips and adjacent areas, the corticobulbar tracts, other supranuclear tracts, the motor nuclei of the cranial nerves (V, VII, IX, X, XII), the cranial nerves themselves, and the muscles involved in speech. Impairment at any level of the effectors results in slowness, weakness, incoordination, or alteration of muscle tone, causing dysfunction in any or all of the basic motor speech processes — respiration, phonation, resonance, articulation, and prosody — the result being designated dysarthria.

Clinical evidence indicates that it is possible to have separate impairment of the central language process (result: aphasia), of the motor speech programmer (result: apraxia of speech), or of the effectors of speech (result: dysarthria). These impairments, as discussed earlier, can occur independently, circumscribed lesions differentially affecting the circuitry subtending each level of function. It is also possible for the lesion to be of such magnitude as to result in simultaneous impairment of two or all three levels of speech-language processing.

Clinical Data Supporting the Models.   When the central language process alone is impaired, we expect to see impairment in all of those functions that enter into and result from the total integrated activity of this process. Studies of groups of aphasic patients confirm the fact that their language dysfunctions cross modalities.

Schuell and Jenkins (1959) administered 29 subtests from the Minnesota Test for Differential Diagnosis of Aphasia to 123 patients consecutively admitted to the Aphasia Division, Neurology Service, Minneapolis Veterans Administration Hospital between June 1954 and April 1957. The subtests assessed auditory comprehension, reading, writing, and speech at various levels of difficulty, employing auditory, visual, and combined presentation of stimuli and requiring various output modes, such as speaking, writing, and gross motor responses. They used Guttman's scale analysis to test for the existence of a single hierarchy of language functions. The results of the study indicated that these language tests were scalable over a wide range of contents and difficulty and over a heterogeneous collection of aphasic patients. The results presented strong evidence compatible with the hypothesis of a single dimension of language deficit present in all aphasia. "It appears to the writers that the obtained results constitute an impressive argument for the consideration of the language deficit in aphasia as a unidimensional trait."

In a subsequent study, Schuell and co-workers (1962) applied factor analysis to the results of the administration of 69 subtests of the Minnesota Test for Differential Diagnosis of Aphasia to 155 aphasic patients at the Minneapolis VA Hospital between June 1955 and June 1958. The results of the factor analysis led to the conclusion that "there is a dimension of general language deficit in aphasia that is not modality specific.... There is no support for the hypothesis of a sensory-motor, a receptive-expressive, or an input-output dichotomy in aphasia. These findings confirm the hypothesis that the general dimension of language impairment isolated by the Guttman technique is essentially the same as the major factor which appeared on the varimax and oblimin solutions in the present factor analysis."

Seventeen years later Powell and associates (1979) added further information about what the Minnesota Test reveals about aphasic impairment. They subjected the Minnesota Test profiles of 86 aphasic patients on variables A (auditory disturbance), B (visual and reading disturbances), C (speech and language disturbances), and D (visuomotor and writing disturbances) to two types of cluster analysis; and they then used factor analysis on test item scores. All three methods of analysis yielded four clusters that reflected only different degrees of severity, which the investigators designated severe, high-moderate, low-moderate, and mild. They did not confirm the existence of the seven "types" of aphasia Schuell and co-workers had described but found that "the seven types can be loosely mapped onto our severity groups." They thus demonstrated the validity of the notion that aphasic patients reveal common multimodality patterns of language dysfunction but vary from each other primarily in terms of the overall severity of their disorder, and they applauded Schuell's later consideration (described by Sefer in Schuell and Sefer, 1973) of a plan to alter her seven-syndrome typology to a severity-based model (mild, moderate, severe).

Jones and Wepman (1961) applied factor analysis to the scores of 168 aphasic subjects on 35 test variables composing the Language Modalities Test for Aphasia. They found "sizable correlations among factors," which probably reflected general language reduction across modalities; their Factor E resembled Schuell and Jenkins' general language factor. In both the Schuell and Jenkins and the Jones and Wepman studies, additional factors were recognized compatible with brain damage, playing some role in aphasic behavior and causing aphasic patients not to act identically in their performances.

Spiegel and colleagues (1965) analyzed the contextual speech of 50 aphasic patients as well as their responses to eight subtests of the Language Modalities Test for Aphasia. They concluded "that victims of aphasia do distribute along a continuum of general language disability, and that they also distribute along other dimensions indicative of specific losses in more specialized language abilities."

Goodglass and Kaplan (1972) applied factor analysis to the scores made by a group of 111 aphasic patients who took the Boston Diagnostic Aphasia Examination with 49 variables. The first factor extracted encompassed naming, auditory comprehension, reading, and writing clusters. They stated, "One would be tempted to call this a severity or, following Schuell and Jenkins, a general language factor," although they chose not to do so.

Similarly, Clark and colleagues (1979) used factor analysis on the scores made by 72 aphasic patients on the Porch Index of Communicative Ability. They derived five factors, four of which were "highly correlated (range, 0.60 to 0.70), suggesting the presence of a general language factor." The factor scores were used to derive six patient groups, which were differentiated essentially by severity of linguistic impairment. "These results appear to indicate that the amount of variance accounted for by a general language impairment dimension clearly outweighs the amount of variance which may be accounted for by specific dimensions."

In spite of the diverse purposes of the four tests used, dissimilarities among the subjects studied, and different methods of analysis, the various sets of data yielded a common finding, which supports the concept of a core of language impairment in aphasia that is not modality-bound. Other investigators have supported this statistically-arrived-at finding. They have reiterated the observation that their aphasic patients manifest language impairment in all modalities.

Having studied 26 aphasic patients in detail, Head (1926) stated: "We have no right to be satisfied with the statement that the patient is unable to speak, read or write. . . . As soon as we examine the clinical phenomenon . . . we find that no one of them is affected alone by any unilateral lesion of the cerebrum; a disturbance of one aspect of speech is invariably associated with some other disorder in the use of language or allied functions."

Weisenberg and McBride (1935) elaborately investigated the performances of 60 aphasic patients. They reported that "expressive disorders free of disturbances in receptive functions or in performances requiring intelligent behavior in language terms were not found among the hundred-odd cases investigated in the selection of the group of aphasic patients." Furthermore:

> The differentiation of types of aphasia according to the various forms of language — speaking, understanding, reading, and writing — is, as Head pointed out, an arbitrary and unsatisfactory procedure, for actual studies do not show that one of these forms is affected to the exclusion of others, or even that the typical case manifests a predominant disturbance in one of those forms. The fact that no "pure" forms of disorder . . . appeared among the patients of this research is in itself a weighty argument against the existence of such forms, for the five-year survey covered a good cross-section of the average run of aphasic patients.

When the language process breaks down, the extremely complicated condition that results is a natural consequence of the
complexity of the process as a whole, of the close functional
interrelationships of the various parts of this process in the course
of their development and in their habitual service, and of the extent
to which language processes have permeated and enriched all
mental functioning.

Although Weisenberg and McBride developed their own fourfold
classification system (predominantly expressive, predominantly receptive, expressive-receptive, amnesic), they discounted the importance of
the apparent distinctions:

> None of the terms is other than descriptive and . . . none does
> more than point out the most marked characteristics of the case.
> Neither the patients of the expressive nor those of the receptive
> group are handicapped solely in expressive functions or solely in
> receptive. The disorders are only *predominantly* expressive or
> receptive; the other processes in either case are always more or less
> affected. . . . Similarly, in the amnesic group, while the fundamen-
> tal difficulty is in the production of words as names, . . . there is
> always some disturbance in the understanding of spoken language
> or printed material.

Wepman's (1951) group of 68 aphasic soldiers undergoing rehabilitation all demonstrated impairment in all language modalities.

Penfield and Roberts (1959) examined a large number of aphasic
patients in connection with their cortical mapping of speech areas
through electrical stimulation. They reported: "In our own experience,
careful testing shows that there are no really pure forms of defect. The
patient who has moderate to severe aphasia may be worse in one
department of speech [language]. But if he is to be called an aphasic he
is rarely, if ever, quite perfect in any department."

Russell and Espir (1961) reported the clinical and anatomic features of 255 penetrating wounds of the brain that caused aphasia.
Through various localization procedures, they delineated the speech
territory in the left hemisphere, wounds in the center of which result in
global aphasia implicating all modalities (their "central aphasia").
They stated, "Injury to the central part of this structure disrupts all
aspects of speech, but small wounds at the periphery of the scaffolding
may lead to a special disorder of one or other speech functions such as
motor aphasia, agraphia, or alexia." These findings are similar to those
of Brown and Simonson (1957), who in a series of 100 cases of aphasia
found that lesions causing global aphasia were usually massive and
involved the midtemporal–anterior parietal region; lesions causing
isolated reading and other defects were situated peripherally.

Rosenberg (1965) reported that all 24 of the aphasic patients he
studied showed problems in all language modalities on the Sklar

Aphasia Scale. "It seems increasingly likely, then, that in past classification, the language deficit in aphasia has merely been called by its major name with a spread of deficits into other areas ignored."

Porch (1967) administered the Porch Index of Communicative Ability to 150 aphasic patients representing varying degrees of communicative involvement. The distribtuion of modality scores indicated that all patients were impaired in all modalities.

Keenan (1968) reviewed data from administration of various tests to aphasic patients. He concluded that recogniton (reception) and recall (production) tasks are simply different ways of eliciting information about language learning, that impairments of both are characteristic of aphasia, that reception is always better than production in aphasic patients, and that deficits in each do not represent different kinds of aphasia but different manifestations of breakdown in language retention.

Goodglass and Hunter (1970), studying the two expressive modalities of speech and writing, observed the same kinds of grammatical errors in both media of expression and concluded that "the formulation of written language is, at least in part, the formulation of spoken language connected to graphic form."

Smith (1971, 1972) has reported on two groups of aphasic patients studied longitudinally (N = 78, 126). He reported that standardized objective measures of language functions revealed impairment in these patients in all four language modalities. Severity of impairment in any single modality generally reflected the severity of overall language impairment.

Zurif and co-workers (1972), studying the ability of Broca's aphasic patients to understand and use grammar, concluded that agrammatism is not an isolated productive deficit: "Agrammatic speech is probably just one externalized aspect of a particular impairment involving all language modalities. . . . There does not seem to be a selective disturbance of performance mechanisms. Rather, since the agrammatic aphasic's tacit knowledge of English syntax appears to be restricted, as is his use of syntax, we may presume that agrammatism reflects a disruption of the underlying language mechanism."

Halpern and colleagues (1973) found that their 10 aphasic patients all showed impairment of all language modalities.

DiSimoni and associates (1975) in their investigation of the practicality of shortening the Porch Index of Communicative Ability (PICA) performed two stepwise regressions using scores from PICA administered to 222 aphasic patients. They found that PICA overall score (based on 18 subtests) was predicted with a high degree of reliability (0.98) by weighted scores on only four subtests (I, VII, D, VI) and by scores on only two items (pencil, knife) on 17 of the subtests (0.99). Correlations between each item score and every other item score and also with overall PICA score ranged from 0.95 to 0.98, showing a high degree of correlation between all language functions measured by this instrument.

Duffy and Ulrich (1976) studied 44 consecutive aphasic patients seen in two rehabilitation hospitals. Following administration of the Minnesota Test for Differential Diagnosis of Aphasia and other tests, the patients were scaled on each of the four modalities from 0 (normal) to 6 (severe impairment). The differences between the ratings for verbal comprehension, speaking, and reading were not significant; writing was significantly more severely impaired than the other three. Correlations between the four sets of ratings were high (0.68 to 0.82), and differences between the correlations were not significant. They also studied individual subject differences between the language modalities: 40 per cent of the 264 comparisons showed no difference between the ratings; 44 per cent showed a difference of one scale point; no more than 20 per cent of the subjects had differences of more than one step. Duffy and Ulrich concluded, "All language modalities tend to be impaired to about the same degree, and the data are compatible with the assertion that there is a strong common factor underlying the impairments in each specific modality."

These studies have dealt with the typical aphasic patients found in hospitals and treatment centers, patients with lesions of variable size and often relatively severe impairment of communication warranting rehabilitation. The Boston Veterans Administration Hospital group has believed that studies of language impairment should not be restricted to this population but should be extended to selected patients with small lesions that produce more selective disorders. Goodglass and Kaplan (1972) have discussed factors that tend to erase evidence for impairment of independent components of language. They state that although various neural subsystems may be selectively vulnerable at certain anatomic points, they are almost certainly intermingled in other areas of the brain. Therefore, the larger the lesion, the greater the effect on many functions. Small lesions producing isolated disorders occur less frequently and therefore have a smaller effect in any study that groups cases together. In order to avoid an overwhelming effect of a general language factor, Goodglass and Kaplan, in building their patient sample for standardization of the Boston Diagnostic Aphasia Examination, selected "a population in which a sufficient number of patients have each symptom in *relatively isolated* (not necessarily pure) form, or show some selectivity in the sparing of certain language functions." They acknowledge that "this smacks of circular reasoning and of data manipulation" but defend their decision, which resulted in a sample with "a greater proportion of selective aphasias than would have been the case if every patient coming through the unit, including all global aphasics, had been tested."

Non-Aphasias. Members of the Boston group have produced a large number of studies of such patients, and they have examined them in such a way as to highlight differences between them rather than likenesses among them. They have used a broadly inclusive definition of aphasia, embracing impairments that other aphasiologists consider to be separate from aphasia. They include under the broad umbrella of aphasia disorders which the models of Wepman and associates (1955, 1960) and Brown (1968) would specifically exclude from designation as examples of aphasia. Some disorders that they consider to be examples of aphasia are language disorders that involve impairment of isolated input or output channels and therefore are fundamentally different from the central integrative disorder designated aphasia. Three examples of "selective" forms of aphasia, which we would consider to be other than aphasia, will be discussed:

Apraxia of Speech. Earlier in this chapter, when the first distinction was made between aphasia as a language disorder and other impairments that are speech disorders, the clinical entity designated apraxia of speech was described. Apraxia of speech, whether called aphemia, anarthria, or phonetic disintegration of speech, is a single-modality disorder; only speaking is implicated. When the disorder occurs in "pure" form, the patient is able to write what he cannot say, understands what he hears, and is able to read with unimpaired comprehension. Treatment of the disorder is direct; it involves helping the patient relearn motor patterns. In contrast, aphasia is a multimodality disorder in which all modalities are impaired to relatively similar degrees. Treatment involves general language stimulation that facilitates reintegration of language functions; treatment of one modality leads to gains in other modalities. In apraxia of speech, general language stimulation shows itself to be irrelevant; it is indeed offensive to the patient, who has no need for bombardment with a variety of linguistic structures; the thing that needs to be treated is his speech programming disorder, whereas in aphasia all modalities warrant treatment, and treatment of each facilitates improvement in the others. Apraxia of speech is a transmissive disorder with a linguistic profile different from that of aphasia and requiring completely different treatment rationale and procedure.

Word Deafness. Isolated auditory verbal agnosia has been described in the literature. A typical clinical example is reported by Wepman and VanPelt (1955). Following a left hemisphere cerebrovascular accident, a foreman in an electronic plant was referred to them as a severe "receptive aphasic" patient. Examination revealed that the patient could not understand what was said to him (" 'word-deafness,' using an old classification system") but showed no involvement of symbolic ability. Therapy was directed specifically at improving auditory recognition. Within 5 months the patient had improved to the point that little of his auditory problem remained, and he returned to his job. The therapy that worked for him was not general language stimulation but direct drill focused on the single-modality input defect.

Alexia Without Agraphia.   Alexia without agraphia ("pure word blindness") has been described by Benson and Geschwind (1969, 1977) as a clinical variety of aphasia, a syndrome with disturbance of a single language modality. In this disorder, infarction (Geschwind, 1962; Geschwind and Fusillo, 1966; Ajax, 1967) or less frequently tumor (Cohen et al., 1976; Turgman et al., 1979) simultaneously damages the left visual cortex (occipital lobe) and the splenium of the corpus callosum. A right homonymous hemianopsia typically results. The intact right visual cortex is separated from the intact left hemisphere central language process by the lesion of the splenium. Patients see words in their intact left visual field but cannot make the associations necessary for identifying the words. They are unable to read; even though they are readily able to write, they cannot after a few moments read what they have written. Clinically these patients show no evidence of language dysfunction other than in reading; their auditory comprehension is unimpaired, they speak fluently and appropriately, they write accurately. Here again is a modality-bound disorder of transmission. Patients with this disorder are not benefited by the general language stimulation that aphasic patients require. Concentration in therapy upon other modalities does not improve the patient's ability to read.

It is inappropriate to consider any of these disorders a form of aphasia, just as it is inappropriate to consider the communication problem attributable to severe hearing loss a form of aphasia. True, these patients, like the hearing impaired, demonstrate difficulty in dealing with certain language units, but their processing of the language code is halted at a different level from that in the case of aphasia. It is not theoretically or clinically useful to consider these disorders to be of the same order as impairments resulting from dysfunction of a central language process. The critical distinction becomes clear, as has been pointed out, when consideration is given to what is effective in rehabilitation.

THE DOMAIN OF APHASIA

We have made three distinctions that help clarify the bounds of the territory to be embraced by the term aphasia. We have separated aphasia, a language disorder, from disorders of speech. We have differentiated aphasia, a language-specific problem, from disorders that may resemble it but in which other aspects of cognition and interaction are also impaired to significant degrees. We have distinguished aphasia, a multimodality disorder resulting from impairment of a central language process, from modality-bound disorders that result from impairment of given input or output transmission channels. With these distinctions in mind, we arrive at a definition of aphasia that specifies what we shall include and what we shall exclude:

> *Aphasia*: Impairment, as a result of brain damage, of the capacity for interpretation and formulation of language symbols; multimodality loss or reduction in efficiency of the ability to decode and encode conventional meaningful linguistic elements (morphemes and larger syntactic units); disproportionate to impairment of other intellective functions; not attributable to dementia, confusion, sensory loss, or motor dysfunction; and manifested in reduced availability of vocabulary, reduced efficiency in application of syntactic rules, reduced auditory retention span, and impaired efficiency in input and output channel selection.

Our definition delineates the common core of language disability of the patients we are discussing in this book. We will use the term without adjectives.

It is acknowledged that patients who meet the criteria established by this definition do not all resemble each other and sound alike. They may be quite different from each other, even as remarkably different as a fast-talking producer of neologistic jargon and an almost speechless patient who struggles to produce a few words. A great many adjectives have been devised which one might apply to highlight these differences. *Dorland's Illustrated Medical Dictionary* (1981) lists 56 different "types" of aphasia. *Stedman's Medical Dictionary* (1976) lists 31 different "types." Neither dictionary exhausts the list of adjectives which one encounters in the literature on aphasia; they oddly omit some of the most common terms used today.

In our opinion, little clinical purpose is served by proliferating adjectives, which are presumed to designate different "types" of aphasia. These adjectives have emerged in part because they are based on different, at times incomplete or biased, observations; they reflect what people look for and believe in. If a person is searching for a term to designate a condition marked by trouble with nouns, he will find it, and he can designate it "nominal aphasia" or "anomia" and throw into shadow all the patient's other problems. If a person is looking for a name for difficulty in use or comprehension of syntax, he will find it, and he can designate it "syntactic aphasia" or "agrammatism," ignoring coexisting lexical problems. Adjectives that have been applied reflect special interests and emphases, different theories of language development and disintegration, emerging theories of neurolinguistic function, and varying anatomic views. Their users tend to apply them simplistically, highlighting aspects of performance that may be prominent but inevitably downgrading or ignoring other aspects of performance that are present. It should be noted that profiles of different "types" of aphasia are never based on the *absence* of impairment in particular modalities but rather on *relative differences* in degrees of impairment between different modalities.

Little is to be gained clinically by splitting aphasia into subgroups; much is to be gained by lumping together patients who share a common core of disability that justifies the adoption of a unified rationale of treatment. The commonalities shared by aphasic patients, even when those patients are divided into allegedly different "types," are impressive. Numerous studies that were designed to discover and delineate *differences* between aphasic types have revealed significant *likenesses* that outweigh the differences. A sampling of studies will be reviewed in order to show why lumping is more reasonable and useful than splitting.

Orgass and Poeck (1966), in a clinical validation of the Token Test, administered it to four patients with motor aphasia, six with sensory aphasia, ten with amnesic aphasia, and six with mixed aphasia. They found no differences in the degree of receptive language impairment between these groups of patients. In a subsequent study, Poeck and co-workers (1972) administered the Token Test to 21 aphasic patients identified as fluent and 13 identified as nonfluent, the classification being based on a rating of 10 spontaneous speech criteria. No significant difference was found between the two groups; low and high error scores occurred with almost equal frequency in both groups; the mean scores for the two groups on each of the five parts of the test and on the total test were not significantly different. "Language understanding, as measured by this test, was equally impaired in both subgroups, in spite of gross differences in the clinical appearance of the aphasic syndrome. . . . Nonfluent aphasics were not superior to fluent ones even in the easier first steps of the test. . . . Thus, our findings confirm the suggestion presented by Orgass and Poeck [1966] that impairment in language understanding, as tested by the Token Test, is common to different clinical types of aphasia." These authors believe that fluent and nonfluent types of aphasia are related to brain lesions of different localization, that is, posterior versus anterior lesions within the language-dominant hemisphere, so "it follows from our results that these different neuronal structures are involved to an equal extent in the psychological processes underlying the performance on the Token Test."

Other studies have confirmed the fact that auditory comprehension is comparably impaired in all "types" of aphasia. Goodglass and colleagues (1970) administered four tests of auditory comprehension (Peabody Picture Vocabulary Test, Directional Prepositions Test, Preposition Preference Test, and Pointing-Span Test) to 7 patients with conduction aphasia, 14 with Broca's aphasia, 19 with anomic aphasia, 10 with Wernicke's aphasia, and 10 with global aphasia. All groups had trouble on one or more of the comprehension tests, even though by definition, and as part of their selection, some were supposed to have good comprehension (Broca's aphasia, "relatively good comprehension"; anomic aphasia, "auditory comprehension good"; conduction aphasia, "good comprehension"). Discriminant function analysis was used to determine how well one could predict that a patient would fall within a given clinical type of aphasia; the prediction was "far from perfect."

Shewan and Canter (1971) presented 42 sentences representing seven different levels of difficulty (in terms of length, vocabulary difficulty, and level of syntactic complexity) to 27 aphasic patients, 9 with Broca's aphasia, 9 with Wernicke's aphasia, and 9 with anomic aphasia. "All groups of subjects showed comparable patterns of decrement in auditory comprehension." The groups, representing different levels of severity of aphasia, were quantitatively but not qualitatively different. "The evident parallelism among aphasic subgroups in comprehension deficits contrasts with the different qualitative verbal output characteristics of these same groups. The language deficits evident in the verbal output of aphasic patients differ both qualitatively and quantitatively. By contrast, receptive deficit for sentences seemed to differ only along a quantitative dimension. Therefore, it is apparent that differential patterns of receptive deficit as found in this investigation cannot be used as a basis for classifying aphasic patients into their respective subgroups." In a subsequent analysis of the errors made by these 27 aphasic patients, Shewan (1976) found that the three clinical types were not significantly different with regard to their patterns of error position, proportions of error with regard to grammatical class, or the rank orderings of errors by grammatical class. "These data support the generalization that various types of aphasics perform similarly in comprehending oral sentences. Quantitatively, comprehension varies among types of aphasia, but the types of errors are similar."

Parisi and Pizzamiglio (1970) administered an original test of the understanding of syntax to 28 patients with Broca's aphasia, 10 with Wernicke's type, 5 with amnesic aphasia, and 17 mixed or global aphasic patients. They found that the groups did not differ with regard to the rank order of difficulty of the items. "The comparison made between the Broca's and Wernicke's groups did not show any difference in the hierarchy of difficulty of syntactic contrasts. . . . The study of syntactic comprehension does not seem to be very useful to characterize one group of aphasics versus the other and the hypothesis of different competences does not seem to be supported by these data." Pizzamiglio and Appicciafuoco (1971) administered an original test of semantic comprehension to two groups of Broca's aphasia and Wernicke's aphasia patients that were matched according to level of auditory comprehension impairment on other tests; "after the patients had been matched according to the severity of their impairment, no significant difference was found between the groups in the present test." Pizzamiglio and co-workers (1976) administered three tests of verbal comprehension (phonetic, semantic, syntactic) to 30 Broca's aphasia and 12 Wernicke's aphasia patients twice 3 months apart to determine patterns of recovery of comprehension. They reported no significant main effect for type of aphasia in their statistical analysis.

Goodglass and others (1979) investigated the ability of aphasic patients to understand an idea presented in a series of syntactically simple propositions versus a single syntactically complex sentence; they tested this with three types of structures, in one situation embedding one simple proposition in another, in another conjoining various syntactic structures, in another building into sentences certain relational attributes such as directionality and with-of agency. Patients heard the sentences and chose one of four pictures in a display to indicate their comprehension. The study's 12 Broca's aphasia patients, 5 Wernicke's aphasia patients, and 5 conduction aphasia patients displayed no group differences on the task; the groups did not differ in their response to the various kinds of grammatical structure.

Albert (1976) tested the short-term memory of aphasic patients by having them point to series of two objects in a group of 18. Some of his 28 aphasic patients had anterior lesions, some had posterior lesions, some had both. He concluded that "a lesion anywhere within this anatomical [perisylvian] region produced a defective auditory short-term memory." The patients with posterior lesions made more errors than those with anterior lesions, but the differences were not statistically significant. "Impaired short-term memory for items and impaired short-term memory for sequences were present regardless of type of aphasia."

Whitehouse and co-workers (1978) showed five Broca's aphasia patients (anterior lesions) and five anomic aphasia patients (posterior lesions) 24 drawings of objects varied systematically to represent a range of form and function (cup, bowl, glass, with and without handles, alone and in context). The patients did not have to name the pictures but were asked to raise their hands to indicate their choice of three multiple-choice foils offered verbally. Results indicated that the two groups could be "broadly differentiated" but "there is some overlap in scores." Goodglass and colleagues (1974) found that three groups of aphasic patients (13 nonfluent, 7 fluent, and 3 unclassified) did equally well on two picture-memory tests in which several of the test foils were confusingly similar to the stimulus words.

Aphasic difficulties with syntactic aspects of language have been found in patients of diverse "types." Studies by Goodglass and Hunt (1958) and Goodglass and Berko (1960) revealed that the relative difficulty of various grammatical markers, identical phonologically but different syntactically, was the same in both fluent and nonfluent aphasic patients. Goodglass and Mayer (1958) asked five agrammatic patients (later designated "motor aphasic") and five nonagrammatic patients (later designated "sensory aphasic") to repeat series of phrases and sentences of each of three levels of length and complexity, scoring them for 10 kinds of errors. The agrammatic patients made more errors but "our study confirms the observation that aphasics of both categories have difficulty with grammatical morphemes."

Goodglass (1973) showed that sentences of various grammatical forms (Wh-questions, imperatives, simple past, simple negative) constitute a hierarchy of difficulty from easier to harder, which applies to all aphasic patients regardless of clinical type. Blumstein and Goodglass (1972) presented aphasic patients with stress contrasts distinguishing nouns from verbs (con'vict versus convict') and nouns from noun phrases (yellowjacket versus yellow jacket), and asked their patients to respond by pointing to corresponding pictures; they found that their nine fluent aphasic patients and eight Broca's aphasic patients showed no difference in the proportion of correct responses. Concluding that pattern of error did not differentiate the two types of patients, they stated,"It is somewhat surprising that there were no differences between the two aphasic groups. . . . The results suggest that regardless of clinical type of aphasia, stress contrasts are preserved."

Gardner and associates (1975) presented to two groups of aphasic patients (13 with anterior lesions, 18 with posterior lesions) 100 pairs of sentences, each pair consisting of one right and one wrong sentence; 50 of the error sentences were syntactically deviant in any of six different ways, and the other 50 error sentences were semantically anomalous in any of seven ways. The stimuli were presented both visually (the patient read the sentences, identified the wrong ones, and marked the errors), and auditorially (the sentences were read aloud and the patients identified the errors). The scores of the two groups of patients did not differ significantly in either condition of presentation, nor were the groups differentiated by their performance on either the syntactically deviant or the semantically anomalous sentences.

Several studies have indicated that difficulty in naming is not characteristic of any particular type of aphasia but characterizes aphasic patients generally. Gardner (1973) had 11 anterior and 11 posterior aphasic patients name a series of pictures that were controlled with regard to the parameters of operativity (discreteness, separateness from surroundings, ease of manipulation, firmness to the touch, availability to several sensory modalities), frequency of occurrence of the words in the language, and pronounceability. No significant differences were found between the groups. The order of difficulty of the stimulus items was the same for both the anterior and the posterior lesion patients, and response latencies were essentially the same for the two groups. Gardner (1974) asked 15 anterior, 15 posterior, and 10 globally aphasic patients (anterior and posterior lesions combined) to demonstrate recognition of and to name 200 items (numbers, letters, faces, colors, animals, objects, number-related signs, printed words, miscellaneous signs). The anterior and posterior lesion patients did no differently on the naming task, confirming that "naming errors have little localizing value." The order of difficulty of the items proved to be the same for all three groups. Similarly, Goodglass and co-workers (1976) asked 13 patients with Broca's aphasia, 8 with Wernicke's aphasia, 12 with conduction aphasia, and 9 with anomic aphasia to name 48 test items. The four groups were not significantly different in their ability to name the items.

Pease and Goodglass (1978) asked 20 aphasic patients (seven with Broca's aphasia, six anomic, five with Wernicke's type, one with transcortical motor aphasia, and one with transcortical sensory aphasia) to name pictures; when they were unable to, they were prompted with six different types of cues. "Regardless of diagnostic category, the same pattern of response across cues was found. Therefore, the apparent differences in diagnostic groups' degree of responsiveness to cuing may constitute primarily a reflection of differences in severity of naming impairment, and may indicate a simple relationship between these two factors in which the more accessible a word is, regardless of the type of aphasia, the more likely it is that it can be elicited by cues." (A finding that challenges the validity of the classification system used was that the so called *anomic* group performed significantly better than both the Broca's aphasia patients and the Wernicke's aphasia patients on the naming task.)

Birbaumer and collaborators (1972) studied the divergent semantic behavior of 50 aphasic patients by asking them to list animals, things you eat, and things you see on the street. The response curves of the 32 fluent and the 18 nonfluent patients showed an "approximately parallel course."

Klor and Ratusnik (1980) studied the breakdown of semantic relations in a sample of 126 aphasic adults. The patients were variously classified as having nonfluent, 66, or fluent aphasia, 60; and Broca's, 66, Wernicke's, 33, or anomic aphasia, 27. Two spontaneous language samples were elicited from each subject, transcribed, and analyzed according to semantic relations categories (nomination, recurrence, nonexistence, action-agent, action-locative, entity-locative, possessor-possessive, entity-attribute, and demonstrative-entity). Quantitative differences in semantic disruption distinguished the various groups, indicating differences between them with regard to amount of verbal output; but no significant qualitative linguistic differences were found between the various aphasic groups. Boone and Friedman (1976) had 12 patients with motor aphasia, 10 with semantic aphasia, 4 with syntactic aphasia, and 4 with jargon aphasia read lists of words written in cursive or printed form and write the same words, presented orally, in cursive or in printing. Results showed "no particular etiologic or type of aphasia group better or worse on the oral reading or writing tasks."

RESOLUTION OF THE CLASSIFICATION PROBLEM

Patients with aphasia emerge from various analyses displaying marked commonalities, which lead us to believe that they share a common impairment. Their disorder is unitary and involves impairment of all aspects of language processing. Yet the patients display certain dissimilarities, which make it tempting to apply different adjectives to tag the differences. However, these labels constitute a difficulty. They turn out to mean different things to different people. Special definitions and "clarifications" of these words are offered; their use without an intervening step of explantion may fail to communicate the user's intent. As we have seen, the use of certain terms regrettably seems to imply that certain undesignated language functions are intact when in actuality they are not. The use of these labels all too often totally fails to convey any *useful* clinical information. Persons who want to know about a patient's language dysfunction usually need clinically practical information about his level of functioning in various modalities, how he manages to respond as well as he does, and whether and at what level one should plan to initiate therapy — information never implicit in any label.

Our choice of action is to designate patients as aphasic without adjectives. Taking into account all the considerations reviewed above, we arrive at a resolution of our terminologic problem:

1. The dichotomies and divisions suggested by the various adjectives are best not considered to be contrasted forms of aphasia but rather aphasia with or without some associated disorder. If the associated disorder is an impairment of the motor speech programmer, the patient will display a restriction of fluency; he is not a different kind of aphasic patient, but he is an aphasic patient with a second problem, apraxia of speech, which must be recognized and dealt with separately in therapy. The associated problem may be in some other transmission channel — auditory, visual, manual — giving a different surface appearance to the symptoms but not altering the basic core of aphasic difficulty.

2. Patients distribute themselves on a continuum of severity. They look much unlike each other when they run the gamut from extremely mild impairment of only the highest levels of communication to global impairment which renders the patient essentially bereft of communication. Not only do patients vary with regard to their overall level of severity, but within certain limits patients display varying degrees of inadequacy of performance in different input and output modalities and on specific tasks that we ask them to perform — naming, repeating, spelling, discriminating between sounds and words, explaining, deciphering. Where the patient falls at the moment on the severity spectrum should not lead us to create an artifactual designation of his having a different *kind* of problem.

3. Patients present themselves for examination and treatment at various stages of recovery. Longitudinal study of patients (see Chapter 3) reveals that patients who originally were markedly different from each other end up seeming much alike. Labels applied early following

onset turn out to be inappropriate at some later period (Leischner, 1960; Goodglass et al., 1964; Kertesz and McCabe, 1977).

Confronted with a specific case, our clinical task involves ascertaining whether the patient demonstrates the core impairment of language processing that would lead us to consider him aphasic; what complicating associated deficits he manifests; how far he has come since the onset of his problem; at what level of function he is performing currently in the various language modalities; what his prospects appear to be for recovery; and when and how we can best intervene to facilitate that recovery.

References

Ajax, E. T.: Dyslexia without agraphia: prognostic considerations. Arch. Neurol., 17:645–652, 1967.

Albert, M. L.: Auditory sequencing and left cerebral dominance for language. Neuropsychologia, 10:245–248, 1972.

Albert, M. L.: Short-term memory and aphasia. Brain Lang., 3:28–33, 1976.

Archibald, Y. M., Wepman, J. M., and Jones, L. V.: Nonverbal cognitive performance in aphasic and nonaphasic brain-damaged patients. Cortex, 3:275–294, 1967.

Aten, J. L., Johns, D. F., and Darley, F. L.: Auditory perception of sequenced words in apraxia of speech. J. Speech Hearing Res., 14:131–143, 1971.

Barton, M. I.: Recall of generic properties of words in aphasic patients. Cortex, 7:73–82, 1971.

Bay, E.: Principles of classification and their influence on our concepts of aphasia. In De Rueck, A. V., and O'Connor, M. (Eds.): Disorders of Language. Boston, Little, Brown, 1964, pp. 122–139.

Benson, D. F., and Geschwind, N.: The alexias. In Vinken, P. J., and Bruyn, A. W. (Eds.): Handbook of Clinical Neurology. Vol. 4. Disorders of Speech Perception and Symbolic Behavior. New York, John Wiley & Sons, 1969, pp. 112–140.

Benson, D. F., and Geschwind, N.: The aphasias and related disturbances. In Baker, A. B., and Baker, L. H. (Eds.): Clinical Neurology. New York, Harper & Row, 1977.

Birbaumer, N., Gloning, I., Gloning, K., and Hift, E.: Sequence analysis of restricted associated response in aphasia. Neuropsychologia, 10:119–123, 1972.

Bliss, L. S., Guilford, A. M., and Tikofsky, R. S.: Performance of adult aphasics on a sentence evaluation and revision task. J. Speech Hearing Res., 19:551–560, 1976a.

Bliss, L., Tikofsky, R. S., and Guilford, A. M.: Aphasics' sentence repetition behavior as a function of grammaticality. Cortex, 12:113–121, 1976b.

Blumstein, S., and Goodglass, H.: The perception of stress as a semantic cue in aphasia. J. Speech Hearing Res., 15:800–806, 1972.

Blumstein, S. E., Cooper, W. E., Goodglass, H., Statlender, S., and Gottlieb, J.: Production deficits in aphasia: a voice-onset time analysis. Brain Lang., 9:153–170, 1980.

Blumstein, S. E., Cooper, W. E., Zurif, E. B., and Caramazza, A.: The perception and production of voice-onset time in aphasia. Neuropsychologia, 15:371–383, 1977.

Boller, F., and Green, E.: Comprehension in severe aphasics. Cortex, 8:382–394, 1972.

Boone, D. R., and Friedman, H. M.: Writing in aphasia rehabilitation: cursive vs. manuscript. J. Speech Hearing Disord., 41:523–529, 1976.

Bricker, A. L., Schuell, H., and Jenkins, J. J.: Effect of word frequency and word length on aphasic spelling errors. J. Speech Hearing Res., 7:183–192, 1964.

Broca, P.: Remarques sur le siège de la faculté du langage articulé suivies d'une observation d'aphémie (perte de la parole). Bull. Soc. d'Anat. (2nd Series), 6:330–337, 1861.

Brookshire, R. H.: Auditory comprehension and aphasia. In Johns, D. F. (Ed.): Clinical Management of Neurogenic Communicative Disorders. Boston, Little, Brown, 1978, pp. 103–128.

Brookshire, R. H.: Recognition of auditory sequences by aphasic, right-hemisphere-damaged and non-brain-damaged subjects. J. Commun. Disord., 8:51–59, 1975.

Brookshire, R. H.: Visual and auditory sequencing by aphasic subjects. J. Commun. Disord., 5:259–269, 1972.

Brown, J.: The problem of repetition: a study of "conduction" aphasia and the "isolation" syndrome. Cortex, 11:37–52, 1975.

Brown, J. R.: A model for central and peripheral behavior in aphasia. Paper presented at Annual Meeting of Academy of Aphasia, Rochester, Minnesota, October, 1968.

Brown, J. R., and Simonson, J.: A clinical study of 100 aphasia patients. I. Observations on lateralization and localization of lesions. Neurology, 7:777–783, 1957.

Burns, M. S., and Canter, G. J.: Phonemic behavior of aphasic patients with posterior cerebral lesions. Brain Lang., 4:492–507, 1977.

Caceres, A., and Maurtua, N.: A propósito de las pruebas de inteligencia y la afasia. Rev. Neuro-psiquiatria, 31:111–121, 1968.

Chapey, R., Rigrodsky, S., and Morrison, E. B.: Aphasia: a divergent semantic interpretation. J. Speech Hearing Disord., 42:287–295, 1977.

Chapey, R., Rigrodsky, S., and Morrison, E. B.: Divergent semantic behavior in aphasia. J. Speech Hearing Res., 19:664–677, 1976.

Charlton, M. H.: Aphasia in bilingual and polyglot patients — a neurological and psychological study. J. Speech Hearing Disord., 29:307–311, 1964.

Clark, C., Crockett, D. J., and Klonoff, H.: Empirically derived groups in the assessment of recovery from aphasia. Brain Lang., 7:240–251, 1979.

Cohen, D. N., Salanga, V. D., Hully, W., Steinberg, M. C., and Hardy, R. W.: Alexia without agraphia. Neurology, 26:455–459, 1976.

Culton, G. L.: Spontaneous recovery from aphasia. J. Speech Hearing Res., 12:825–832, 1969.

Darley, F. L., Aronson, A. E., and Brown, J. R.: Differential diagnostic patterns of dysarthria. J. Speech Hearing Res., 12:246–269, 1969a.

Darley, F. L., Aronson, A. E., and Brown, J. R.: Clusters of deviant speech dimensions in the dysarthrias. J. Speech Hearing Res., 12:462–496, 1969b.

Darley, F. L., Aronson, A. E., and Brown, J. R.: Motor Speech Disorders. Philadelphia, W. B. Saunders Co., 1975.

Deal, J. L.: Consistency and adaptation in apraxia of speech. J. Commun. Disord., 7:135–140, 1974.

Deal, J. L., and Darley, F. L.: The influence of linguistic and situational variables on phonemic accuracy in apraxia of speech. J. Speech Hearing Res., 15:639–653, 1972.

Denny-Brown, D.: Physiological aspects of disturbances of speech. Aust. J. Exp. Biol. Med. Sci., 43:455–474, 1965.

De Renzi, E., and Vignolo, L. A.: The Token Test: a sensitive test to detect receptive disturbances in aphasia. Brain, 85:665–678, 1962.

De Renzi, E., Faglioni, P., Savoiardo, M., and Vignolo, L. A.: The influence of aphasia and of the hemispheric side of the cerebral lesion on abstract thinking. Cortex. 2:399–420, 1966.

DiSimoni, F. G., Darley, F. L., and Aronson, A. E.: Patterns of dysfunction in schizophrenic patients on an aphasia test battery. J. Speech Hearing Disord., 42:498–513, 1977.

DiSimoni, F. G., Keith, R. L., Holt, D. L., and Darley, F. L.: Practicality of shortening the Porch Index of Communicative Ability. J. Speech Hearing Res., 18:491–497, 1975.

Dorland's Illustrated Medical Dictionary. 26th ed. Philadelphia, W. B. Saunders Co., 1981.

Duffy, R. J., and Ulrich, S. R.: A comparison of impairments in verbal comprehension, speech, reading, and writing in adult aphasics. J. Speech Hearing Disord., 41:110–119, 1976.

Duffy, R. J., Duffy, J. R., and Pearson, K. L.: Pantomime recognition in aphasics. J. Speech Hearing Res., 18:115–132, 1975.

Dunlop, J. M., and Marquardt, T. P.: Linguistic and articulatory aspects of single word production in apraxia of speech. Cortex, 13:17–29, 1977.

Ettlinger, G., and Moffett, A. M.: Learning in dysphasia. Neuropsychologia, 8:465–474, 1970.

Flowers, C. R.: Proactive interference in short-term recall by aphasic, brain-damaged non-aphasic, and normal subjects. Neuropsychologia, 13:59–68, 1975.

Freeman, F. J., Sands, E. S., and Harris, K. S.: Temporal coordination of phonation and articulation in a case of verbal apraxia: a voice onset time study. Brain Lang., 6:106–111, 1978.

Gainotti, G., and Lemmo, M. A.: Comprehension of symbolic gestures in aphasia. Brain Lang., 3:451–460, 1976.

Gardner, H.: The contribution of operativity to naming capacity in aphasic patients. Neuropsychologia, 11:213–220, 1973.

Gardner, H.: The naming and recognition of written symbols in aphasic and alexic patients. J. Commun. Disord., 7:141–153, 1974.

Gardner, H., and Denes, G.: Connotative judgements by aphasic patients on a pictorial adaptation of the semantic differential. Cortex, 9:183–196, 1973.

Gardner, H., Denes, G., and Zurif, E.: Critical reading at the sentence level in aphasia. Cortex, 11:60–72, 1975.

Gardner, H., Zurif, E. B., Berry, T., and Baker, E.: Visual communication in aphasia. Neuropsychologia, 14:275–292, 1976.

Geschwind, N.: The anatomy of acquired disorders of reading. In Money, J. (Ed.): Reading Disability: Progress and Research Needs in Dyslexia. Baltimore, Johns Hopkins University Press, 1962, pp. 115–129.

Geschwind, N.: The varieties of naming errors. Cortex, 3:97–112, 1967.

Geschwind, N., and Fusillo, M.: Color-naming defects in association with alexia. Arch. Neurol., 15:137–146, 1966.

Glass, A. V., Gazzaniga, M. S., and Premack, D.: Artificial language training in global aphasics. Neuropsychologia, 11:95–103, 1973.

Goodglass, H.: Studies on the grammar of aphasics. In Goodglass, H., and Blumstein, S. (Eds.): Psycholinguistics and Aphasia. Baltimore, Johns Hopkins University Press, 1973, pp. 183–215.

Goodglass, H., and Berko, J.: Agrammatism and inflectional morphology in English. J. Speech Hearing Res., 3:257–267, 1960.

Goodglass, H., and Hunt, J.: Grammatical complexity and aphasic speech. Word, 14:197–207, 1958.

Goodglass, H., and Hunter, M.: A linguistic comparison of speech and writing in two types of aphasia. J. Commun. Disord., 3:28–35, 1970.

Goodglass, H., and Kaplan, E.: Disturbance of gesture and pantomime in aphasia. Brain, 86:703–720, 1963.

Goodglass, H., and Kaplan, E.: The Assessment of Aphasia and Related Disorders. Philadelphia, Lea and Febiger, 1972.

Goodglass, H., and Mayer, J.: Agrammatism in aphasia. J. Speech Hearing Disord., 23:99–111, 1958.

Goodglass, H., Barton, M. I., and Kaplan, E.: Sensory modality and object-naming in aphasia. J. Speech Hearing Res., 11:488–496, 1968.

Goodglass, H., Denes, G., and Calderon, M.: The absence of covert verbal mediation in aphasia. Cortex, 10:264–269, 1974.

Goodglass, H., Gleason, J. B., and Hyde, M. R.: Some dimensions of auditory language comprehension in aphasia. J. Speech Hearing Res., 13:595–606, 1970.

Goodglass, H., Quadfasel, F. A., and Timberlake, W. H.: Phrase length and the type and severity of aphasia. Cortex, 1:133–153, 1964.

Goodglass, H., Blumstein, S. E., Gleason, J. B., Hyde, M. R., and Statlender, S.: The effect of syntactic encoding on sentence comprehension in aphasia. Brain Lang., 7:201–209, 1979.

Goodglass, H., Kaplan, E., Weintraub, S., and Ackerman, N.: The "tip-of-the-tongue" phenomenon in aphasia. Cortex, 12:145–153, 1976.

Halpern, H., Darley, F. L., and Brown, J. R.: Differential language and neurologic characteristics in cerebral involvement. J. Speech Hearing Disord., 38:162–173, 1973.

Halpern, H., Keith, R. L., and Darley, F. L.: Phonemic behavior of aphasic subjects without dysarthria or apraxia of speech. Cortex, 12:365–372, 1976.

Head, H.: Aphasia and Kindred Disorders of Speech. Vol. 1. New York, Macmillan, 1926.

Hecaen, H.: Introduction à la Neuropsychologie. Paris, Larousse, 1972.

Howes, D.: Application of the word-frequency concept to aphasia. In De Rueck, A. V. S., and O'Connor, M. (Eds.): Disorders of Language. Boston, Little, Brown, 1964, pp. 47–75.

Itoh, M., Sasanuma, S., Hirose, H., Yoshioka, H., and Ushijima, T.: Abnormal articulatory dynamics in a patient with apraxia of speech: X-ray microbeam observation. Brain Lang., 11:66–75, 1980.

Itoh, M., Sasanuma, S., and Ushijima, T.: Velar movements during speech in a patient with apraxia of speech. Brain Lang. 7:227–239, 1979.

Itoh, M., Sasanuma, S., Tatsumi, I. F., and Kobayashi, Y.: Voice onset time characteristics of apraxia of speech. Ann. Bull. Res. Inst. Logoped. Phoniat. U. of Tokyo, 13:123–132, 1979.

Johns, D. F., and Darley, F. L.: Phonemic variability in apraxia of speech. J. Speech Hearing Res., 13:556–583, 1970.

Jones, L. V., and Wepman, J. M.: Dimensions of language performance in aphasia. J. Speech Hearing Res., 4:220–232, 1961.

Keenan, J. S.: The detection of minimal dysphasia. Arch. Phys. Med. Rehabil., 52:227–232, 1971.

Keenan, J. S.: The nature of receptive and expressive impairments in aphasia. J. Speech Hearing Disord., 33:20–25, 1968.

Keenan, J. S., and Brassell, E. G.: Comparison of minimally dysphasic and minimally educated subjects in a sentence writing task. Cortex, 8:93–105, 1972.

Kertesz, A., and Benson, D. F.: Neologistic jargon: a clinicopathologic study. Cortex, 6:362–386, 1970.

Kertesz, A., and McCabe, P.: Recovery patterns and prognosis in aphasia. Brain, 100:1–18, 1977.

Kinsbourne, M., and Warrington, E. K.: Jargon aphasia. Neuropsychologia, 1:27–37, 1963.

Klee, A.: Akinetic mutism: review of the literature and report of a case. J. Nerv. Ment. Dis., 133:536–553, 1961.

Klor, B. M., and Ratusnik, D. L.: Semantic relations in aphasic adults. Clinical Aphasiology Conference Proceedings 1980. Minneapolis, BRK Publishers, 1980.

Lambert, W. E., and Fillenbaum, S.: A pilot study of aphasia among bilinguals. Canad. J. Psychol., 13:28–34, 1959.

LaPointe, L. L., and Johns, D. F.: Some phonemic characteristics in apraxia of speech. J. Commun. Dis., 8:259–269, 1975.

Lebrun, Y., and Hoops, R. (Eds.): Recovery in Aphasics. Atlantic Highlands, New Jersey, Humanities Press, 1976.

Leischner, A.: Zur Symptomatologie und Therapie der Aphasien. Nervenarzt, 31:60–67, 1960.

Lenneberg, E. H.: Biological Foundations of Language. New York, John Wiley & Sons, 1967.

Marshall, R. C.: Word retrieval of aphasic adults. J. Speech Hearing Disord., 41:444–451, 1976.

Martin, A. D.: Some objections to the term apraxia of speech. J. Speech Hearing Disord., 39:53–64, 1974.

Martin, A. D., and Rigrodsky, S.: An investigation of phonological impairment in aphasia, Part I. Cortex, 10:317–328, 1974.

Martin, A. D., and Rigrodsky, S.: An investigation of phonological impairment in aphasia, Part II. Distinctive feature analysis of phonemic commutation errors in aphasia. Cortex, 10:329–346, 1974.

Mayo Clinic: Clinical Examinations in Neurology. 4th Ed. Philadelphia, W. B. Saunders Co., 1976.

Meyers, R.: Semantic dilemmas in neurology, psychology, and general semantics. Gen. Semantics Bull., 10–11:53–54, 1952–53.

Mohr, J. P., Pessin, M. S., Finkelstein, S., Funkenstein, H. H., Duncan, G. W., and Davis, K. R.: Broca aphasia: pathologic and clinical. Neurology, 28:311–324, 1978.

Noll, J. D., and Hoops, H. R.: Aphasic grammatical involvement as indicated by spelling ability. Cortex, 3:419–432, 1967.

Orgass, B., and Poeck, K.: Clinical validation of a new test for aphasia: an experimental study of the Token Test. Cortex, 2:222–243, 1966.

Orgass, B., Hartje, W., Kerschensteiner, M., and Poeck, K.: Aphasie und nichtsprachliche Intelligenz. Nervenarzt, 43:623–627, 1972.

Parisi, D., and Pizzamiglio, L.: Syntactic comprehension in aphasia. Cortex, 6:204–215, 1970.

Pease, D. M., and Goodglass, H.: The effects of cuing on picture naming in aphasia. Cortex, 14:178–189, 1978.

Penfield, W., and Roberts, L.: Speech and Brain Mechanisms. Princeton, New Jersey, Princeton University Press, 1959.

Pizzamiglio, L., and Appicciafuoco, A.: Semantic comprehension in aphasia. J. Commun. Dis., 3:280–288, 1971.

Pizzamiglio, L., Appicciafuoco, A., and Rozanno, C.: Recovery of comprehension in aphasic patients. In Lebrun, Y., and Hoops, R. (Eds.): Recovery in Aphasics. Atlantic Highlands, New Jersey, Humanities Press, 1976, pp. 163–167.

Poeck, K., Kerschensteiner, M., and Hartje, W.: A quantitative study on language understanding in fluent and nonfluent aphasia. Cortex, 8:299–304, 1972.

Porch, B. E.: The Porch Index of Communicative Ability. Palo Alto, California, Consulting Psychologists Press, 1967.

Powell, G. E., Clark, E., and Bailey, S.: Categories of aphasia: a cluster-analysis of Schuell test profiles. Br. J. Disord. Commun., 14:111–122, 1979.

Rochford, G.: A study of naming errors in dysphasic and in demented patients. Neuropsychologia, 9:437–443, 1971.

Rosenbek, J. C., Wertz, R. T., and Darley, F. L.: Oral sensation and perception in apraxia of speech and aphasia. J. Speech Hearing Res., 16:22–36, 1973.

Rosenberg, B.: The performance of aphasics on automated visuo-perceptual discrimination, training, and transfer tasks. J. Speech Hearing Res., 8:165–181, 1965.

Rosenberg, B., and Edwards, A. E.: The performance of aphasics on three automated perceptual discrimination programs. J. Speech Hearing Res., 7:295–298, 1964.

Russell, W. R., and Espir, M. L. E.: Traumatic Aphasia. London, Oxford University Press, 1961.

Schlanger, P. H., Geffner, D., and DiCarrado, C.: A comparison of gestural communication with aphasics: pre- and post-therapy. Paper presented at annual convention of American Speech and Hearing Association, Las Vegas, Nevada, 1974.

Schuell, H.: Aphasic difficulties understanding spoken language. Neurology, 3:176–184, 1953.

Schuell, H.: Clinical observations on aphasia. Neurology, 4:179–189, 1954.

Schuell, H., and Jenkins, J. J.: Comment on "Dimensions of language performance in aphasia." J. Speech Hearing Res., 4:295–299, 1961a.

Schuell, H., and Jenkins, J. J.: Reduction of vocabulary in aphasia. Brain, 84:243–261, 1961b.

Schuell, H., and Jenkins, J. J.: The nature of language deficit in aphasia. Psychol. Rev., 66:45–67, 1959.

Schuell, H., and Sefer, J.: Differential Diagnosis of Aphasia: Revised. Minneapolis, University of Minnesota Press, 1973.

Schuell, H., Jenkins, J. J., and Carroll, J. B.: A factor analysis of the Minnesota Test for Differential Diagnosis of Aphasia. J. Speech Hearing Res., 5:349–369, 1962.

Schuell, H., Jenkins, J. J., and Jiménez-Pabón, E.: Aphasia in Adults: Diagnosis, Prognosis, and Treatment. New York, Harper & Row, 1964.

Schuell, H., Jenkins, J., and Landis, L.: Relationship between auditory comprehension and word frequency in aphasia. J. Speech Hearing Res., 4:30–36, 1961.

Schuell, H., Shaw, R., and Brewer, W.: A psycholinguistic approach to study of the language deficit in aphasia. J. Speech Hearing Res., 12:794–806, 1969.

Shane, H. C., and Darley, F. L.: The effect of auditory rhythmic stimulation on articulatory accuracy in apraxia of speech. Cortex, 14:444–450, 1978.

Shankweiler, D., and Harris, K. S.: An experimental approach to the problem of articulation in aphasia. Cortex, 2:277–292, 1966.

Shankweiler, D., Harris, K. S., and Taylor, M. L.: Electromyographic studies of articulation in aphasia. Arch. Phys. Med. Rehabil., 49:1–8, 1968.

Shewan, C. M.: Error patterns in auditory comprehension of adult aphasics. Cortex, 12:325–336, 1976.

Shewan, C. M., and Canter, G. J.: Effects of vocabulary, syntax, and sentence length on auditory comprehension in aphasic patients. Cortex, 7:209–226, 1971.

Sklar, M.: Sklar Aphasia Scale. Beverly Hills, California, Western Psychological Services, 1966.

Smith, A.: Diagnosis, Intelligence, and Rehabilitation of Chronic Aphasics: Final Report. Ann Arbor, University of Michigan, 1972.

Smith, A.: Objective indices of severity of chronic aphasia in stroke patients. J. Speech Hearing Disord., 36:167–207, 1971.

Spiegel, D. K., Jones, L. V., and Wepman, J. M.: Test responses as predictors of free-speech characteristics in aphasia patients. J. Speech Hearing Res., 8:349–362, 1965.

Spinnler, H., and Vignolo, L. A.: Impaired recognition of meaningful sounds in aphasia. Cortex, 2:337–348, 1966.

Square, P. A.: Auditory perceptual abilities of patients with apraxia of speech. Ph.D. Dissertation, Kent, Ohio, Kent State University, 1981.

Stedman's Medical Dictionary. 23rd Ed. Baltimore: Williams and Wilkins, 1976.

Thurston, J. R.: An empirical investigation of the loss of spelling ability in dysphasics. J. Speech Hearing Disord., 19:344–349, 1954.

Trost, J. E.: Patterns of articulatory deficits in patients with Broca's aphasia. Ph.D. Dissertation, Evanston, Illinois, Northwestern University, 1970.

Trost, J. E., and Canter, G. J.: Apraxia of speech in patients with Broca's aphasia: a study of phoneme production accuracy and error patterns. Brain Lang., 1:63–79, 1974.

Turgman, J., Goldhammer, Y., and Braham, J.: Alexia, without agraphia, due to brain tumor: a reversible syndrome. Ann. Neurol., 6:265–268, 1979.

Van Dongen, H., Luteijn, F., and Van Harskamp, F.: De vergelijkbaarheid van een WAIS, een verkorte GIT en een Raven IQ in een neurologische patientengroup. Ned. Tijdschr. Psychologie Grensgebieden, 27:631–641, 1972.

Voinescu, I., Vish, E., Sirian, S., and Maretsis, M.: Aphasia in a polyglot. Brain Lang., 4:165–176, 1977.

Waller, M. R., and Darley, F. L.: Effect of prestimulation on sentence comprehension by aphasic subjects. J. Commun. Disord., 12:461–479, 1979.

Waller, M. R., and Darley, F. L.: The influence of context on the auditory comprehension of paragraphs by aphasic subjects. J. Speech Hearing Res., 21:732–745, 1978.

Watamori, T. S., and Sasanuma, S.: The recovery process of a bilingual aphasic. J. Commun. Disord., 9:157–166, 1976.

Watamori, T. S., and Sasanuma, S.: The recovery processes of two English-Japanese bilingual aphasics. Brain Lang., 6:127–140, 1978.

Weinstein, E. A., and Lyerly, O. G.: Personality factors in jargon aphasia. Cortex, 12:122–133, 1976.

Weinstein, E. A., Lyerly, O. G., Cole, M., and Ozer, M. N.: Meaning in jargon aphasia. Cortex, 2:155–187, 1966.

Weinstein, S.: Deficits concomitant with aphasia or lesions of either cerebral hemisphere. Cortex, 1:154–169, 1964.

Weisenberg, T., and McBride, K. E.: Aphasia: A Clinical and Psychological Study. New York, Commonwealth Fund, 1935.

Welman, A.: Brain tumor patients tested with the Wechsler-Bellevue scale. Dis. Nerv. Syst., 25:746–751, 1964.

Wepman, J. M., Recovery from Aphasia. New York, Ronald Press, 1951.

Wepman, J. M., and Van Pelt, D.: A theory of cerebral language disorders based on therapy. Folia Phoniatr., 7:223–235, 1955.

Wepman, J. M., Bock, R. D., Jones, L. V., and Van Pelt, D.: Psycholinguistic study of aphasia: a revision of the concept of anomia. J. Speech Hearing Disord., 21:468–477, 1956.

Wepman, J. M., Jones, L. V., Bock, R. D., and Van Pelt, D.: Studies in aphasia: background and theoretical formulations. J. Speech Hearing Disord., 25:323–332, 1960.

Wertz, R. T., Collins, M., Weiss, D., Brookshire, R. H., Friden, T., Kurtzke, J. F., and Pierce, J.: Veterans Administration Cooperative Study on Aphasia: preliminary report on a comparison of individual and group treatment. Paper presented at 54th Annual Convention, American Speech and Hearing Association, San Francisco, 1978.

Whitehouse, P., Caramazza, A., and Zurif, E.: Naming in aphasia: interacting effects of form and function. Brain Lang., 6:63–74, 1978.

Winchester, R. A., and Hartman, B. T.: Auditory dedifferentiation in the dysphasic. J. Speech Hearing Disord., 20:178–182, 1955.

Yorkston, K. M., and Beukelman, D. R.: An analysis of connected speech samples of aphasic and normal speakers. J. Speech Hearing Disord., 45:27–36, 1980.

Ziegler, F. J., Imboden, J. B., and Rodgers, D. A.: Contemporary conversion reactions: III. Diagnostic considerations. J.A.M.A., 186:307–311, 1963.

Zurif, E. B., Caramazza, A., and Myerson, R.: Grammatical judgments of agrammatic aphasics. Neuropsychologia, 10:405–417, 1972.

2 · APPRAISAL AND PREDICTION

Purposes of Language Appraisal
  Differential Diagnosis
  Determination of Level of Functional
    Communication
  Localization of Brain Lesion
What to Look for in the Appraisal
of Aphasia
  Sampling a Spectrum of Language
    Behavior
    Selection of input/output tasks
    Assessing divergent language
      behavior
    A sample of contextual speech
    Parallel tasks in different modalities
    Noting success as well as failure
    The ability to self-correct
  Other Communicative Behavior
  Nonlanguage Behavior
  History and Psychosocial Information
    Medical information
    Premorbid level of language function
    Personality characteristics
    The patient's home language practices
    Family opinions and practices
    Patient's social interaction
Tests for Evaluation of Aphasia
Guiding Principles in Aphasia Evaluation
  Testing Enough
  The Attitude of the Examiner
  Consistency of Administration
  Quantification of Results
  When All Else Fails
Predictions Based upon Appraisal Data
  Initial Level of Severity of the Aphasia
  Patterns of Test Performance
  Associated Speech Problems
  Specific Language Behaviors
References

"Our methods of examination are questions which we put to nature,
and the answers will depend on how the questions are put."

EBERHARD BAY

PURPOSES OF LANGUAGE APPRAISAL

Any of several purposes may be served in appraising a patient's
language functions:

Differential Diagnosis. It is necessary to determine whether a
patient's language dysfunction is aphasia or something else. Is his
language impairment disproportionate to his impairment in other areas

of intellectual function — that is, is he aphasic? — or is his language dysfunction one aspect of, a feature rooted in, a more comprehensive "thinking" disorder? Is the patient demented, confused, neurotic, psychotic? Does he, because of some more serious disorder, faultily apply language in problem solving and social interaction? Or is his communication impaired because of some single-modality input or output problem of nonsymbolic nature — that is, does he demonstrate an agnosia or an apraxia or some limitation of sensory input or motor output that impedes his communication? All of the distinctions that must be made for appropriate application of the label of aphasia, as suggested in Chapter 1, must be made.

Recognition of differential patterns of language impairment also provides at least rough information about the nature and extent of the cerebral lesion. Identification of the patient's problem as aphasia denotes a focal lesion, whereas identification of the problem as dementia or confusion is indicative of a more diffuse lesion or of multifocal lesions.

Determination of Level of Functional Communication. How severe is the breakdown of ability to process the language code? What length and complexity of message can the patient decode as he listens and reads? What length and complexity of message can he encode into speech or writing? This interest in the patient's ability to process language is a continuing concern and motivates serial appraisals of performance levels during recovery. A longitudinal series of such samples can reveal what recovery is occurring spontaneously, what changes are appearing in response to treatment, what the effects of medication and other adjunctive therapy may be, and what setbacks in language function occur that may be traceable to seizures, extension of a neoplasm, or recurrent vascular episodes.

The primary purpose in obtaining such information initially and at subsequent intervals is to provide a reasonable basis for the design and implementation of an individual treatment program for the patient. On the basis of the appraisal one determines the modalities of most efficient input and output, the level of response of which the patient is capable, at what levels he succeeds, and at what levels he fails. One can then plan a program of stimulation in order to facilitate optimal input and make possible maximum response and improvement.

Localization of Brain Lesion. Detailed information about language performance may provide some hint regarding the locus of a patient's cerebral lesion. Some investigators in aphasiology, past and present, have been less interested in aphasia as a disorder per se or in the aphasic patient as a focus of rehabilitation efforts and have been more concerned with using aphasia as a vehicle for studying the brain or the mechanisms of acquisition and organization of language or some other goal. The relationship between language behavior and brain anatomy has been pursued for the past 150 years; investigators observe a set of clinical symptoms, study the brain of the patient in some way, and conclude that a given behavior or cluster of behaviors is correlated with impairment of a given anatomic area. As Brown (1975) and Rubens (1977) have pointed out, the value of such enterprises is vitiated by the notorious inconsistency of brain organization from subject to subject.

The importance of language data for the purpose of localization of brain lesions was significantly decreased by the development of advanced electrophysiologic and radiologic techniques. These days if one wants to know the location of lesion, a brain scan or computed tomography (Mazzochi and Vignolo, 1979; Kertesz et al., 1979; Naeser et al., 1981a, 1981b) provides objective information that does not require an inferential leap. Lacking such information, neurologists and others may use the information provided by a language appraisal to arrive at a gross estimate of anatomic site of lesion.

This chapter is primarily devoted to the second of the above purposes, namely, determination of level of functional communication. The kinds of testing to be described and the tests that are mentioned as available for clinical use are largely designed for evaluation of a patient's current level of language function, but some have been used to delineate differences between clinical groups. Regrettably, tests designed to accomplish several purposes may not accomplish any of them ideally, including differential diagnosis. Nevertheless, procedures have been designed to use some of these tests to make differential diagnostic determinations.

One might think from its title that Schuell's Minnesota Test for Differential Diagnosis of Aphasia (Schuell, 1965) is an instrument to separate patients with aphasia from those with other language disorders. However, in fact the only persons other than aphasic patients studied by Schuell during the test standardization process were normal subjects. These normal persons made few errors in comparison with the aphasic patients, their random occurrence indicating primarily limitations of education. Schuell's special meaning of "differential diagnosis" was the placement of aphasic patients within subgroups on the basis of patterns of performance and prognosis for recovery.

An abbreviated adaptation of the Minnesota Test was used (Halpern et al., 1973), as reported in Chapter 1, to discover differential performances of four groups of patients: aphasic, demented, apraxic, and confused. Scores on various subtests yielded information about auditory retention span, auditory comprehension, reading comprehension, naming, writing to dictation, arithmetic, and oral expression, which was scored to reflect correctness of syntax, adequacy of response, relevance of response, and fluency. The four groups performed differently, the aphasic patients showing the greatest language impairment. Adequacy of oral expression, auditory comprehension, arithmetic, syntax, and naming were impaired in all four disorders and failed to differentiate the groups. The aphasic group displayed considerable impairment of auditory retention and fluency. The demented group showed impaired reading comprehension and, to a lesser extent, impaired auditory retention, but relevance was not subnormal. The apraxia of speech group was marked primarily by lack of fluency. The patients with confused language showed decided impairment of reading comprehension and writing to dictation but were best differentiated from the others by confabulation and the frequent lack of relevance of their bizarre responses.

DiSimoni and co-workers (1977) administered this test in somewhat expanded form to still another group, 27 chronic schizophrenic patients. The performance of these patients was quite dissimilar from that of aphasic patients and could be differentiated from the performances of the other groups as well. Schizophrenic patients were most deviant with regard to the relevance of their responses and their reading comprehension, while naming, syntax, and adequacy of oral expression were essentially normal. It was concluded that the performance of these patients gradually deteriorates, probably first in the direction of the pattern shown by confused patients, ultimately toward that shown by patients with dementia.

The Porch Index of Communicative Ability (PICA) has been used to differentiate certain groups. Porch (1971a) presents several profiles that differentiate certain groups from those who display the typical profiles of "aphasia without complications." In its purest form, the profile of apraxia of speech has very low scores on the four verbal subtests (I, IV, IX, XII) with other aspects of language processing being relatively intact. Profiles of patients with severe dysarthria closely resemble those of apraxic patients, but the verbal subtest scores rarely drop below the 4 level since dysarthric patients can generate a variety of speech sounds, although perhaps these are unintelligible. Patients illiterate before onset of aphasia can be distinguished by PICA profiles; they reject the reading and writing tests, so scores on subtests V, VII, A, B, C, and D are at the 5 level; if an illiterate patient is severely aphasic when tested early, there may be no evident disproportion, but with recovery from aphasia reading and writing subtest scores remain disporportionately low in comparison with the rest of the profile. Finally, patients with bilateral hemisphere involvement are distinguished by a reversal of the relationship between auditory and visual test scores usually seen in aphasic patients. Bilaterally damaged patients find visual tasks (VIII and XI) more difficult than auditory tasks (VI and X), whereas aphasic patients have more difficulty with the auditory than the visual tasks; bilaterally damaged patients also do less well gesturally and graphically than verbally.

Watson and Records (1978) have used the PICA to differentiate patients with senile dementia from aphasic patients. On graphic tests, demented patients did worse on subtests E and F (visual stimulation) than on subtests C and D (auditory stimulation), whereas aphasic patients did better on the visual than on auditory tests. Also noted was the dementia group's poor performance on subtest F (copying geometric forms) and a decline on subtest V (reading).

Porec and Porch (1977) have described how patients perform when deliberately feigning aphasia. Among the differentiating features are the use of infantile responses (childlike articulation patterns and infantile grammatical forms); inconsistency of aberrant behavior across or within subtests; overdoing an incorrect response such as overuse of letter reversals; too much phonetic sophistication; yielding to time pressure and giving some response rather than remaining unable to respond at the end of allotted time; and substituting more difficult words when simulating trouble remembering frequently occurring words.

Keenan and Brassell (1972) have shown how a test of writing five sentences to dictation can differentiate between aphasic patients and persons who are poorly educated. Nearly three fourths of the responses produced by the poorly educated group (education below fourth grade) were either essentially correct or characterized by simple misspellings, but over three fourths of the responses of the aphasic group had more serious errors that altered or destroyed the meaning of the sentences. Only aphasic patients made errors of omission of content words.

It can be seen, then, that some aphasia tests provide clues to differentiate aphasia from at least some other kinds of problems, but it is also evident that a test designed to determine level of functional communication requires the patient to engage in some tasks that reveal little of differential diagnostic importance; most tests are loaded with nondifferentiating material. Even if one could detect which subtests are most telling, it would seem that use of this information would depend on one's clinical judgment and the amount of one's clinical experience, and decisions might be unreliable.

One way to improve differential diagnostic procedures would be to start out with a battery of tests more wide-ranging than tests designed specifically for aphasia. Chédru and Geschwind (1978) did this and were able to select tasks that best characterized patients in acute confusional states. Orgass and Poeck (1969) made a preliminary application of such a procedure in a study of aphasia "by psychometric methods," using discriminant analysis to determine what variables predict membership in a diagnostic group and the respective weights of those variables.

Orgass and Poeck studied 18 patients with left hemisphere damage, six with right hemisphere lesions, and 26 with bilateral hemisphere damage to see how well some selection of tests could identify the 15 aphasic patients within this total group. They put together three groups of tests: (1) tests of intelligence and memory, including the German version of the Wechsler Adult Intelligence Scale (WAIS), two tests of verbal learning of paired associates, three tests of verbal retention, and Benton's Visual Retention Test; (2) tests of abilities frequently impaired in aphasia, including copying a 60 syllable paragraph and 10 single rare words, three subtests involving writing to dictation, and some arithmetic tasks; (3) some tests originally conceived to differentiate aphasic from nonaphasic patients, including Head's hand-eye-ear test and the Token Test. They correlated the obtained test results and grouped the most highly correlated scores into 11 variables. They ranked the 50 subjects on these variables, summed the ranks, then developed a new set of ranks from one to 50 on the basis of these sums. They divided the total group of ʾ50 into the poorest, medium, and highest scores. The Token Test and the WAIS Verbal score best differentiated the three levels of subjects. They compared the scores of aphasic and nonaphasic subjects using the Mann-Whitney U Test and obtained z values and levels of significance; there were no significant differences between the two groups except on the copying task. Since the aphasic patients did more poorly than the other patients on even nonverbal tests, the investigators wondered whether the aphasic patients had a lower general intelligence level, so they correlated all scores with WAIS Full-Scale IQ, Verbal IQ, and Performance IQ; all tests were found to be related to a certain degree to general intelligence. Orgass and Poeck ended up selecting 15 aphasic and 15 nonaphasic subjects matched for age, education, and side of brain lesion. All test differences were now significant except for the copying task and the Benton Visual Retention Test. The most significant differences between the two groups were on the Token Test, arithmetic, Verbal IQ, Head test, and writing to dictation. These variables were combined stepwise: Token Test plus arithmetic; then Token Test plus arithmetic plus Verbal IQ; then Token Test plus arithmetic plus Verbal IQ plus Head test; and so forth. The maximum differentiation between the two groups was reached on the basis of four variables: Token Test, arithmetic, Verbal IQ, and the Head test. Using more variables did not improve the discriminating power of the battery but reduced it. The total score on this four-part battery corresponded closely to clinical diagnosis; only two of the 15 aphasic patients would have been erroneously classified as nonaphasic. The total score proved to be better than any of its single components in discriminating between groups.

Tests for differential diagnosis of aphasia based upon this model and extending the work of Orgass and Poeck regrettably are still not available. Tests are needed that are trimmed down to those components that allow most precise differentiation of aphasic patients from other groups of patients with which they might be confused.

WHAT TO LOOK FOR IN THE APPRAISAL OF APHASIA

Sampling a Spectrum of Language Behavior.   In general terms, the clinician is interested in a patient's ability to process the arbitrary language code for communication. More specifically, how well can a patient decode (interpret) the language that he hears and reads? How well can he encode (formulate and express) his ideas into the symbol system in order to share those ideas with others? Still more specifically, the clinician wants to know how efficiently the patient recognizes, retains, and comprehends various kinds of input — auditory, visual, and tactile; how well he integrates and interprets this input and formulates some

Table 2–1   Optional Inputs and Outputs that Might Be Combined in Language Evaluation

STIMULUS	RESPONSE MODALITY	TYPE OF RESPONSE
Auditory		
Speech sound		Imitate (repeat, copy)
Word		
Word series		Name
Phrase		
Sentence		Complete a sentence
1-step, 2-step	Speak	
Complex		Spell
Short-long		
Paragraph		Answer questions
Visual		Retell
Nonlinguistic:		
		Describe
Object		
Photograph		Explain
Realistic drawing		
Line drawing	Write	List
Scene		
		Point
Linguistic:		
		Match
Letter		
Number		Sort
Word		
Sentence		Execute a task
Paragraph		
		Calculate
Tactile	Gesture	
Olfactory		
Taste		
Combinations		

sort of response to it; and how well he produces various types of output — oral, graphic, and gestural — both imitatively and spontaneously.

It can be seen from Table 2–1 that the spectrum of possible stimuli is broad, and the types of possible responses using three response modalities are numerous, involving several levels of complexity. To illustrate this in terms of a single modality, reading, the following choices are available: visual stimuli can be presented in a range of print sizes from large to small; the patient may be asked to point to letters named by the examiner; to match one set of letters to another set; to name the letters indicated by the examiner; to point to words named by the examiner; to read designated words aloud; to read the words as completions of open-ended sentences spoken by the examiner; to read words and define them; to match words to corresponding pictures; to copy the words in writing; to read sentences and answer the questions or execute the actions requested by them; to read sentences and respond yes or no; to read sentences and choose answers from multiple choices presented in writing or orally by the examiner; to read sentences and repeat them aloud or write them down; to read a paragraph and answer questions about it orally or in writing; or to state what was in a paragraph or write a précis of it, including as many salient details as possible. Each response can be evaluated in varying degrees of detail to provide information about accuracy, completeness, promptness, and efficiency.

Selection of Input/Output Tasks.   It is apparent that the administration of any given test item involves not just one modality but at least two — the input modality and the response modality. One is continually faced with the contamination of evidence of the patient's capacity to receive a given stimulus input by limitations of his capacity to respond in given ways, a danger recognized by Weisenberg and McBride (1935), who warned, "Defects in expression . . . may make it hard to determine how much the patient has understood. . . . Studies of expression in speech or writing must be independent of the extent to which the patient has understood, and studies of comprehension must involve responses such as checking a word or drawing a line, which are as little as possible influenced by the patient's expressive defects." We should follow their advice and keep the response mode extremely simple on a given input task, or we should use a number of tasks permitting alternative modes of response so as to arrive at a conclusion that we have adequately tested an input modality and not simply produced an artifact of output modality disability. Using the previously cited example of testing the patient's ability to read, when failure results, it is important to know whether it is due to impaired visual language processing or to something else — a visual acuity or field defect, a visual form agnosia, impaired auditory comprehension, difficulty in formulation and oral expression of ideas, or motor dysfunction in writing. The examiner must test the patient in enough ways to confirm a conclusion that the problem is indeed one of visual language processing.

The dangers of too simplistic an approach to testing are pointed out by Sidman and co-workers (1971). They emphasize the importance of ruling out input deficit as an explanation for subnormal performance, taking steps to show that a patient can, under some circumstances, respond normally to the same stimulus; for example, if the patient is unable to name a letter, he may still be able to write it or to match similar letters. Similar testing can rule in or rule out a specific output dysfunction. "If input and output are intact, a subnormal performance that involves the intact elements must, by exclusion, fall into the relational category — a deficient stimulus-response relationship. . . . By evaluating different responses to the same stimulus, and the same response to different stimuli, one can identify subnormal performance as an input, output, or relational deficit. . . . Only by rigorously applying the method of logical practice of testing all combinations of each available input and output can relational deficits be identified and analyzed."

A further consideration in designing tasks for evaluation is that one would like to have the patient's test performance as reflective as possible of how the patient performs in real life rather than having it consist of a set of artificial, classroom-like performances bearing little relationship to his mode of communication with family and friends. Some tasks that might be selected give direct insight into the patient's ability to function in activities of everyday life; these tasks seem more "relevant" or "valid" than some that require language activities rarely found in everyday life. One might therefore prefer to have the patient read road signs, follow recipes, answer the telephone, and tell about a family event because such tasks seem more "real" than spelling words aloud, thinking of all possible words that begin with a given letter within one minute, indicating by gestures how certain implements are used, or even naming pictures and objects.

However, some apparently artificial and nonrealistic tasks constitute "shortcuts" in language appraisal that may save time and provide objective information about a patient's performance. A task such as confrontation naming of objects and pictures is probably such a shortcut to evaluation of word-finding ability, which is less conveniently and objectively tested by having the patient describe a picture or converse spontaneously about a topic. Such a seemingly unrealistic test as the Token Test (DeRenzi and Vignolo, 1962), in which a person points to or manipulates colored shapes in response to instructions of increasing length and complexity, is highly revealing, discriminating effectively between language-impaired and non–language-impaired patients.

Whatever tasks are to be administered must include enough items to guarantee reliable estimates of the patient's capacity. It is not true that the results of aphasia testing are necessarily unreliable. Porch (1967), Schuell (1965), and others who have devised standardized procedures for testing have disposed of that myth; the variability more usually lies in the examination or the examiner. When tested in the same way repeatedly, aphasic patients demonstrate quite consistent behavior. From day to day a patient may pass or fail different items within a subtest, but his overall performance in terms of percentage correct is reasonably stable. Tasks should be designed, therefore, to include a generous number of items so as to allow for diurnal variability within a representative sample of behavior.

If one were to exhaust the optimal combinations outlined in Table 2–1 and try to evaluate comprehensively every conceivable type of language stimulus coupled with every possible mode of response, the result would be a test battery so complicated and lengthy as to be impractical and unbearable for the patient. As a necessary alternative, one resorts to a sampling of the various combinations of modes of input and output in order to estimate a patient's ability to cope with language, short enough to fall within the practical time limits of a clinical situation but comprehensive enough to uncover major and minor deficits in communicative behavior and allow differential diagnosis of aphasia from nonaphasic language disorders. Clinicians can develop their own battery of subtests to accomplish these goals, and they have a number of commercially available tests to draw upon, some of which are described below. Some of these tests resemble each other in their sampling of performance in the various modalities, but they vary in degree of comprehensiveness, standardization of procedure, and quantification of results.

Assessing Divergent Language Behavior. The language tasks referred to in the preceding section are what might be called "convergent" in nature. Chapey and associates (1977) have pointed out that most testing is based upon the assumption that aphasia is a convergent semantic disorder. Many of the usual procedures built into the tests to be described later "require a subject to converge upon a predetermined correct answer, which is intimately linked to the stimulus. Each item presented — whether it is highly stimulus-response bound or if it requires more spontaneous responses — taps the patient's ability to converge upon what he knows in a more or less mechanical way." The patient engages in a narrow search of memory storage in order to produce "a single solution or the one conventionally best response." But there is another aspect of language behavior suggested by Guilford's (1967) model of cognitive behavior: divergent language behavior. "Divergent behavior involves the generation of logical alternatives from given information where emphasis is on variety, quantity, and relevance of output from the same source. It is concerned with the generation of logical possibilities, with the ready flow of ideas, and with the readiness to change the direction of one's response. Divergent

behavior is the ability to provide ideas in situations where a prolifera-
tion of ideas on some topic is required. Such behavior necessitates the
use of a broad search of memory storage, so that multiple possible
solutions to a problem can be formulated." Guilford (1967) developed
tests to evaluate divergent semantic behavior, open-ended tests that do
not have a single correct answer — for example, to list things that are
soft and fluffy, to think of problems anyone might have in eating lunch,
to list what would happen if people no longer needed sleep. Responses
can be scored for fluency (the number of ideas produced) or flexibility
(the variety of ideas suggested).

Chapey and colleagues (1976) have demonstrated that aphasic
patients are less fluent and less flexible on such tasks than are normal
subjects. They concluded that "aphasia should be redefined as an
inability to generate a number and a variety of logical semantic
alternatives to given information as well as an inability to converge
upon semantic (lexical and syntactic) final products." It is this paucity
of ideas that led Wepman (1972, 1976) to call aphasia a thought process
disorder, in which thinking fails as a "catalyst for verbal expression."

It seems important to include in our sampling of the spectrum of
language behavior from the aphasic patients we assess a measure of
their divergent as well as their convergent semantic behavior. This may
be done by using the type of tests suggested by Guilford (1967) or
others: list everything conceivable that rolls; list everything that might
be used to make music; list the things used in cooking. One might
adopt the Verbal Expression subtest items in the Illinois Test of
Psycholinguistic Abilities (Kirk et al., 1969) and ask the patient to list
everything he can think of about each of four subjects — a ball, a block,
an envelope, and a button. Some commercially available aphasia tests
include subtests of this type. For example, the Boston Diagnostic
Aphasia Examination (Goodglass and Kaplan, 1972) includes a test of
"fluency in controlled association," an animal naming test adapted
from a similar test in the Stanford-Binet Examination. The patient is
instructed, "I want to see how many different animals you can call to
mind and name for about a minute, while I count them. Any animals
will do; they can be from the farm, the jungle, the ocean, or house pets.
For instance, you can start with dog." This test appears also in the
Western Aphasia Battery (Kertesz, 1979). Another test for divergent
semantic behavior is the Word Fluency Measure suggested by Borkowski and co-workers (1969) and included in the Neurosensory
Center Comprehensive Examination for Aphasia (Spreen and Benton,
1977). The patient is asked to list as many words as he can think of in
one minute beginning with a letter of the alphabet specified by the
examiner, and the procedure is repeated three or four times. (See the
review of this test in Darley, 1979, pages 243–246.)

A Sample of Contextual Speech. A comprehensive clinical

evaluation of communication status requires scrutiny of performance in all language modalities, but as Keenan and Brassell (1974) observed, "An overall judgment of a person's communicative ability is almost universally based on his conversational speech. The patient's family seldom mentions or even seems aware of the patient's comprehension difficulties. . . . This layman's focus on speech as a global indicator of communication ability seems to be justified." A complete evaluation of the patient's communicative performance should therefore include a generous sample of his contextual speech, a sample that goes well beyond the single-word responses elicited on a naming or a sentence completion task. One should determine with what speed and flexibility the patient can formulate and express ideas, how well he structures his sentences, the volume of words and ideas that he generates, and the fluency that characterizes his prosody.

One may elicit such a sample in various ways. One may ask the patient to define words, explain proverbs, or answer commands such as "Tell me three things every good citizen should do," "Tell me some of the things that you have done today," "Tell me a bit about where you live and what you do at home," or "Take me on a guided tour through your home." A sequence of tasks built into the Boston Diagnostic Aphasia Examination includes (1) an informal exchange of questions and answers, (2) open-ended conversation about familiar topics, such as "What kind of work were you doing before you became ill?" or "What happened to bring you to the hospital?" designed to elicit at least 10 minutes of conversation, and (3) the presentation of a picture (the Cookie Theft picture) with the request to "tell everything you see going on in this picture," designed to elicit approximately one minute's worth of speech.

Such a contextual speech sample can be evaluated in several ways. The following simple clinical scale of speech performance used by Keenan and Brassell (1974) captures critical information about the length and complexity of messages that the patient is able to convey orally:

> *Good speech performance:* The patient frequently uses meaningful sentences that are five or more words long. He produces many multisentence comments with no more than minor hesitancies or misarticulations.
> *Fair speech performance:* The patient's speech is characterized principally by the use of two- to four-word phrases and sentences, most of which are appropriate and grammatically normal. There may be many hesitancies and minor articulation errors.
> *Poor speech performance:* The patient's speech is mostly limited to single words (not counting jargon), automatic speech, vocal inflections, and gestures. In some cases speech may be fluent but irrelevant to environmental stimuli.

Benson (1967) used the set of scales listed in Table 2–2 for evaluating the speech output of aphasic patients and dividing them

Table 2–2 Variables and Rating Scales for Evaluation
of the Fluency of Contextual Speech

1. Word Choice			6. Pauses	
Nominal or fragments of words	−1		Many	1
Normal	0		Medium	2
Many relational words, cliché, etc.	+1		Normal	3
2. Rate of Speaking			**7. Prosody**	
Very slow (0–50 wpm)	1		Marked disturbance	1
Slow (51–90 wpm)	2		Slight disturbance	2
Normal (>90 wpm)	3		Normal	3
3. Articulation			**8. Verbal Paraphasias**	
Marked dysarthria	1		Many	1
Moderate dysarthria	2		Some	2
Normal	3		None	3
4. Phrase Length			**9. Phonemic Paraphasias**	
Predominantly 1–2 word phrases	1		Many	1
Predominantly 3–4 word phrases	2		Some	2
Predominantly >4-word phrases	3		None	3
5. Effort			**10. Perseveration**	
Marked	1		Severe	1
Moderate	2		Moderate	2
None	3		None	3

From Benson, D. F.: Fluency in aphasia: correlation with radioactive scan localization. Cortex, 3:373–394, 1967.

into two main groups. One group produces nonfluent, sparse, effortful, perseverative speech with many pauses, disturbances of rhythm, abnormal pronunciations, short phrases, and word substitutions; these patients make a low score on this scale, with a total close to 10. A second group of fluent speakers produce a great deal of speech easily with little pausing, normal rhythm, and a lack of perseveration, lack of abnormal pronunciation, and lack of word and speech sound substitutions, earning scores closer to 30.

Goodglass and Kaplan (1972) designed a rating scale profile of speech characteristics that is reproduced in Figure 2–1. Six speech features are rated on a seven-point scale in which 1 stands for maximum and 7 stands for minimum abnormality. A seventh scale of auditory comprehension is included. To supplement this profile of speech characteristics, they designed a severity rating scale based primarily upon speech performance but in part upon auditory comprehension, reproduced in Table 2–3.

Yorkston and Beukelman (1980) have developed a procedure for quantifying such contextual speech samples in a different way. Their procedure involves three measures: one is a measure of amount of

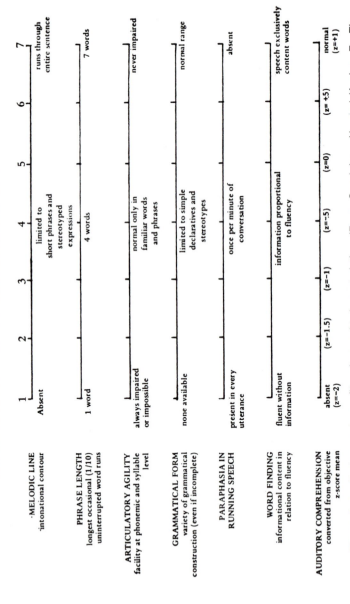

Figure 2–1. Rating scale profile of speech characteristics. (From Goodglass, H., and Kaplan, E.: The Assessment of Aphasia and Related Disorders. Philadelphia, Lea & Febiger, 1972.)

Table 2-3 Aphasia Severity Rating Scale

---

0. No usable speech or auditory comprehension.

1. All communication is through fragmentary expression; great need for inference, questioning and guessing by the listener. The range of information which can be exchanged is limited, and the listener carries the burden of communication.

2. Conversation about familiar subjects is possible with help from the listener. There are frequent failures to convey the idea, but patient shares the burden of communication with the examiner.

3. The patient can discuss *almost all everyday problems* with little or no assistance. However, reduction of speech and/or comprehension makes conversation about certain material difficult or impossible.

4. Some obvious loss of fluency in speech or facility of comprehension, without significant limitation on ideas expressed or form of expression.

5. Minimal discernible speech handicaps; patient may have subjective difficulties which are not apparent to listener.

From Goodglass, H., and Kaplan, E.: The Assessment of Aphasia and Related Disorders. Philadelphia, Lea & Febiger, 1972.

information conveyed, the so-called "content unit" — a grouping of information always expressed as a unit by normal speakers performing the task (in this case description of the Cookie Theft picture); two measures of efficiency include speaking rate in syllables per minute (total number of syllables contained in each speech sample divided by number of minutes occupied by the task), and the rate at which information is conveyed, that is, number of content units per minute. Using these measures they compared the performance of 50 aphasic speakers with that of 48 normal adult speakers (age range, 19 to 49 years) and a group of 30 normal geriatric adults (age range, 58 to 93 years). They found an inverse relationship between severity of aphasia and amount of information conveyed, although mild and high-moderate aphasic speakers tended to communicate as much information as normal speakers. Both measures of efficiency differentiated groups of mild and high-moderate aphasic speakers from normal speakers and also differentiated low-moderate from mild aphasic speakers.

Golper and co-workers (1980) have suggested an expansion of the analysis developed by Yorkston and Beukelman. They propose the tabulation of occurrences of certain performance deviations outlined by Logan (1976):

> Sequence interrupters: the use of non-contentive utterances which interrupt a word or a grammatical string, such as "uh," "well," "and so," "you see," etc.
> Incomplete phrases or phrase revisions, such as "She had her arm . . . but she is not looking."
> Incomplete words or word revisions, such as "This is a ch . . . stool."

Morphosyntactic deviations: the use of any non-standard structure, word-agreement, or grammatical form, such as: "That children is falling off the stool" or "She put her hand up to her hand for her mouth."

Phonemic errors, including substitutions, omissions, or unintelligible phonemes, such as "tookie" for "cookie."

Golper and associates found significantly more frequent occurrences of these performance deviations among aphasic patients than among right hemisphere–damaged patients and normal geriatric speakers.

Parallel Tasks in Different Modalities.   It will be useful in designing the language tasks and the materials for administering them to include parallel sets of items that permit comparison of the patient's performance on identical items in different modes of stimulus and response. The same set of pictures may be used for testing auditory recognition (patient points to pictures when examiner names them) and confrontation naming (patient names each picture). The ability of the patient to spell words orally may be contrasted with his ability to spell them in writing. The output produced in an oral description of a picture can be compared with the written description of the same picture. The patient's grasp of salient details in a paragraph which he hears read by the examiner can be contrasted with his grasp when he reads the same paragraph silently. One can use a limited number of items, such as the 10 objects used in the Porch Index of Communicative Ability (Porch, 1967), to learn a great deal about how a patient performs when given different amounts and kinds of information. Building such parallel procedures into the test will help determine the relative intactness of alternative modalities in deciding the most efficient approaches in therapy.

Noting Success as Well as Failure.   Obviously the kind of testing discussed so far will yield considerable information about the severity of a patient's deficits in various language modalities. But the evaluation should tell more than what the patient cannot do. It should also reveal how the patient manages to respond and what successes he has in using compensatory mechanisms to communicate. It is useful to know that a patient fails 75 per cent of the items in a 20-item subtest when his responses are scored as right or wrong, but it is equally useful to know whether the patient overcomes some of those failures when the stimulus is repeated, when it is presented at a slower rate with insertion of pauses between phrases, or when a cue or prompt is presented as a response facilitator. It is likewise useful to know whether, when the patient is given more time, he self-corrects an initial error, and whether he uses supplementary techniques, such as gestures, to convey more exactly what cannot be uttered precisely.

Davis and Leach (1972) have demonstrated the usefulness of scaling patient's responses rather than simply scoring them right or wrong. They used a four-point scale to evaluate certain gross features of patients' responses, a six-point scale to evaluate syntactic features of response, and a three-point scale to evaluate the phonologic components of responses. They believed that such a system captured much more information, allowed one to select features of response to work on in therapy, and permitted a more objective and complete basis for charting progress.

Porch (1967, 1971c) has highlighted the inadequacies of many conventional test procedures, particularly the loss of significant information when patient responses are scored correct or incorrect. A major contribution he has made to the appraisal of aphasia is his development of multidimensional scoring. He points out that most of the characteristics of a patient's performance can be subsumed under five dimensions: accuracy, responsiveness, completeness, promptness, and efficiency. Accuracy refers to whether the response is correct or incorrect. Responsiveness has to do with how much stimulation or information the patient needs before he can respond accurately. Completeness denotes whether the patient is able to make only a partial response or can complete the assigned task in its entirety. Promptness reflects the latency of the patient's response and relative need for more processing time. Efficiency relates to the facility of the peripheral communicative mechanism and the amount of distortion of the response in speech or writing due to impairment of motor control. Combining these five aspects of patient response, Porch developed a 16-level multidimensional scoring scale, reproduced in Table 2–4. Each response made by the patient to a test item is scaled and assigned a number from 1 to 16. Instead of jotting down on the margin of the test observations of how the patient managed to perform, such details of performance are built into the scoring of every item. Analysis of the test results allows one to determine just what compensatory mechanisms the patient can use, how he responds to a repetition, whether the provision of an additional cue is helpful, and whether he recognizes and corrects his errors. As Porch points out, the benefits of such a scoring system are numerous: "First, it describes the nature of the patient's response with considerable sensitivity and descriptiveness. Equally important, the characteristics of the patient's response enter into the scoring and modify it. . . . The clinical features of the patient's behavior are quantified and affect the test means. For this reason, as the patient's behavior changes his test scores also change. This close correlation between behavior and test scores is not true of other scoring systems. For instance, in using a plus-minus scoring system, a patient could get all responses on the subtests correct even though he required repetitions of the instructions, manifested self-corrective and delayed responses, and had distortions in his output. On retests he would again score all pluses and, therefore, show no apparent change even though he had in the meantime resolved all of these abnormal approaches to achieving a response." Another benefit is that "in order to decide

Table 2–4 Multidimensional Scoring Scale

SCORE	LEVEL	DESCRIPTION
16	Complex	Accurate, responsive, complex, immediate, elaborative response to test item.
15	Complete	Accurate, responsive, complete, immediate response to test item.
14	Distorted	Accurate, responsive, complete response to test item, but with reduced facility of production.
13	Complete-Delayed	Accurate, responsive, complete response to the test item which is significantly slow or delayed.
12	Incomplete	Accurate, responsive response to test item which is lacking in completeness.
11	Incomplete-Delayed	Accurate, responsive, incomplete response to test item which is significantly slowed or delayed.
10	Corrected	Accurate response to test item self-correcting a previous error without request or after a prolonged delay.
9	Repetition	Accurate response to test item after a repetition of the instructions by request or after a prolonged delay.
8	Cued	Accurate response to test item stimulated by a cue, additional information, or another test item.
7	Related	Inaccurate response to test item which is clearly related to or suggestive of an accurate response.
6	Error	Inaccurate response to the test item.
5	Intelligible	Intelligible response which is not associated with the test item, for example, perseverative or automatic responses or an expressed indication of inability to respond.
4	Unintelligible	Unintelligible or incomprehensible response which can be differentiated from other responses.
3	Minimal	Unintelligible response which cannot be differentiated from other responses.
2	Attention	Patient attends to test item but gives no responses.
1	No Response	Patient exhibits no awareness of test item.

From Porch, B. E.; Multidimensional scoring in aphasia testing. *J. Speech Hearing Res., 14:*776–792, 1971.

which of the 16 categories of response best describes the patient's response, the scorer must be sensitive to all these differences" and one's clinical awareness is increased. In addition, the reduction of descriptions of the patient's responses to single numbers is mechanically efficient and simplifies analysis of the data. When observers are adequately trained in the use of the procedure, high interscorer reliability results.

The multidimensional scoring system is an integral part of the Porch Index of Communicative Ability. Its usefulness is so great that clinicians have adapted it to other testing procedures (e.g., the Revised Token Test; see McNeil and Prescott, 1978). It can be applied to many testing procedures or test batteries so as to guarantee that useful information about how the patient manages to respond is not lost.

The Ability to Self-Correct. Level 10 of the Porch multidimensional scoring scale indicates that the patient recognized an error and spontaneously corrected it. This is a dimension of behavior of which particular note should be taken. Wepman (1958) pointed out that "the ability to recognize and self-correct errors made in language production, which is a commonplace in the behavior of the unimpaired speaker or writer, is defective to some degree in almost every aphasic adult patient." He related this inability to the indicator of brain pathology revealed on Rorschach test protocols which Piotrowski (1937) called "impotence," giving a response in spite of recognizing its inadequacy and being unable to withdraw or improve it. Aphasic patients distribute themselves along what might be visualized as a continuum of insight into one's errors, ability to self-criticize, and ability to correct. Wepman devised a self-correction scale, presented in Table 2–5. This scale can be used to record the severity of the defect upon initial evaluation and on subsequent evaluations, and it can be used to trace changes over time. On the basis of his clinical experience, Wepman concluded that "it is the movement through this continuum that seems of such importance to rehabilitation. The failure to move from one level to another is thought to be a bad prognostic sign, while speed of movement should be a good sign for recovery. . . . Thus, a

Table 2–5 Self-Correction Scale

Level 1. Fails to recognize errors made in any modality.
Cannot recognize errors when they are pointed out and therefore cannot correct them.

Level 2. Fails to recognize errors in any modality. Can recognize them when they are pointed out, but cannot correct them.

Level 3. Fails to recognize errors in *either* speech or writing. Can recognize errors when pointed out, but cannot correct them.

Level 4. Fails to recognize errors in *either* speech or writing. Can recognize the errors when pointed out and can correct them with assistance.

Level 5. Recognizes errors made in *both* speech and writing. Cannot correct them without assistance.

Level 6. Recognizes errors in *both* speech and writing. Can correct errors in one without assistance, but not in both.

Level 7. Recognizes errors made in *both* speech and writing. Can correct them without assistance most of the time but only with considerable effort and even then with some mistakes.

Level 8. Recognizes errors made in both speech and writing. Corrects them easily without assistance. May subvocalize as a means of self-correction before exposing his speech efforts.

From Wepman, J. M.: The relationship between self-correction and recovery from aphasia. J. Speech Hearing Disord., 23:302–305, 1958.

patient who begins his therapy at a very low level, but who succeeds in rather rapid order in going from one stage to another is likely to be the more successful patient. In contrast, the patient who begins at a somewhat higher original level, but who fails to make much change in his ability to be self-critical, is likely to plateau and reach a lower level of eventual spontaneous language."

Other Communicative Behavior. In the definition of aphasia presented in Chapter 1, the first distinction made was between aphasia and two kinds of motor speech disorders: dysarthria and apraxia of speech. The differentiating characteristics of dysarthria are summarized on pages 8 and 9, and those of apraxia of speech are reviewed on pages 10 to 15. The initial appraisal of the patient should include test procedures that would allow one to determine whether or not the patient thought to be aphasic also presents an associated motor speech disorder. Guidelines for the examination of motor dysfunction are presented in Chapter 4 of *Motor Speech Disorders* (Darley et al., 1975), and detailed information about the components of a comprehensive motor speech examination are presented on pages 86 to 98 of that chapter.

Some patients who display language dysfunction display this not in isolation but rather as a component of a more comprehensive "thinking" disorder of which aberrant language function is but one aspect. In such patients, one observes faulty application of language in problem solving and social interaction. It was pointed out in Chapter 1 (pages 22 to 28) that it is important to recognize whether the problem being dealt with is language-specific (aphasia) or is distributed as well in other cognitive areas. Observations are necessary to distinguish aphasic patients, then, from patients with senile and presenile dementia, confused patients, and patients with various psychiatric disorders, as outlined on pages 23 to 28 of Chapter 1. An appraisal adequate to make distinctions between aphasia and these other disorders may require considerable time and the efforts of such other professionals as clinical psychologists, neurologists, and psychiatrists. The initial evaluation may be designed, however, to include at least some appraisal of cognitive processes that go beyond language use alone. It will probably be useful to include a battery of questions about general information, items about which even poorly educated subjects might have some information (when Christmas is celebrated, how many states there are in the United States, where the United States capital is, who discovered America, who the president is, who the president was before him, and so forth). Tests should probably be included of mental and written calculation graduated from easy to harder items involving all arithmetic processes. One may want to include a test of the patient's recognition of absurdities. A subtest in which the patient is asked to explain the general meaning of proverbs may be useful, the purpose being to see whether the patient can generalize and develop an abstract statement of the truth expressed in the proverb or whether his analysis remains on a concrete level. One should also include orientation questions about the identity of the patient, his age, his home town, and the present day, month, year, and locale, as well as reasons why he is where he is currently.

It would be hoped that tests would also be arranged early for determination of the integrity of the patient's sensory input mechanism. A neurologist or neuro-ophthalmologist can supply critical information about the visual acuity of the patient and the presence and characteristics of any visual field defect that might significantly influence his performance on aphasia testing and his reception of therapy materials. A hearing loss may constitute a significant additional handicap to the communicative integrity of aphasic patients. Street (1957) found that 88 per cent of the 90 aphasic patients she studied had hearing losses, 55 per cent with speech frequency losses affecting two or more frequencies in the range from 125 to 2000 Hz, 45 per cent with losses in higher frequencies. Similarly, Miller (1960) found a high frequency of sensorineural losses in the 3 to 8 kHz range in aphasic patients as well as other brain-damaged patients. Karlin and associates (1959) reported a lower incidence of hearing loss in aphasic patients and in fact concluded that hearing loss may be present in the same proportion in aphasic and nonaphasic patients, the loss being due to age rather than to brain damage.

With regard to procedures for the audiometric testing of aphasic patients, Ludlow and Swisher (1971) tested out alternative methods of conducting pure-tone audiometry. They found that less severely aphasic patients performed equally well on both ascending and descending approaches; however, with more severe aphasia a descending approach resulted in the obtaining of lower hearing levels, whereas an ascending approach resulted in more response variability and the recording of less sensitive hearing levels. Their recommendation is to use a descending approach with aphasic patients, terminating testing as soon as three responses occur at one hearing level for a test frequency. Mencher (1967) demonstrated good reliability of conventional pure-tone audiometry with 40 aphasic patients and almost equally good reliability using electrodermal audiometry. He stated, "The successful use of the EDR instrumentation to test the auditory sensitivity of an aphasic patient, in spite of the severity of his condition, suggests that the EDR procedure can be successfully employed with patients who cannot be examined by conventional methods."

Nonlanguage Behavior.   During the evaluation, observations can be made of the patient's behavior, which help one judge the test's reliability, estimate prognosis, and decide whether the patient is currently amenable to a program of language rehabilitation. Many patients with acquired language dysfunction are older persons, and almost all of them will have had or have been suspected of having damage to the brain resulting in various kinds of cerebral dysfunction. They typically present impairments of health and a wide range of emotional reactions to their situation. Observations concerning the following will be useful in conduct of the examination, evaluation of the results of it, and the making of decisions based upon it:

Is the responsiveness of the patient impaired by reduced alertness? Does he appear to be generally obtunded? A patient with organic brain syndrome or a patient emerging from coma following stroke or trauma may demonstrate reduced awareness of what is going on and be unable to relate to the examiner and focus upon stimulus materials presented to him. A conclusion that the behavior represents aphasia should be delayed, since the impaired responsiveness is to the total environment and not simply to language stimuli within it. Valid language testing with reliable results cannot be expected until the patient is in touch with his surroundings and able to interact with the examiner and to respond consistently to stimuli.

Is the patient depressed? Severe depression may cause the patient to become almost as unresponsive as does being obtunded. The patient may look at the examiner blankly, respond with inordinate delays, or respond not at all and be unable to explain why he cannot respond. Once again, an accurate analysis of language status must await a time when the patient's mood is elevated and cooperation is better. Patients who have suffered a cerebral insult may show heightened emotionality and emotional lability. Patients with bilateral hemispheric damage may demonstrate pseudobulbar crying or laughing that interrupts test performance. A patient may be sensitive to the fact that he is experiencing unusual difficulty in performing what are obviously simple tasks; this realization may at times overwhelm him and cause him to break down. The patient may perceive in the testing situation a threat to his self-esteem and his intellectual intactness; he may display panic and frustration; he may react so strongly as to reject the testing situation as a threat not to be endured. One may observe whether the offering of words of reassurance, an explanation of why language testing is being done, or a shift to a less threatening task restores the patient's emotional equilibrium so that he can cooperate. Other brain-damaged patients may lack insight and seem too cheerful and unconcerned about their situation, even demonstrating euphoria.

Is the patient's general physical condition such as to make participation in language evaluation difficult? Does he appear cachectic? Is he quickly fatigued by the tasks given him? Perhaps the deleterious effect of fatigue has been overemphasized in descriptions of aphasic behavior; nevertheless, it should be recognized that patients in the early stages of recovery from a stroke and elderly patients may find a language evaluation tiring. It is known that patients perform less well on aphasic tests following fatiguing exercise (Marshall and King, 1973) and that they generally perform better in the morning than later in the day (Tompkins et al., 1980).

Are there sensory or motor obstacles to normal response? Does an associated hemiplegia prevent the patient from using his preferred hand in gesturing or writing? Is the patient willing to use the nonpreferred hand in writing and how well does he use it? Is there apparent neglect of space to the right or to the left as the patient examines materials, suggesting a right or left homonymous hemianopsia? Does the patient use glasses and do they seem to help him? Does he use a hearing aid and is it working? Is there evidence that he misses low-intensity speech input?

History and Psychosocial Information.   The amount of information about the patient one should try to collect depends upon how soon after onset the language evaluation is being done. Some areas of information indicated here are irrelevant if the testing is being conducted shortly after the onset event, for they relate to the ways the patient and his family and associates have learned to cope with aphasia. Other information is useful with every patient as one tries to understand what kind of person the patient is and how his characteristics and interests may relate to rehabilitation activities.

Medical Information.   Determine the date of onset of the problem and the reported etiology. What is the patient's present medical status? In addition to the aphasia are there known associated sensory or motor problems? Is there a seizure disorder? Does he complain of headaches? How often do these occur? Does he seem unusually fatigable? How much sleep does he get daily? Does he spend most of the day resting or is he usually active? Does he walk around the house and does he get outside? What progress has he made in recovery of language to date? Has any aphasia therapy been scheduled to date?

Premorbid Level of Language Function.   How far did the patient go in school? Has he studied any particular subjects since leaving school? Has he maintained an interest in intellectual pursuits? What has been the patient's occupation? Has he enjoyed his work? Would he like to return to it and does he expect to? Has he indicated concern that he may not be able to? What hobbies and other interests did he have outside of his job, and does he still show an interest in these? What did he formerly do for recreation? What clubs, fraternal organizations, or other groups did he belong to? How active has he been in them and is he active now? Was the patient much of a reader? Did he like to read books, magazines, newspapers? What parts of the newspaper did he formerly like to read? What kind of motion pictures did he like to see? What were his radio and TV listening/watching habits? Did he write letters to family members and others? Did he like card games? Which ones has he played?

Personality Characteristics.   Prior to onset of aphasia was the patient an extrovert or more of an introvert? Was he a happy-go-lucky type or was he a worrier who tended to be depressed at times? Was he sensitive to criticism and to the opinion of others or did he tend to be tough-minded, unbothered by others' opinions? Was he compulsive in his habits, perfectionistic, or fairly easygoing? Has the patient's personality changed? In what way? Does he ever lose his temper or become emotional? Does he become upset when family members try to help him with something? Is he depressed or anxious about his condition, or is he perhaps too cheerful and unconcerned about it? Does he trust his ability and judgment? Has he indicated in any way that he desires to do something about his aphasia?

The Patient's Home Language Practices.   Does the patient try to talk at home? Does he initiate conversations himself without first being addressed by someone else? Does he try to use sentences or only words or only gestures? When he wants something, does he ask for it or try to ask for it or does he just point? Does he use the right words? Does the family understand him, or is he difficult to understand because he mixes up the words or misarticulates them? In speaking sentences, does he omit little words such as "if," "of," "the," and "and"? Can he recall the names of people and things around the house? Is his speech halting or fluent? Can he offer greetings and farewells? Can he follow simple requests and instructions or does he seem not to understand what is said to him? Can he carry out more complicated instructions? Does he seem to understand when someone tells him about an incident or about something in the newspaper? On what basis does the informant believe that he understands? How much does the patient read now? What does he read? How well does he apparently understand what he reads, hears on the radio, or watches on television? How well does he write? Can he make change for sums of money? Does he play card games? How well? Does he have a sense of direction? Does he distinguish between right and left? Does he know where he is? Does he know the day and the date?

Family Opinions and Practices.   Does the family understand what aphasia is? Have they read about it? Do family members include the patient in their conversation or as a rule pay little attention to him? Do they let him talk for himself or try to talk for him? Do they try to help him by supplying words when he has trouble expressing himself? Do they anticipate his needs and wishes or try to guess what he wants? Do they correct him when he misspeaks? How do they feel about the patient and his situation? Have they ever in his presence expressed opinions about his condition and his present characteristics? Do they become angry or impatient with him or criticize him? How do they act when he becomes angry or upset? Do they try to reason with him or scold him or leave him alone and hope that he will get over it? Do they or does he for any reason feel guilty about his condition or the causes of it? Are they optimistic or pessimistic about the outcome? When he has difficulty doing something such as dressing himself, do they help him or allow him to do it for himself and assist him only when he asks for help? Do they think it would be a good idea to allow him to do as many things as possible for himself? Do they seem overly solicitous?

Patient's Social Interaction. Is the patient interested in his family and friends? Does he try to occupy a role in the family circle? Does he ask about financial and other family concerns? Does he try to carry on his former household activities? Did he formerly spend much time with members of the family and does he now take an interest in them? If he has children or grandchildren, does he play with them? Does he like to see his friends? How often does he see them? Has he indicated that he would like them to visit him or that he would prefer that they not visit him? When there are visitors in the home, does he seem interested in what they are saying? Does he understand and laugh at jokes? Does he try to carry on conversations with visitors? How well does he succeed?

TESTS FOR EVALUATION OF APHASIA

A number of tests are commercially available for appraisal of the communication problems of aphasic patients. A selected group of the more useful tests are described below. It is to be noted that what is presented is a brief description of each test, not a critical evaluation of it. Some of these tests have been critically evaluated in the book *Evaluation of Appraisal Techniques in Speech and Language Pathology* (Darley, 1979). Such appraisals indicate the purposes of the tests; review details of their administration, scoring, and interpretation; and present an analysis of test adequacy in terms of standardization procedures, reliability, various types of validity, and clinical strengths and weaknesses.

The first seven tests described are designed to assess performance in all language modalities.

The Porch Index of Communicative Ability (PICA). A limited sample of language behavior is quantified. The trained examiner rates performance of 10 items in each of 18 subtests on a 16-point multidimensional scale encompassing aspects of completeness, accuracy, promptness, responsiveness, and efficiency of the patient's communicative attempts. An overall test score is obtained together with separate scores on verbal, gestural, and graphic subtests. Percentile scores indicate how a patient compares with a large standardizing sample of aphasic patients. (Author: Bruce E. Porch. Publisher: Consulting Psychologists Press, 577 College Avenue, Palo Alto, CA 94306.)

The Minnesota Test for Differential Diagnosis of Aphasia (MTDDA). Exhaustive testing in major areas of possible disturbance is provided by 47 subtests: 9 subtests of auditory recognition, retention, and comprehension; 9 of visual and reading performance; 15 of oral function and oral expression; 10 of visual motor and writing skills; and 4 of numerical concepts and arithmetic processes. Subtests range in length from five to 32 items. A clinical rating scale from 0 to 6 can be used to quantify performance in areas of comprehension, reading, speaking, and writing. The test provides for classification of patients into one of five major and several minor groups. A short form of the test (Schuell, 1957) was devised consisting of selected subtests from the longer battery found to have high diagnostic and prognostic value; Schuell (1966) later regretted publication and general use of the short test, as she felt it was not reliable or comprehensive enough. (Author: Hildred Schuell. Publisher: University of Minnesota Press, Minneapolis, MN 55455.)

The Boston Diagnostic Aphasia Examination (BDAE). Comprehensive exploration of a wide range of communication skills is accomplished with a battery of 31 subtests and an evaluation of conversational speech that yields seven additional scores, plus supplementary groups of 13 language and 14 nonlanguage tests. Z-scores can be derived that allow comparison of subtest scores with the performances of a standardized group. Patient profiles that the authors consider to be characteristic of each syndrome of the "classic" classification system of aphasia (Broca, Wernicke's, anomic, conduction) are presented. (Authors: Harold Goodglass and Edith Kaplan. Publisher: Lea and Febiger, 600 Washington Square, Philadelphia, PA 19106.)

Western Aphasia Battery (WAB). Composed in large part of a selection of subtests from the BDAE, the WAB has four oral language subtests (spontaneous speech, comprehension, repetition, and naming) upon which an Aphasia Quotient (AQ) is based. Additional tests of reading, writing, praxis, drawing, block design, calculation, and portions of the Raven's Colored Progressive Matrices can be combined to yield a Performance Quotient (PQ). AQ and PQ combined provide the Cortical Quotient (CQ) as a summary of cognitive function. (Author and publisher: Andrew Kertesz, M.D., Department of Clinical Neurological Sciences, University of Western Ontario, London, Ontario, Canada N6A4V2.)

Aphasia Language Performance Scales (ALPS). Four ten-part subtests cover the modalities of listening, talking, reading, and writing. Each subtest permits scaling of performance within the modality from 1 to 10, different levels of performance being defined in terms of message length and complexity (single words, phrases, sentences, multisentence groups). Test instructions emphasize using the clinician-patient relationship to elicit the patient's best responses. (Authors: Joseph S. Keenan and Esther G. Brassell. Publisher: Pinnacle Press, P.O. Box 1122, Murfreesboro, TN 37130.)

Neurosensory Center Comprehensive Examination for Aphasia (NCCEA). This examination consists of 20 language subtests and four control subtests of visual and tactile function designed to detect deficits that might affect performance on the language tests. One can construct a profile of percentile scores for performance on all parts of the test corrected for age and educational level. (Authors: Otfried Spreen and Arthur L. Benton. Publisher: Neurosensory Laboratory, University of Victoria, British Columbia, Canada.)

Sklar Aphasia Scale. Four major language skills are evaluated: auditory decoding, visual decoding, oral encoding, graphic encoding. A percentage of impairment profile is drawn for classification of the patient in the categories of no impairment or mild, moderate, severe, and total or global impairment. (Author: Maurice Sklar. Publisher: Western Psychological Services, 12031 Wilshire Blvd., Los Angeles, CA 90025.)

The next two tests are designed to discern how well the patient functions in communicative activities of everyday life:

Functional Communication Profile (FCP). In informal interaction with the patient in a conversational situation the clinician rates his ability to use residual communication skills in 45 activities. Ratings are made on a nine-point scale; a percentage score can be derived to indicate the general language ability of the patient. (Author: Martha T. Sarno. Publisher: Institute of Rehabilitation Medicine, New York University Medical Center, 400 East 34th Street, New York, NY 10016.)

Communicative Abilities in Daily Living (CADL). In interview and role-playing situations the examiner evaluates the patient's ability to handle 68 different communicative tasks involving various levels of listening, reading, writing, and speaking. Responses are rated on a three-point scale (0 = communications fail; 1 = communications somewhat successful; 2 = communications successful). (Author: Audrey L. Holland. Publisher: University Park Press, 233 East Redwood Street, Baltimore, MD 21202.)

The following tests are designed to evaluate performance in given modalities:

The Token Test. This highly discriminating test is designed to detect minimal auditory comprehension deficits. It uses 20 tokens — two shapes, two sizes, and five colors — arranged before the patient, who is given progressively longer and more complex instructions to manipulate them. Part I requires the processing of two bits of information; Part II, three bits; Part III, four bits; Part IV, six bits; Part V, linguistically more complex tasks. Materials and response demands are simple; the patient must grasp the significance of each word in each completely nonredundant message. (Authors: Ennio DeRenzi and Luigi A. Vignolo. Not published commercially but easily made by any clinician.) An abbreviated version of the Token Test has been proposed by DeRenzi and Faglioni (1979). A commercial form of the original test is available with appropriate norms for children in the form of *The Token Test for Children*. (Author: Frank DiSimoni. Publisher: Teaching

Resources Corporation, 100 Boylston Street, Boston MA 02116.) An expansion of the Token Test into ten 10-item subtests with multidimensional scoring is commercially available as the *Revised Token Test*. (Authors: Malcolm R. McNeil and Thomas E. Prescott. Publisher: University Park Press, 233 East Redwood Street, Baltimore, MD 21202.) A modification of the Token Test, which requires the patient to describe what the clinician has done in manipulating the tokens, has been proposed as the *Reporter's Test* (DeRenzi and Ferrari, 1978).

The Word Fluency Test. The patient is required to list within one minute all the words he can think of beginning with a designated letter. Four letters are tested. Various modifications and norms for the test are available (Darley, 1979, pp. 243–246). (Authors: John G. Borkowski, Arthur L. Benton, and Otfried Spreen. Not commercially available except as a subtest in the NCCEA.)

Reading Comprehension Battery for Aphasia. Ten subtests comprehensively cover single-word comprehension, functional reading for everyday activities, recognition of synonyms, sentence comprehension, paragraph comprehension, and comprehension of various morphosyntactic structures. Analysis of severity of reading impairment and specific patterns of deficit provides a guide to the focus of therapy. (Authors: Leonard L. LaPointe and Jennifer Horner. Publisher: C.C. Publications, Inc., P.O. Box 23699, Tygard, OR 97223.)

Auditory Comprehension Test for Sentences (ACTS). Each of 42 sentences graduated systematically in length, vocabulary difficulty, and syntactic complexity is read aloud to the patient, who indicates comprehension by pointing to the correct picture among four foils. Scoring reflects promptness, correctness, and perseveration of responses. (Author: Cynthia M. Shewan. Publisher: Biolinguistics Clinical Institutes, P.O. Box 11356, Chicago, IL 60611.)

GUIDING PRINCIPLES IN APHASIA EVALUATION

Testing Enough. It is important that when we size up a patient's ability to handle language we test him far enough. One can draw seriously erroneous conclusions about a patient's language performance by sampling it too sketchily. All too often medical practitioners base their impressions about a patient's language upon his automatic or reactive responses to everyday, repetitiously asked questions such as "How are you?" and "How do you feel?" and repetitiously offered commands such as "Close your eyes," "Stick out your tongue," and "Wiggle your toes." Incomplete examinations frequently lead the unwary examiner to the conclusion that the patient "understands everything." Schuell and co-workers have said, "Somehow or other this is something people always say about aphasic patients, particularly when they have no speech and even when they cannot comprehend instructions as simple as 'Put the spoon in the cup'. . . . Sometimes when the patient makes an obvious error the speaking person ascribes it to his own difficulty in communicating with the aphasic patient. This is a very curious phenomenon" (Schuell et al., 1964). It has already been pointed out that any given function being tested should be tested with enough items to allow for diurnal variability and provide a reliable estimate of performance.

Steps should be taken to make sure that enough "top" has been built into the evaluation. Especially with patients whose aphasia is relatively mild or who are well on their way to recovery, tasks should be administered that are demonstrably discriminating between normal and impaired performance. The Token Test and the Reporter's Test were particularly designed in order to reveal "latent aphasia," to uncover difficulties of language processing that might escape casual exploration.

Within a given subtest, one should include items representing a range of difficulties. In a confrontation naming test, for example, one should include highly familiar and commonly used items but also less common items, the names of which are used less frequently. One might test the naming of "hand" and "fingers" but also "thumb," "nail," "knuckles," "wrist," and "palm"; in addition to testing the naming of "watch," one might include "stem," "second hand," and "numerals"; in addition to identification of "coat," one might have the patient name "sleeve," "buttons," and "lapel." In oral and written tests of spelling a range of difficulty may similarly pick up lesser degrees of aphasic impairment.

The Attitude of the Examiner. It was dramatically demonstrated by Stoicheff (1960) that the attitudinal "set" established by different kinds of instructions given to patients causes significant variation in their performance. Patients subjected to an encouraging condition in which they received from the examiner favorable feedback, expressions of approval, and predictions of success did significantly better than a matched group of patients subjected to a discouraging condition in which they received negative feedback and were reminded of how poorly they had done before and would probably continue to do.

It would be desirable in the evaluation situation to try to ensure that one is eliciting an optimum performance from the aphasic patient. We should let patients know that we are interested in them, expect them to do well, and appreciate their best efforts. Insofar as the instructions permit in administration of standardized tests, we can provide positive feedback and let the patient know when he is succeeding or at least when he is making efforts that we appreciate and commend. The examiner should indicate throughout the test that he is interested in the patient's performance; there should be no hint of inattention or indifference; signs of impatience when the patient is slow in responding should not be allowed to appear. The clinician should maintain a friendly, encouraging, and optimistic attitude, not daunt the patient with a too efficient or bellicose or critical demeanor.

Consistency of Administration. When serial administrations of aphasia tests are needed to follow a patient's recovery, meaningful interpretation of results requires that the same administration procedures be adhered to consistently. Given items should be administered in the same way from test situation to test situation; uniform scoring

Table 2–6 Scales for Quantifying Aphasic Patients' Responses in Four Modalities

Auditory comprehension	*Spoken language*
0 No information.	0 No information.
1 No observable impairment.	1 No observable impairment.
2 Follows radio program or general discussion with only minimal difficulty.	2 Converses easily with only occasional difficulty.
3 Follows ordinary conversation with little difficulty.	3 Conversational speech with mild impairment of formulation or fluency.
4 Follows most conversation but sometimes fails to grasp essentials.	4 Some conversational speech but marked difficulty expressing long or complex ideas.
5 Follows simple conversations but requires repetition.	5 Ready communication with single words and short phrases.
6 Follows brief statements with considerable repetition.	6 Expresses needs and wishes in limited or defective manner.
7 Usually responds inappropriately because he did not understand.	7 No functional speech.
Reading	*Written language*
0 No information.	0 No information.
1 No observable impairment.	1 No observable impairment.
2 Reads average adult materials with only minimal difficulty.	2 Can write acceptable letter with only minimal errors.
3 Reads paper and short magazine articles.	3 Spontaneous writing present with mild impairment of spelling and formulation.
4 Reads simple sentences and simple paragraph materials.	4 Can write short easy sentences spontaneously and to dictation.
5 Reading vocabulary of 100 or more words; reads some phrases and sentences.	5 Spelling vocabulary of 100 or more words; can write some phrases and sentences.
6 Matches words to pictures and some spoken to printed words.	6 Can write name and a few words to dictation.
7 No functional reading.	7 No functional writing.

From Schuell, H.: A re-evaluation of the short examination for aphasia. J. Speech Hearing Disord., *31*:137–147, 1966.

procedures should be used. The goal is to ensure that any change recorded in the level of performance from test to test is attributable to patient's variability and not to examiner's inconsistency. It behooves the examiner, therefore, to adhere strictly to the instructions prescribed by the designers of the various tests. These vary in explicitness and rigor. The examiner should be consistently rigorous even if the designer does not stress it, restraining himself throughout the test from inserting irrelevant though well-meant comments that might influence the patient's level of behavior.

Quantification of Results. Some of the tests described previously have built into them a system of quantification of results so that statistical manipulation of test scores is facilitated and convenient reference for serial studies is provided. If no such quantification is provided in the test, one may still impose quantification on the results. Whatever the test or tests used, the examiner may convert his impressions about the patient's performance to a scale of adequacy using numbers and descriptive terms that can communicate to others information about the patient's level of performance. The scale suggested by Schuell (1966) (see Table 2–6) allows assigning of a number from 0 to 7 with accompanying descriptive explanations to each of the modalities of language processing. A somewhat different scale with the same purpose has been suggested by Kaplan (1959).

When All Else Fails. Sometimes the application of standardized testing procedures fails to yield what the examiner believes is an adequate picture of what the patient can do in language processing. After a trial of standardized procedures, the clinician may decide to abandon them and engage in some other kind of interaction with the patient that may yield information about his capacity to respond. No test is sacred, and no test or combination of tests will necessarily accomplish what needs to be accomplished with a given patient at a given moment in his recovery. One may turn to informal interaction with the patient, engaging with him in some sort of activity, such as television watching, card playing, magazine or catalogue examination, or joke-cracking to try to stimulate the patient and elicit evidence of understanding and use of language. The limits of what might work in language evaluation are set only by the limits of one's imagination and creativity.

PREDICTIONS BASED UPON APPRAISAL DATA

Now that evaluation has spelled out the patient's language deficits and how he manages to respond, what predictions can be made about his eventual recovery from aphasia? What facts implicit in the initial test data provide clues to the eventual outcome? Several kinds of information have been found to have prognostic value.

Table 2–7   Percentages of Aphasic Patients Classified
According to Initial Severity Who Were Judged to Be Much
Improved or Improved in Three Language Modalities
After Treatment

	MODALITY		
LEVEL OF SEVERITY	Speech	Reading	Writing
Severe	65	58	60
Moderate	100	94	100
Mild	100	93	89

From Butfield, E., and Zangwill, O. L.: Re-education in aphasia: a review of 70
cases. J. Neurol. Neurosurg. Psychiatry, 9:75–79, 1946.

Initial Level of Severity of the Aphasia.   Over a dozen studies of
changes made by aphasic patients over time are in agreement that the
level of severity of communication impairment soon after onset is a
significant indicator of how far recovery will progress. The more severe
the initial impairment, the lower the level of recovery ultimately
attained by the patient.

Butfield and Zangwill (1946) judged the progress made by a group
of 70 aphasic patients who received language rehabilitation, rating
their terminal language functions as "much improved," "improved,"
or "unchanged"; these ratings were relative rather than absolute, being
based on unlike degrees of original impairment. Table 2–7 shows the
percentages of patients in three severity groups — severe, moderate,
and mild — who were judged to be "much improved" or "improved"
in three modalities following treatment. It can be seen that much lower
percentages attained these levels of recovery among those initially
judged to be severe than those among those judged to be moderate or
mild. In general, from 90 to 100 per cent of the patients in the mild and
moderate groups showed these levels of improvement, while only 65
per cent of the severely affected patients showed these levels of
improvement in speech, 58 per cent in reading, and 60 per cent in writing.

In his study of the recovery from aphasia of 68 patients with
traumatically incurred aphasia, Wepman (1951) described 10 of them
as falling in the category of "global aphasia," in whom "all language
forms are seriously affected to the degree that it is impossible to use one
of the preceding categories [expressive aphasia, receptive aphasia,
expressive-receptive aphasia]." These were his most severely affected
patients, having the lowest starting points in reading, writing, spelling,
mathematics, and speech. Although they made more gains than the 11
patients in the receptive group, they still attained "the lowest level of
accomplishment" of all the groups. Although the global group was the
most homogeneous in terms of ability at the beginning of training, after
rehabilitation there was great divergence: "Some of the subjects in this

group were at the very bottom of the total distribution, while others were almost at the top." As a group, then, their ultimate level of attainment was lower than that of each of the other groups, but some individual members of this very severe group made significant gains, just as did members of the other groups.

Mitchell (1958) reported on 31 treated aphasic patients. Four of them were "totally aphasic and made no profitable improvement under observation."

Using the MTDDA, Schuell and associates (1964) studied the nature and severity of language dysfunction of a large number of aphasic patients who were judged to be stable neurologically. The profiles of performance and the patterns of recovery shown by the patients led them to develop a classification system composed of five major and two minor categories. They were able to classify 96 per cent of the patients into the five major categories:

Group 1.   Simple aphasia.

Group 2.   Aphasia with cerebral involvement of visual processes.

Group 3.   Aphasia with sensorimotor involvement affecting speech.

Group 4.   Aphasia with scattered findings, usually including both visual involvement and dysarthria.

Group 5.   An irreversible aphasic syndrome.

Table 2–8 shows the mean percentages of error for 69 subjects in five major categories on five sections of the MTDDA.

Table 2–8   Mean Percentages of Error on Five Sections of the MTDDA for 69 Aphasic Subjects Grouped into Five Major Categories

Group		Auditory Tests (N 9)	Reading Tests (N 6)	Language Tests (N 14)	Writing Tests (N 8)	Arithmetic Tests (N 8)
Group 1	Initial	21	24	27	32	14
(N 17)	Final	9	12	12	16	5
Group 2	Initial	24	43	25	57	26
(N 16)	Final	12	26	14	37	15
Group 3	Initial	35	39	87	65	36
(N 14)	Final	24	26	45	48	23
Group 4	Initial	43	54	51	72	43
(N 22)	Final	29	43	36	60	36
Group 5	Initial	89	86	93	98	77
(N 4)	Final	67	81	84	98	55
Nonaphasic Subjects (N 50)		2	4	1	6	2

From Schuell, H., Jenkins, J. J., and Jiménez-Pabón, E.: Aphasia in Adults: Diagnosis, Prognosis, and Treatment. New York, Hoeber, 1964.

It can be seen that patients in Group 1 presented a mild aphasia in comparison with the other categories and made about equal recovery in all modalities. Recovery was substantial although not complete. "The majority of Group 1 patients . . . went home to work on their own, until more recovery had taken place. They were able to talk and to listen and to read and to write, and they knew how to work independently to obtain continued improvement."

Patients in Group 2 resembled those in Group 1 in terms of their mildly impaired listening, speech, and arithmetic abilities, but displayed marked problems in discrimination, recognition, and recall of learned visual symbols, resulting in higher levels of error in reading and writing tests. Substantial recovery was observed in all modalities.

Patients in Group 3 showed a higher level of error in all modalities, with marked difficulty in writing and particularly in speech. The markedly disproportionate difficulty in speech was reduced as a result of therapy, and improvement occurred in all modalities.

Group 4 patients showed still higher levels of impairment in listening, reading, writing, and arithmetic, with less marked impairment of speech than Group 3. Both visual and motor processes were almost always involved in these patients, and there were other signs of generalized brain damage, including impairment of recent memory, confusion, and emotional lability. Recovery of language was limited. "Scattered or generalized brain damage and the presence of many adverse physiological and psychological conditions . . . imposed limitations upon recovery. . . . Drive toward recovery, and capacity for intensive and persistent effort, was always diminished, and this was usually a limiting factor."

Group 5 patients presented a picture of severe impairment in all modalities, amounting to almost complete loss of functional language skills. Gains as a result of therapy were small, and patients did not achieve functional speech, reading, or writing. "We are . . . forced to the conclusion that there is a degree of cerebral damage that is incompatible with recovery of functional language skills." This, then, is an irreversible aphasic syndrome compatible with large focal lesions.

Schuell and co-workers demonstrated by longitudinal studies of patients who presented the characteristics described that classification into a given group carries with it a built-in prognosis. Particularly noteworthy is the limited recovery evidenced by the more severely affected groups — Group 4 patients with scattered or generalized brain damage and Group 5 patients with extensive focal lesions. It should be pointed out that test data upon which classification was based were not gathered immediately post onset but rather after the patients were judged to be neurologically stable (generally about 3 months post onset).

Leischner and Linck (1967) reported the results of therapy with two groups of aphasic patients, a group of 46 patients originally described by Leischner (1960) and a second group of 70 patients. These patients reflected a wide range of ages, degrees of severity of aphasia, and etiologies, the largest single group having aphasia of vascular origin. A six-point scale was used to rate the outcome of therapy. Twenty of the 46 patients (43 per cent) in the first study, and 30 of the 70 patients (43 per cent) in the second study made "small improvement," "slight improvement," or "no improvement." Analysis of the outcome of treatment in terms of the "types" of aphasia that patients presented at onset indicated that two thirds of those in the second study who made negligible or no improvement were classified as having "total aphasia," meaning that "there was a disturbance of all functions of speech — spontaneous speech, speech flow, word finding, understanding speech, writing, and reading." The investigators searched for explanations "outside the actual disturbance of speech" to explain the relative nonimprovement of these patients and implicated the personality of the patient, associated somatic and psychic diseases, and excessively long delay between onset of aphasia and treatment; but it is impressive that such a large percentage of those who made little progress were initially globally aphasic.

Sands and colleagues (1969) observed a group of 30 treated aphasic patients during a follow-up period after termination of therapy. They considered differences between scores on the FCP administered at the time of initial pretreatment evaluation, at discharge from treatment, and at a reevaluation 4 to 12 months later. They concluded from their comparison of the three scores that "the higher intake score predicts a higher outcome score. Conversely, the lower the intake score, the poorer is the prognosis for recovery. In the high-gain group the average intake FCP score was 38.3 per cent. In the low-gain group the average intake score was 17.2 per cent. Thus, the severity of language impairment at initial evaluation is a moderately good predictor of the amount of recovery that may be expected."

Sarno and co-workers (1970) reported the results of therapy with 31 stroke patients (age range, 46 to 83 years), all described as patients with severe expressive-receptive aphasia in whom aphasia had commenced 3 to 144 months prior to treatment. Their severe aphasia was defined operationally as an overall FCP score of less than 31 per cent; at the outset, these patients had essentially no speech and little understanding of it; some could say a few words and understand some simple commands. The patients were assigned to one of three treatment groups (programmed instruction, nonprogrammed instruction, no treatment) for variable periods. Evaluation at termination of treatment revealed no significant differences among the three treatment conditions, and the improvement shown in all groups was negligible. The investigators concluded: "The fact that speech therapy, of either type, did not affect language recovery in this study is no doubt related to the severity of their aphasia."

Kenin and Swisher (1972) studied a group of 15 "Broca's aphasic patients" (mean age, 58 years). They administered the NCCEA twice, once at the time of initial contact and a second time within 6 weeks to 3 months; during the interim all patients received therapy. On initial contact the patients were also evaluated with the FCP. The study revealed that all patients improved, but to unequal degrees: "As would be expected, patients considered to be most severely impaired as rated on the FCP during initial evaluation tended to have fewer positive changes and more stationary results on tests than the less severe aphasics, who showed the reverse trend, that of fewer stationary changes and more positive changes."

The clinical records of 39 aphasic patients were studied by Keenan and Brassell (1974) in an effort to correlate factors noted in their initial examination with their subsequent progress in communication. Three nonlanguage and five language variables were studied. A clinical scale of speech performance based on the patient's most characteristic conversational responses was used to classify terminal communicative performance as "good," "fair," or "poor." The patients' initial performance levels in the four language modalities — listening, talking, reading, and writing — were classified on three-point scales analogous to the speech performance scale. Initial listening performance level was rated as follows: when patients' speech comprehension was limited to following single-item instructions ("Point to the door"), listening was rated poor; if they could follow an instruction involving a series of three items or a simple relationship among items ("Put the quarter under the paper"), their listening was rated fair; if they could follow a complex, multisentence instruction ("Pick up the pencil and the little key. Then give them to me along with the paper"), listening was rated good. Initial reading performance was rated as follows: patients who showed comprehension of nothing more complex than single nouns were rated poor; if they followed instructions such as "Knock on the table," they were rated fair; if they correctly executed longer printed instructions such as "Put your finger on each s in this sentence," reading was rated good. Talking performance level consisted of a judgmental rating with the three-point scale. For determination of writing performance level, patients were asked to write the names of objects and describe simple and complicated actions; those who could not get past the single-word level were rated poor; if they wrote an intelligible and grammatical phrase, they were considered fair; if they wrote adequate legible sentences, they were rated good.

Two of the four modality performance levels — listening and talking — were found to be related significantly to the patient's terminal speech performance. When correlated with initial listening performance, the distributions of the terminally poor speakers and the fair and good speakers were significantly different. Of 17 patients whose initial listening performance was poor, 12 (70 per cent) had poor terminal speech and five had fair or good terminal speech; of 22 patients whose initial listening performance was fair or good, five had poor terminal speech, and 17 (77 per cent) completed therapy with fair or good speech. Similarly, patients' initial speech performances were significantly related to their terminal speech performances. Of 28 patients with poor speech initially, 17 had poor speech at the conclusion of therapy. All 11 patients whose speech was good or fair at initial evaluation were dismissed with good speech.

In contrast, correlation of both initial reading and initial writing performance levels with terminal speech performance failed to reach significance. The investigators concluded that initial listening level and initial talking level provide useful information to predict ultimate speech performance with a fairly high degree of accuracy, but initial reading and writing performances are not similarly useful for prediction.

Holland and Sonderman (1974) provided programmed instruction to a group of 24 aphasic patients. The training task was based on the Token Test, and improvement and errors were analyzed to evaluate the training. Severity of the patients' aphasia was rated on the basis of their clinical behavior and the results of initial Token Test and MTDDA scores: mild, 4; mild to moderate, 6; moderate, 5; moderate to severe, 3; and severe, 6. Results of the study indicated that patients rated as having mild or mild to moderately severe aphasia showed significant improvement; in contrast, those rated as having moderate, moderate to severe, or severe aphasia failed to show significant improvement.

The possible influence of each of 19 variables conceivably related to recovery from aphasia was studied by Gloning and co-workers (1976) in a study of 107 aphasic patients (mean age, 39 years) who after initial evaluation were retested after 7 days and again after approximately 18 months. All patients had aphasia of traumatic or vascular etiology. Multiple linear regression analysis was performed to determine which variables were significantly related to outcome. One of the four variables found to have a significant negative influence was "severe aphasia." Patients were judged to present severe aphasia "if verbal communication between examiner and patient was completely lacking." Patients with severe aphasia recovered significantly less completely than patients not so described initially.

Another study of prognostic factors in recovery from aphasia was reported by Messerli and associates (1976). They studied a group of 53 patients (age range, 17 to 74 years) with aphasia of vascular or traumatic etiology, all of whom had "benefitted from speech therapy or ... been subjected to neuro-psychological treatment." Among other things, the investigators related initial severity of aphasia to the level of communication reached at the end of therapy. The oral expression, repetition, comprehension, writing, and reading of the patients were evaluated, and on the basis of these evaluations their overall language impairment was rated as "very severe," "severe," "moderate," or "light." A significant relationship was found between the severity of the aphasia and the level of communication reached at the end of therapy. The investigators concluded: "The severity of aphasia influences to a large extent the amount of residual disorders of language. The severe aphasic patients rarely recovered their previous verbal capacities completely even though it is among these patients that we find the longest periods of therapy. This explains why we do not find any significant relationship between the duration of therapy and the level of communication reached at the end of that period."

In his study of aphasia due to focal disorders of cerebral circulation, Kohlmeyer (1976) made observations about patients of various "types" and levels of severity of aphasia. One conclusion that he drew pertained to patients with "global aphasia," which he defined as having "no useful language left." His conclusion was that "the spontaneous recovery from global aphasia is always limited, whether there is an occlusion of middle cerebral artery or not."

Kertesz and McCabe (1977), in their study of the recovery patterns of aphasic patients, correlated the initial severity of aphasia, measured by the initial Aphasia Quotient (AQ) levels on the WAB, and the outcome, measured by the final AQ levels in the study. They reported: "The initial severity of aphasia and final outcome in the stable CVA's [N = 30] was found to be significantly correlated (r = 0.849). In other words, severely affected aphasics recovered to a lesser extent and reached a lower level of speech function than mildly affected ones. . . . One should qualify that 'outcome,' as we used it, should not be considered final, but we chose the test values beyond 12 months post onset to represent outcome for practical purposes. This was felt to be justified by the relatively little improvement with a few exceptions beyond this point. Caution should be exercised when individual prognosis is given because of these exceptions." They also commented on the progress of 22 patients designated "global aphasics," "who understand little or nothing and speak only in stereotyped utterances." They concluded that globally aphasic patients "show limited recovery as a rule."

Hanson and Cicciarelli (1978) scheduled serial administrations of the PICA to a group of 13 aphasic patients (mean age, 56 years). The first PICA was administered from 8 to 64 days post onset (mean, 33 days) and PICAs were subsequently administered about every 6 weeks, with a range of three to nine administrations. Therapy was conducted throughout the period of the study. It was found that the amount and level of improvement demonstrated by these patients were significantly related to the initial severity of their aphasia. The patients with the highest initial overall PICA scores attained the highest peak scores (r =

0.87). It was also noted that those with the lowest initial scores made a greater amount of change ($r = -0.67$). For example, whereas the patient who scored highest initially moved during therapy from the 83rd to the 99th percentile on the PICA, the patient who scored lowest initially moved from the 15th to the 50th percentile. So patients who had more ground to regain tended to regain more ground than those who had less ground to regain, but the more severely affected patients attained lower terminal levels than did those whose aphasia was initially less severe.

In their study of the differential effects of treatment and nontreatment in a total group of 281 aphasic patients, Basso and co-workers (1979) reported the effect of overall initial severity of aphasia on improvement of language function. In each of four separate analyses of the language modalities studied (oral expression, auditory verbal comprehension, writing, reading) a significant relationship was found between the amount of improvement and the initial severity. Their main finding was that formal language rehabilitation has a positive effect on the ability to communicate, but they added, "At the same time, our results also showed that the beneficial influence of treatment is counterbalanced to a certain extent by the negative (and equally significant) effect of two other factors, that is, time since onset and overall severity of aphasia. These factors significantly influenced the subsequent course of nontreated as well as that of treated patients. The practical implication of such contrasting effects is that all three variables should be taken into consideration before formulating a prognosis."

Patterns of Test Performance.   In Chapter 4, data from treatment studies will be reviewed showing the relationship between initial patterns of aphasic performance (usually abbreviated as "types of aphasia") and the outcome of treatment. We will see that Wepman (1951) found that patients with predominantly expressive difficulty improved most and attained the highest level of achievement, whereas those with predominantly receptive difficulty improved least. In contrast, Vignolo (1964) felt that expressive disorders had a more negative effect on recovery and a poorer prognosis. But other investigators (Leischner, 1960; Messerli et al., 1976; Gloning et al., 1976; Basso et al., 1974, 1979) found that all "types" have an essentially equal chance of recovery (see pp. 180–181). These data will not be detailed here further. Other data will be reviewed which suggest how early patterns of performance may indicate ultimate recovery.

Gloning and associates (1976) studied 107 patients with aphasia of traumatic or vascular etiology, first arriving at a diagnosis of aphasia on the results of a screening test and the judgment of a neurologist, then securing a baseline aphasia examination after 7 days, and administering a final examination after approximately 18 months. Using a modified multiple linear regression analysis, they related each of 19 selected variables to the outcome as measured by the final examination. One of the two variables found to have a positive influence on the prognosis was "improvement of aphasia within 1 week," meaning "improvement within the week subsequent to the first examination." The investigators clarified this finding as follows: "In most patients it may reflect the role of spontaneous recovery. But there are two aphasics with long-lasting illness (two years' and 19 years' duration of aphasia) in whom aphasia was markedly improved after one week of intensive speech therapy."

The recovery patterns of 36 aphasic patients were studied by Kertesz and McCabe (1977). They administered the WAB to the patients within a period of 0 to 6 weeks post onset, subsequently retested them at 3 and 6 months, and then at yearly intervals. They divided their group, using taxonomic principles, into several subgroups on the base of fluency, comprehension, repetition ability, and naming ability. Statistical analysis revealed significant differences in recovery rates (not extent of recovery) between the various types of aphasia so classified. Globally aphasic patients (those who understood little or nothing and spoke only in stereotyped utterances) showed limited recovery. Patients with impaired fluency but good comprehension (identified as having Broca's or motor aphasia) showed the highest recovery rates. Patients who made many phonemic paraphasic errors but displayed fair fluency and good comprehension but poor repetition (identified as conduction aphasic patients) likewise showed high recovery rates. Patients with limited comprehension and varying degrees of jargon behavior (identified as Wernicke's aphasic patients) displayed two patterns of recovery. Those who used more jargon improved little and continued to use fluent jargon for many months; those who had less severe comprehension difficulty and used less jargon improved more rapidly. Patients whose primary difficulty was in naming (identified as anomic aphasic patients) had the mildest language impairment initially and often recovered completely.

Kertesz and McCabe present further information about the outcome in various types of aphasia in a group of 47 patients followed for a year or longer (average follow-up, 28.6 months). Language performance on the last test was rated as poor, fair, good, or excellent. "Almost all of the global aphasics remained poor. Broca's and Wernicke's aphasics showed a wider range of outcome; some patients with Wernicke's aphasia remained severely incapacitated for a long time; some recover well. Broca's aphasics have an intermediate outlook just about evenly divided between fair and good recovery. Anomic, conduction, and transcortical aphasics have a uniformly good prognosis, the majority of cases showing excellent recovery."

An investigation specifically designed to study the recovery over a 3-month period of patients with different patterns of receptive and expressive deficits has been reported by Lomas and Kertesz (1978).

They selected 31 patients with aphasia of cerebrovascular etiology (age range, 31 to 82 years), administered the WAB initially within 30 days post onset, and administered a retest at or around 3 months post onset with no intervening aphasia therapy. Two tests were used for classification of the patients into four groups: the patients' speech samples, consisting of oral responses to six simple questions and their description of a picture, were rated on a 10-point scale of fluency of spontaneous speech (fluency in terms of prosody, jargon, telegraphic speech, word-finding difficulty, neologisms, and paraphasias); these ratings were used as a measure of expressive ability. On a test of auditory word discrimination, the patients pointed to objects, pictures, or body parts on request; their response scores were used as a measure of receptive ability. The median value for each task (based on 31 patients) was made the cutoff point between "high" (good) and "low" (poor) scores. With each patient's scores defined as either high or low on each of these tasks, each was placed into one of four groups: Low Fluency/Low Comprehension (N = 13), Low Fluency/High Comprehension (N = 5), High Fluency/Low Comprehension (N = 5), and High Fluency/High Comprehension (N = 8). "By describing an aphasic group purely on the basis of their language scores it was felt that some of the ambiguities of the more frequently used historical terms might be avoided while maintaining the distinction between predominantly expressive or receptive disorders."

All patients were administered eight tasks from the WAB: two comprehension tasks (yes/no questions and sequential commands); oral imitation (repetition of words, phrases, and sentences); and five expressive tasks (word fluency in producing as many animal names as possible in one minute; orally naming objects; information content rated on a 10-point scale applied to spontaneous speech in the form of the patients' responses to simple questions and their description of a picture; sentence completion; and responsive speech involving single-noun responses to simple questions). The measure of recovery was the difference in scores between initial and second testings, designated the recovery score for each of the eight tasks. The statistical procedure used controlled for initial severity so that "the degree of recovery for any aphasic or language task is not simply attributable to the amount of 'space' available for their improvement."

The relative degrees of recovery of the four groups as represented by their overall mean recovery scores on all eight language tasks are shown in Figure 2–2. The Low Fluency/Low Comprehension group improved significantly less than the other three groups, and the Low Fluency/High Comprehension group improved significantly more than the other three groups.

Furthermore, the four groups showed different patterns of recovery, as summarized in Figure 2–3. In the Low Fluency/Low Comprehension group (Fig. 2–3A), only comprehension and imitation

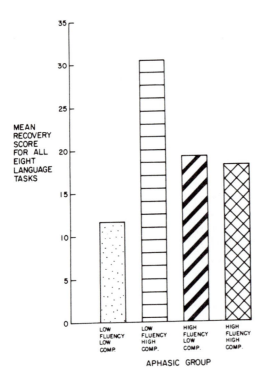

Figure 2–2. Mean recovery scores (score on eight language tasks at 3 month testing minus score at initial testing with initial severities statistically controlled) of four groups of untreated aphasic patients, as reported by Lomas and Kertesz. (From Lomas, J., and Kertesz, A.: Patterns of spontaneous recovery in aphasic groups: a study of adult stroke patients. Brain and Language, 5:388–401, 1978.)

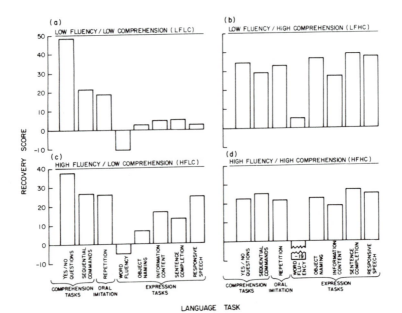

Figure 2–3. Recovery scores on eight language tasks of four groups of untreated aphasic patients, as reported by Lomas and Kertesz. (From Lomas, J., and Kertesz, A.: Patterns of spontaneous recovery in aphasic groups: a study of adult stroke patients. Brain and Language, 5:388–401, 1978.)

showed recovery scores significantly different from zero. Nonimitative expressive tasks showed little or no improvement.

The Low Fluency/High Comprehension group (Fig. 2–3B) demonstrated significant recovery on all language tasks except word fluency. Comprehension, imitation, and expression showed equal and appreciable improvement.

The High Fluency/Low Comprehension group (Fig. 2–3C) exhibited a recovery score significantly different from zero on comprehension and imitation tasks and also on the responsive speech task. Lesser degrees of improvement were shown on other expression tasks except object naming and word fluency. "This pattern is very similar to that of the Low Fluency/Low Comprehension group, suggesting that an initial impairment in comprehension gives rise to most marked improvement in imitation and comprehension tasks. . . . The additional recovery of some expressive ability. . . does not match the level of improvement seen in these tasks for a group with relatively intact comprehension and impaired fluency."

The High Fluency/High Comprehension group (Fig. 2–3D) earned recovery scores significantly different from zero on all language tasks except word fluency, which deteriorated in this group. The across-the-board improvement observed in comprehension, imitation, and expression was not, however, of the same magnitude as seen in the Low Fluency/High Comprehension group.

The investigators drew the following conclusions from their data: "These results would seem to suggest that the degree of initial comprehension deficit is an important prognostic indicator. Those aphasic groups with a high initial level of comprehension (Low Fluency/High Comprehension and High Fluency/High Comprehension) showed across-the-board improvement with the exception of Word Fluency. In contrast, those groups with a low initial level of comprehension (Low Fluency/Low Comprehension and High Fluency/Low Comprehension) showed only a selective improvement in language functions with appreciable increases in scores occurring largely for the comprehension and imitation tasks. It appears, then, that initial level of comprehension may predict the extent of expressive language recovery. Only those groups initially high on comprehension showed appreciable improvements in expressive language. All groups showed improvement in receptive language and repetition."

As noted earlier in this chapter, Schuell and co-workers (1964) showed that appraisal information obtained with a comprehensive aphasia test such as the MTDDA yielded five major profiles of aphasic dysfunction, combining levels of severity and modality patterns of involvement; these groupings carry with them a prediction regarding ultimate recovery. Porch has suggested several ways in which information gathered with another test, the PICA, can be used for making predictions about the level of recovery from aphasia. Four of these methods that use performance on the PICA administered early post onset to predict performance at a later date will be reviewed.

In the PICA test manual, Porch (1971a) described use of the Nine-High percentile and the Nine-Low percentile. One selects the patient's nine highest subtest scores, adds them, divides the total by nine, and using a table of recovery curve percentiles (Porch's Appendix E) finds the closest score to the Nine-High mean in the column headed "Highs"; the percentile in the adjacent column is the percentile equivalent for the Nine-High score. Similarly, one calculates the

RECOVERY CURVE PERCENTILES, LEFT HEMISPHERE DAMAGE (N =280)

%	Highs	OA	Lows
//	//	//	//
97	14.96	14.46	13.95
96	14.95	14.33	13.72
95	14.93	14.21	13.49
94	14.91	14.12	13.83
93	14.89	14.03	13.17
92	14.88	13.95	13.01
91	14.86	13.86	12.85
90	14.84	13.77	12.69
89	14.83	13.68	12.53
88	14.80	13.59	12.38
87	14.77	13.50	12.22
86	14.75	13.41	12.07
85	14.73	13.32	11.91
84	14.70	13.25	11.80
83	14.67	13.18	11.69
82	14.65	13.11	11.58
81	14.62	13.04	11.47
80	14.59	12.97	11.36
79	14.57	12.89	11.22
78	14.54	12.81	11.07
77	14.52	12.72	10.93
76	14.49	12.64	10.78
75	14.47	12.56	10.64
74	14.43	12.48	10.52
73	14.40	12.40	10.40
72	14.36	12.33	10.28
71	14.33	12.25	10.16
70	14.29	12.17	10.04

Predicted OA %ile at 6 MPO — 96

Predicted OA at 6 MPO — 93 / 92

Predicted OA at 6 MPO — 74 / 73 → 14.33

OA at One MPO — 70

Figure 2–4. Use of the HOAP method to predict PICA performance at 6 months post onset for a patient at 70th percentile 1 month post onset. (From Wertz, R. T., Deal, L., and Deal, J.: Prognosis in aphasia: investigation of the High-Overall Prediction (HOAP) method and the Short-Direct or HOAP Slope method to predict change in PICA performance. In Clinical Aphasiology Conference Proceedings 1980. Minneapolis, BRK Publishers, 1980, pp. 164–172.)

percentile equivalent for the average of the nine lowest subtest scores. The difference between the high and the low percentiles, called the High-Low gap, "represents the potential dynamic range of the patient's communicative system" (Porch, 1971b). "Unless there are other complications this difference. . .should be erased by treatment. A zero High-Low gap after the patient's condition has stabilized generally means that he has reached maximum benefit from his treatment" (Porch, 1971a).

An extension of this procedure, called the High-Overall Prediction method (HOAP), is described by Wertz and co-workers (1980) as a procedure to use data from a PICA administered approximately 1 month post onset to predict overall performance at 6 months post onset. "The clinician finds the patient's Overall PICA score at 1 month post onset in the percentile table, moves laterally in the table to the 'Highs' column, selects the High raw score, re-enters the Overall column, moves upward until the selected High score is found, and selects the corresponding percentile to represent the patient's predicted performance at 6 months post onset. For example [Fig. 2–4],. . .if a patient obtains a PICA Overall score of 12.25 (71st percentile) at 1 month post onset, the clinician enters the percentile table Overall column (OA) and locates the adjacent 'High' score, which is 14.33. Re-entering the Overall column, the clinician moves upward to find a raw score of 14.33. Once located, the raw score is converted to the corresponding percentile (96th percentile), and this becomes the patient's predicted performance at 6 months post onset."

Another method, the Short-Direct or HOAP Slope method, uses the HOAP Slope graph provided by Porch (Fig. 2–5). A PICA is administered within the first month post onset and the Overall score is computed and converted to a percentile. Quoting Wertz and colleagues (1980), "Utilizing the HOAP Slope sheet, the clinician finds the patient's appropriate months post onset (MPO) column, locates the patient's Overall percentile in the MPO column, and moves parallel up the nearest HOAP Slope to find the patient's predicted performance at points in time up to 6 months post onset. For example [Fig. 2–5],. . .a PICA Overall score of 12.25 obtained at one MPO converts to the 71st percentile. Entering the one MPO column and moving downward to the HOAP Slope at the 70th percentile, the clinician then moves parallel along this slope to predict 85th percentile performance at three MPO and 96th percentile performance at six MPO." Porch cautioned that both methods are most accurate when applied to patients with aphasia of thromboembolic etiology.

Wertz and associates (1980) have reported on the accuracy of prediction of both methods. They used the results of two administrations of the PICA within the first 6 months post onset to a group of 85 patients who had had a single left-hemisphere thromboembolic cerebrovascular accident (CVA). One prediction group (one MPO predict-

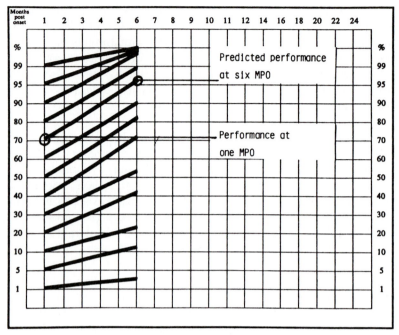

Figure 2–5. Use of HOAP Slope method to predict PICA Overall percentile at 6 months post onset for a patient with 12.25 Overall score at 1 month post onset. (From Wetz, R. T., Deal, L., and Deal, J.: Prognosis in aphasia: investigation of the High-Overall Prediction (HOAP) method and the Short-Direct or HOAP Slope method to predict change in PICA performance. *In* Clinical Aphasiology Conference Proceedings 1980. Minneapolis, BRK Publishers, 1980, pp. 164–172.)

ing six MPO) was used to test the HOAP method; three prediction groups (one MPO predicting three MPO, one MPO predicting six MPO, and three MPO predicting six MPO) were used to test the HOAP Slope method.

With regard first to the HOAP method, the mean Overall percentile predicted by this method at six MPO was the 72nd. The mean Overall percentile actually obtained by the group of 63 patients (age range, 36 to 79 years) was the 67th. The correlation between predicted and obtained performance was 0.75. The differences between predicted and obtained scores for individual patients ranged from −40 to +27 percentile units. If one designated a 10-percentile change in PICA Overall percentile as a clinically significant change, the HOAP method predicted accurately (that is, obtained scores within plus or minus 10 percentile points of those predicted) for 49 per cent of the sample; it underpredicted (obtained scores were greater than 10 percentile units) for 40 per cent; and it overpredicted (obtained scores were greater than −10 percentile units) for 11 per cent.

The HOAP Slope method predicted a mean Overall percentile of 56 for the one MPO predicting three MPO group; a mean percentile of

59 was actually obtained; prediction was accurate for 67 per cent of the patients. For the one MPO predicting six MPO group, 71st percentile mean performance was predicted, and 67th percentile mean performance was obtained; prediction was accurate for 52 per cent of this group. For the three MPO predicting six MPO group, 76th percentile mean performance was predicted, and 66th percentile mean performance was obtained; prediction was accurate for 42 per cent of this group.

The investigators concluded, "Our results suggest that the HOAP and the HOAP Slope methods for predicting improved PICA performance are more promising than practical. Neither method placed more than 67 per cent of the patients in any of our prediction groups within plus or minus ten percentile units of the PICA score obtained. Group predictions were more accurate than individual predictions. While correlations between predicted scores and scores obtained were significant, the range of misprediction for individual patients was frightening."

A statistical technique for predicting change in aphasia has been suggested by Porch and co-workers (1980). Using data available on a group of 144 patients with aphasia of vascular etiology, they employed a stepwise multiple regression procedure to predict change in severity of aphasia at 3, 6, and 12 months post onset based on performance at 1, 3, and 6 months post onset. The predictors incorporated into their formulae were PICA Gestural, Verbal, and Graphic subtest scores and age. "The most consistent significant predictor of recovery from aphasia was the PICA Gestural mean. It was included in all six of the predictive equations. In fact, the PICA Gestural mean at one MPO was the single significant predictor for predicting the PICA Overall score at 12 MPO. The PICA Graphic mean was included as a predictor in four of the six predictive equations. The PICA Verbal mean was included in three of the six equations. Age was included in only two of the six equations. . . . Age,. . . in the sample we studied, was less important for predicting recovery than the three measures of language behavior. Thus, a patient's language performance may be more important in developing a prognosis than age."

To determine the relationship between the predicted PICA Overall score and the Overall score actually obtained by each prediction group, multiple correlation coefficients were computed. Correlations ranged from 0.74 to 0.94, all values being significant. Predictions over shorter durations (for example, one MPO to three MPO and three MPO to six MPO) and for periods when improvement is more stable (for example, three MPO to 12 MPO and six MPO to 12 MPO) yielded large correlation values. Predictions over longer periods or during a period of rapid change yielded smaller correlation values.

Their report constitutes an attempt to evaluate a method of predicting change in aphasia rather than the production of a specific set of predictive equations that have immediate application. Their findings suggested that "it is possible to generate formulae which convert an aphasic patient's language behavior into a fairly accurate prognosis for eventual change in communicative ability."

Associated Speech Problems. Contradictory evidence concerning the negative influence of certain expressive speech difficulties on recovery from aphasia has been reported by several investigators. In the earliest of the three studies by the Milan group on recovery from aphasia, Vignolo (1964) drew the conclusion on the basis of changes in 69 aphasic patients that expressive disorders have a poorer prognosis and greater negative effect on overall recovery than receptive disorders. "The factor limiting recovery of oral expression is to be found within expression itself." Examining the individual case data, he observed that total inability to communicate through oral speech was in itself a poor prognostic sign, although not absolute. "The hypothesis may be advanced that one specific expressive symptom, *anarthria*, [may] be responsible for limiting expressive recovery. Anarthria is characterized by severe reduction in the flow of speech, marked phonemic disorders of expression — such as elisions or substitutions of phonemes — and articulatory difficulties, usually accompanied by oral apraxia." (Presumably his "anarthria" is the equivalent of our "apraxia of speech.") Vignolo attempted to test the hypothesis but had to conclude, "There are hints that anarthria has a negative influence on recovery of expression, but we cannot demonstrate it unequivocally because we cannot isolate anarthria from other variables (time from onset, in particular)." Subsequently, Basso and Vignolo (1969) likewise stated that, "Other things being equal, the presence of phonemic articulatory disorders has a poor prognostic significance."

In the third of the Milan studies, Basso and co-workers (1979) obtained no data that would support this hypothesis. The expressive difficulties implicit in the term "nonfluent," presumably similar to the behavior called "anarthria," were found not to influence the outcome of aphasia recovery significantly in either treated or untreated patients.

Thomsen (1975) reported on a group of 12 patients who became aphasic as a result of severe closed head trauma (mean age, 25.5 years). They were tested informally during the first few weeks following injury and then had a comprehensive follow-up aphasia examination an average of 33 months later (range, 12 to 50 months). At the time of this re-evaluation, eight of the 12 patients still had symptoms of aphasia, one severe. "None of the four patients with dysarthria. . .made a full recovery." And Thomsen adds, "The presence of and degree of concomitant neuropsychological disorders were most important for the final outcome."

Similarly, Keenan and Brassell (1974) have suggested a negative prognostic influence of dysarthria. They studied the clinical records of

39 aphasic patients and correlated factors noted in their initial examination with their subsequent progress in communication, their terminal communicative performance being rated as "good," "fair," or "poor." Patients were classified according to degree of articulation difficulty observed on initial examination. Motor speech impairment, "chiefly apraxia and some dysarthria," was classified as "minimal," "mild," or "severe." (Patients rated as having severe impairment usually had unintelligible speech and showed marked difficulty imitating vowels, simple words, or numerals; patients whose conditions were rated mild produced effortful and often distorted speech but were usually understood; those with still less prominent difficulty were rated as having minimal impairment.) Results showed that "14 of the 16 patients who began with marked difficulty imitating vowels or simple common words continued to have poor speech. Of the 23 patients who initially had mild or minimal impairment of motor speech, 20 had at least fair speech at the termination of therapy." Statistical analysis revealed significantly different distributions of incidence of initial motor speech impairment among the three terminal speech groups.

In their study of 19 variables conceivably related to recovery from aphasia, Gloning and colleagues (1976) included among the variables severe dysarthria (judged to be present in patients who were totally unable to speak or at least 50 per cent of whose utterances were unintelligible) and severe oral apraxia (patient unable to stick out his tongue or open his mouth on command or in imitation without paresis of such degree as to account for this incapacity). In the 107 aphasic patients studied (mean age, 39 years) severe dysarthria was found to have a significant negative prognostic effect on recovery, but severe oral apraxia did not.

Specific Language Behaviors. Several investigators who have studied aphasic patients longitudinally and tested them serially have reported that certain language behaviors or changes in language behavior appear to have prognostic value.

Schuell did not believe that reliable prediction could be based upon testing very early post onset. Her recommendation was that testing for prediction should be done at approximately 3 months, when patients' conditions have become neurologically stable. It was her observation that in such stabilized patients, those who failed ultimately to recover functional speech were patients who made errors in recognition of common words spoken by the examiner (Schuell, 1953, 1955). She called this behavior "auditory verbal agnosia" and considered it to be a prognostic sign when it persisted this long. One might say that such behavior is a kind of abbreviated index of the behavior often identified as global aphasia, with severe impairment of all modalities and limited recovery.

Wepman (1958) has pointed out that the ability to recognize and self-correct errors "is defective to some degree in almost every aphasic adult patient. The severity of the defect and its effect upon the patient is felt to be one of the best indicators of the extent of the language problem." Wepman believed that it was useful to chart the patient's degree of insight and ability to self-correct errors. He designed the Self-Correction Scale, presented earlier (Table 2–5). He summarized the value of such observations thus: "The time it takes a particular patient to move from one level of the ability to self-correct to another is felt to be an excellent indicator of the prognosis for the patient." He presented no data in support of this conclusion, but based it, as have other clinicians, upon observation of language change in aphasic patients.

Changes in language behavior during the earliest weeks post onset were charted by Culton (1968, 1969). He administered eight tasks involving all language modalities to a group of 11 "recent" aphasic patients. He tested them initially less than 30 days post onset and readministered the test battery at 2-week intervals over a period of 2 months. He drew the following conclusions: Poor recovery of language is indicated when subjects are initially unable to point to pictures of objects after having been given the names of the objects (Schuell's auditory verbal agnosia) and when a few weeks after onset the patients remain unable to write words to dictation. He thought that prognosis was good for subjects who exhibited large amounts of spontaneous recovery on oral encoding tasks, such as naming and answering simple questions, and who progressively improved in their ability to write words to dictation even though initially they made no correct responses on this task.

In the study whose design was described earlier, Keenan and Brassell (1974) used as one of the five language variables which they related to the patients' terminal communicative performance what they called speech stimulability, defined as "the relative effectiveness of measures taken to improve a patient's speech responses." When their patients produced speech errors during the initial examination, they were provided with prompts or cues, such as related words, phrases, or sentences, or they were given correct responses to read aloud or to imitate; sometimes they were asked only to try again. The degree to which these attempts at correction resulted in improved responses was scaled as "not effective," "effective to a limited extent," or "rapidly and significantly effective." Results indicated that this variable was significantly related to terminal speech outcome. Of the 14 patients for whom stimulation was not effective, 13 were reported to have poor speech at the terminal examination; all 12 for whom stimulation was very effective finished with good speech. Of 25 patients who showed some speech stimulability, four had poor terminal speech and 21 had fair or good terminal speech.

In their study of the changes in language performance of 107 aphasic patients over a period of approximately 18 months, Gloning and co-workers (1976) included among the 19 variables conceivably related to recovery five variables that were specific speech behaviors: severe jargon (production of utterances of consistent jargon lasting at least 2 minutes during the examination), severe paraphasia (if 50 per cent or more of the patient's utterances consisted of phonologic, verbal, neologistic, or unclassifiable substitutes), severe disturbance of repetition (inability to repeat correctly combinations of at least two syllables), lack of verbal spontaneity (when spontaneous initiation of speech was completely absent), and severe disorders of verbal comprehension (lack of response to commands "with the exception of the elementary commands such as opening the mouth or shaking hands"). Only one of these variables was found to have significant negative prognostic value — namely, severe disturbance of repetition.

It is apparent that certain appraisal data obtained in the early period post onset provide significantly useful predictors of the probable outcome of recovery in aphasia. First, the evidence is incontrovertible that, in general, the more severe the aphasia initially, the less likely the patient is to regain functional communication. Patients who are initially severely aphasic, including those often designated as having global aphasia, may make measurable gains and indeed may advance many percentile points on a scale of communication adequacy; but the best expectation is that they will not attain levels of achievement in communication comparable to those whose initial severity is less. Observations made of individual exceptional cases would cause one to temper the absoluteness of such a prediction, but as a general rule, patients who are still severely aphasic a month or two post onset cannot be expected to regain normal language function.

Patterns of aphasic dysfunction in the various modalities observed on initial testing also provide some indication of projected relative degrees of recovery. Higher degrees of initial auditory comprehension generally constitute a favorable prognosis for significant recovery in all modalities. Greater initial impairment of auditory comprehension generally portends poorer recovery of expressive skills, although there may be significant improvement in comprehension and the ability to make imitative responses.

Specific language behaviors that suggest limited ultimate recovery include the persistence of jargon, associated usually with persistent impairment of auditory comprehension; early and persistent inability to recognize the import of single spoken words (auditory verbal agnosia); persistent inability to write single words to dictation; and severe impairment of ability to repeat words. Behaviors that suggest a favorable prognosis include a significant degree of early spontaneous recovery, especially on such expressive tasks as naming and answering questions; rapid increase in insight and the ability to self-correct errors; and the ability to respond better when further stimulated or encouraged.

Profiles of test performance derived from given tests such as the

MTDDA and the PICA can be used to predict outcome. Such predictions, though fairly accurate for groups of patients, involve considerable error when applied to individual patients.

REFERENCES

Basso, A., and Vignolo, A. L.: Come se imposta rieducazione del linguaccio nell'afasia: utilita di una analisi qualitativa dell'eloquio patologico. Europa Medicophys., 5:140–160, 1969.

Basso, A., Capitani, E., and Vignolo, A. L.: Influence of rehabilitation on language skills in aphasic patients. Arch. Neurol., 36:190–196, 1979.

Basso, A., Faglioni, P., and Vignolo, A. L.: Etude controlée de la réeducation du langage dans l'aphasie: comparaison entre aphasiques traités et non-traités. Rev. Neurol. (Paris), 131:607–614, 1975.

Benson, D. F.: Fluency in aphasia: correlation with radioactive scan localization. Cortex, 3:373–394, 1967.

Borkowski, J. G., Benton, A. L., and Spreen, O.: Word fluency and brain damage. Neuropsychologia, 5:135–140, 1967.

Brown, J.: The problem of repetition: a study of "conduction" aphasia and the "isolation" syndrome. Cortex, 11:37–52, 1975.

Butfield, E., and Zangwill, O. L.: Re-education in aphasia: a review of 70 cases. J. Neurol. Neurosurg. Psychiatry, 9:75–79, 1946.

Chapey, R., Rigrodsky, S., and Morrison, E. B.: Divergent semantic behavior in aphasia. J. Speech Hearing Res., 19:664–677, 1976.

Chapey, R., Rigrodsky, S., and Morrison, E. B.: Aphasia: a divergent semantic interpretation. J. Speech Hearing Disord., 42:287–295, 1977.

Chédru, F., and Geschwind, N.: Disorders of higher cortical functions in acute confusional states. Cortex, 8:395–411, 1972.

Culton, G. L.: Spontaneous recovery from aphasia. Ph.D. Dissertation, Denver, Colorado, University of Denver, 1968.

Culton, G. L.: Spontaneous recovery from aphasia. J. Speech Hearing Res., 12:825–832, 1969.

Darley, F. L. (Ed.): Evaluation of Appraisal Techniques in Speech and Language Pathology. Reading, Massachusetts, Addison-Wesley, 1979.

Darley, F. L., Aronson, A. E., and Brown, J. R.: Motor Speech Disorders. Philadelphia, W. B. Saunders, 1975.

Davis, N., and Leach, E.: Scaling aphasics' error responses. J. Speech Hearing Disord., 37:305–313, 1972.

DeRenzi, E., and Faglioni, P.: Examination for aphasic disturbances of oral comprehension by means of an abbreviated version of the Token Test. Aphasia-Apraxia-Agnosia, 1:12–25, 1979.

DeRenzi, E., and Ferrari, C.: The Reporter's Test: a sensitive test to detect expressive disturbances in aphasics. Cortex, 14:279–293, 1978.

DeRenzi, E., and Vignolo, L. A.: The Token Test: a sensitive test to detect receptive disturbances in aphasics. Brain, 85:665–678, 1962.

DiSimoni, F. G., Darley, F. L., and Aronson, A. E.: Patterns of dysfunction in schizophrenic patients on an aphasia test battery. J. Speech Hearing Disord., 42:498–513, 1977.

Gloning, K., Trappl, R., Heiss, W. D., and Quatember, R.: Prognosis and speech therapy in aphasia. In Lebrun, Y., and Hoops, R. (Eds.): Recovery in Aphasics. Atlantic Highlands, New Jersey, Humanities Press, 1976, pp. 57–64.

Golper, L. E. A., Thorpe, P., Tompkins, C., Marshall, R. C., and Rau, M. T.: Connected language sampling: an expanded index of aphasic language behavior. In Clinical Aphasiology Conference Proceedings 1980. Minneapolis, BRK Publishers, 1980, pp. 174–186.

Goodglass, H., and Kaplan, E.: The Assessment of Aphasia and Related Disorders. Philadelphia, Lea & Febiger, 1972.

Guilford, J.: The Nature of Human Intelligence. New York, McGraw-Hill Book Company, 1967.

Halpern, H., Darley, F. L., and Brown, J. R.: Differential language and neurologic characteristics in cerebral involvement. J. Speech Hearing Disord., 38:162–173, 1973.

Hanson, W. R., and Cicciarelli, A. W.: The time, amount, and pattern of language improvement in adult aphasics. Br. J. Disord. Commun., 13:59–63, 1978.

Holland, A. L., and Sonderman, J. C.: Effects of a program based on the Token Test for teaching comprehension skills to aphasics. J. Speech Hearing Res., 17:589–598, 1974.

Kaplan, L. T.: A descriptive continuum of language responses in aphasia. J. Speech Hearing Disord., 24:410–412, 1959.

Karlin, I. W., Eisenson, J., Hirschenfang, S., and Miller, M. H.: A multievaluational study of aphasic and non-aphasic right hemiplegic patients. J. Speech Hearing Disord., 24:369–379, 1959.

Keenan, J. S., and Brassell, E. G.: Comparison of minimally dysphasic and minimally educated subjects in a sentence writing task. Cortex, 8:93–105, 1972.

Keenan, J. S., and Brassell, E. G.: A study of factors related to prognosis for individual aphasic patients. J. Speech Hearing Disord., 39:257–269, 1974.

Kenin, M., and Swisher, L.: A study of pattern of recovery in aphasia. Cortex, 8:56–68, 1972.

Kertesz, A.: Aphasia and Associated Disorders: Taxonomy, Localization, and Recovery. New York, Grune & Stratton, 1979.

Kertesz, A., and McCabe, P.: Recovery patterns and prognosis in aphasia. Brain, 100:1–18, 1977.

Kertesz, A., Harlock, W., and Coates, R.: Computer tomographic localization, lesion size, and prognosis in aphasia and nonverbal impairment. Brain Lang., 8:34–50, 1979.

Kirk, S. A., McCarthy, J. J., and Kirk, W. D.: The Illinois Test of Psycholinguistic Abilities. Revised Ed. Urbana, Illinois, University of Illinois Press, 1969.

Kohlmeyer, K.: Aphasia due to focal disorders of cerebral circulation: some aspects of localization and of spontaneous recovery. In Lebrun, Y., and Hoops, R. (Eds.): Recovery in Aphasics. Atlantic Highlands, New Jersey, Humanities Press, 1976, pp. 79–95.

Leischner, A.: Zur Symptomatologie und Therapie der Aphasien. Nervenarzt, 31:60–67, 1960.

Leischner, A., and Linck, H. A.: Neuere Erfahrungen mit der Behandlung von Aphasien. Bericht über die Rehabilitation von 70 Aphasien. Nervenarzt, 38:199–205, 1967.

Loban, W.: Language Development: K through 12. Champaign, Illinois, National Council of Teachers of English Report #18, 1976.

Lomas, J., and Kertesz, A.: Patterns of spontaneous recovery in aphasic groups: a study of adult stroke patients. Brain Lang., 5:388–401, 1978.

Ludlow, C. L., and Swisher, L. P.: The audiometric evaluation of adult aphasics. J. Speech Hearing Res., 14:535–543, 1971.

Marshall, R. C., and King, P. S.: Effects of fatigue produced by isokinetic exercise on the communicative ability of aphasic adults. J. Speech Hearing Res., 16:222–230, 1973.

Mazzochi, F., and Vignolo, L. A.: Localization of lesions in aphasia: clinical CT scan correlations in stroke patients. Cortex, 15:627–654, 1979.

McNeil, M. R., and Prescott, T. E.: Revised Token Test. Baltimore, University Park Press, 1978.

Mencher, G. T.: The reliability of electrodermal audiometry with aphasic adults. J. Speech Hearing Res., 10:328–332, 1967.

Messerli, P., Tissot, A., and Rodriguez, J.: Recovery from aphasia: some factors of prognosis. In Lebrun, Y., and Hoops, R. (Eds.): Recovery in Aphasics. Atlantic Highlands, New Jersey, Humanities Press, 1976, pp. 124–134.

Miller, M. H.: Audiologic evaluation of aphasic patients. J. Speech Hearing Disord., 25:333–339, 1960.

Mitchell, J.: Speech and language impairment in the older patient. Geriatrics, 13:467–476, 1958.

Naeser, M. A., Hayward, R. W., Laughlin, S. A., and Zatz, L. M.: Quantitative CT scan studies in aphasia. I. Infarct size and CT numbers. Brain Lang., 12:140–164, 1981a.

Naeser, M. A., Hayward, R. W., Laughlin, S. A., Becker, J. M. T., Jernigan, T. L., and Zatz, L. M.: Quantitative CT scan studies in aphasia. II. Comparison of the right and left hemispheres. Brain Lang., 12:165–189, 1981b.

Orgass, B., and Poeck, K.: Assessment of aphasia by psychometric methods. Cortex, 5:317–330, 1969.

Piotrowski, Z.: The Rorschach inkblot method in organic disturbances of the central nervous system. J. Nerv. Ment. Dis., 86:527–537, 1937.

Porec, J. P., and Porch, B. E.: The behavioral characteristics of "simulated" aphasia. In Clinical Aphasiology Conference Proceedings 1977. Minneapolis, BRK Publishers, 1977, pp. 297–301.

Porch, B. E.: The Porch Index of Communicative Ability. Vol. 1. Theory and Development. Palo Alto, California, Consulting Psychologists Press, 1967.

Porch, B. E.: The Porch Index of Communicative Ability. Manual, Vol. 2. (Rev. Ed.) Palo Alto, California, Consulting Psychologists Press, 1971a.

Porch, B. E.: PICA Talk Newsletter No. 4. Palo Alto, California, Consulting Psychologists Press, 1971b.

Porch, B. E.: Multidimensional scoring in aphasia testing. J. Speech Hearing Res., 14:776–792, 1971c.

Porch, B. E., Collins, M., Wertz, R. T., and Friden, T. P.: Statistical prediction of change in aphasia. J. Speech Hearing Res., 23:312–321, 1980.

Rubens, A. B.: The role of changes within the central nervous system during recovery from aphasia. In Sullivan, M., and Kommers, M. S. (Eds.): Rationale for Adult Aphasia Therapy. Lincoln, Nebraska, University of Nebraska Press, 1977, pp. 28–43.

Sands, E., Sarno, M. T., and Shankweiler, D.: Long-term assessment of language function in aphasia due to stroke. Arch. Phys. Med. Rehabil., 50:202–206, 222, 1969.

Sarno, M. T., Silverman, M., and Sands, E.: Speech therapy and language recovery in severe aphasia. J. Speech Hearing Res., 13:607–623, 1970.

Schuell, H.: Aphasic difficulties understanding spoken language. Neurology, 3:176–184, 1953.

Schuell, H.: A short examination for aphasia. Neurology, 7:625–634, 1957.

Schuell, H.: A re-evaluation of the short examination for aphasia. J. Speech Hearing Disord., 31:137–147, 1966.

Schuell, H.: Diagnosis and prognosis in aphasia. Arch. Neurol. Psychiatry, 74:308–315, 1955.

Schuell, H.: Differential Diagnosis of Aphasia with the Minnesota Test. Minneapolis, University of Minnesota Press, 1965.

Schuell, H., Jenkins, J. J., and Jiménez-Pabón, E.: Aphasia in Adults: Diagnosis, Prognosis, and Treatment. New York, Hoeber, 1964.

Sidman, M., Stoddard, L. T., Mohr, J. P., and Leicester, J.: Behavioral studies of aphasia: methods of investigation and analysis. Neuropsychologia, 9:119–140, 1971.

Spreen, O., and Benton, A. L.: Neurosensory Center Comprehensive Examination for Aphasia. Victoria, British Columbia, University of Victoria, 1977.

Stoicheff, M. L.: Motivating instructions and language performance of dysphasic subjects. J. Speech Hearing Res., 3:75–85, 1960.

Street, B. S.: Hearing loss in aphasia. J. Speech Hearing Disord., 22:60–67, 1957.

Thomsen, I. V.: Evaluation and outcome of aphasia in patients with severe closed head trauma. J. Neurol. Neurosurg. Psychiatry, 38:713–718, 1975.

Tompkins, C. A., Marshall, R. C., and Phillips, D. S.: Aphasic patients in a rehabilitation program: scheduling speech and language services. Arch. Phys. Med. Rehabil., 61:252–254, 1980.

Vignolo, L. A.: Evolution of aphasia and language rehabilitation: a retrospective exploratory study. Cortex, 1:344–367, 1964.

Watson, J. M., and Records, L. E.: The effectiveness of the Porch Index of Communicative Ability as a diagnostic tool in assessing specific behaviors of senile dementia. In Clinical Aphasiology Conference Proceedings 1978. Minneapolis, BRK Publishers, 1978, pp. 93–105.

Weisenberg, T., and McBride, K. E.: Aphasia: A Clinical and Psychological Study. New York, Commonwealth Fund, 1935.

Wepman, J. M.: Aphasia therapy: A new look. J. Speech Hearing Disord., 37:203–214, 1972.

Wepman, J. M.: Aphasia: language without thought or thought without language? ASHA, 18:131–136, 1976.

Wepman, J. M.: Recovery from Aphasia. New York, Ronald Press, 1951.

Wepman, J. M.: The relationship between self-correction and recovery from aphasia. J. Speech Hearing Disord., *23*:302–305, 1958.

Wertz, R. T., Deal, L., and Deal, J.: Prognosis in aphasia: investigation of the High-Overall Prediction (HOAP) method and the Short-Direct or HOAP Slope method to predict change in PICA performance. *In* Clinical Aphasiology Conference Proceedings 1980. Minneapolis, BRK Publishers, 1980, pp. 164–172.

Yorkston, K. M., and Beukelman, D. R.: An analysis of connected speech samples of aphasic and normal speakers. J. Speech Hearing Disord., *45*:27–36, 1980.

3 · THE NATURAL HISTORY OF APHASIA

The Period of Spontaneous Recovery
Changing Profiles of Recovery
  Modality Shifts
  Changes in "Type" of Aphasia
Prognostic Factors Related to Recovery
  Etiology of Aphasia
  Site and Extent of Lesion
  General Health and Associated
    Sensory and Motor Deficits
  Age
  Sex
  Psychosocial Factors
References

"Most intelligent patients begin to train themselves very soon."

THEODORE H. WEISENBURG AND KATHERINE E. MCBRIDE

Although severely aphasic patients — those identified as globally aphasic — may constitute an exception, it is commonly expected that aphasic patients will display some remission of their language dysfunction without intervention of formal therapy. What is the course of that recovery? What are the temporal limits of the stage of spontaneous recovery? How do the several language modalities change over time and what are the consequent alterations in patients' profiles of language behavior? What factors (other than those implicit in the test data reviewed in Chapter 2) have some prognostic value concerning outcome?

THE PERIOD OF SPONTANEOUS RECOVERY

The early period post onset of aphasia is commonly known as the stage of spontaneous recovery. It was probably Butfield and Zangwill (1946) who first used the term in reporting on the "reeducation" of 70 patients with aphasia. They regretted the fact that "we possess no definite standards whereby to assess spontaneous recovery of cerebral function as opposed to the effect of reeducation. This is a particular disadvantage in the study of traumatic cases in which, as is well known, spontaneous recovery is to be expected much more frequently than in cases of cerebral disease." They did not document this "well-known" fact concerning the differential prognosis for traumatic and cerebral disease etiologies, nor did they document their stated conviction concerning the limits of the period of spontaneous recovery: "In view of the fact that spontaneous improvement is in general liable to be both limited and slow after 6 months, it is permissible to ascribe

110

the greater part at least of any improvement made by the patients in Group 2 [patients whose treatment began more than 6 months post onset] to reeducation."

In his report of the treatment of 68 soldiers with traumatically incurred aphasia, Wepman (1951) quoted an unpublished manuscript by Luria ("Topical syndromes of traumatic aphasia") in which two distinct stages of recovery were defined: the initial stage, in which both permanent and temporary language problems and personality deviations are observed, and a residual stage (beginning 6 months post onset) with persistent language and personality problems. Luria reported that 43 per cent of 394 patients with left hemisphere lesions showed residual signs requiring reeducation or psychotherapy, the other 57 per cent of the patients having recovered spontaneously during the initial 6-month period. In a later book (1963), Luria again referred to the residual period as beginning 6 to 7 months after onset of aphasia, but still later (1970), he described the residual stage as occurring 2 to 5 months after trauma.

In the first of the three reports from Milan concerning the effects of language rehabilitation in aphasia, Vignolo (1964) included information about 27 patients who received no treatment, but who, like 42 other treated patients, were tested twice within a period of no less than 40 days. He concluded that "spontaneous evolution does exist and it is in the direction of improvement and restitution of function." He based his conclusion upon the fact that 14 of the untreated aphasic subjects demonstrated improvement in their language behavior, as reflected in the second examination in comparison with the first; one patient changed for the worse; 12 patients demonstrated no change between examinations. Vignolo further reported that the percentage of patients who improved decreased as the time interval post onset increased. With regard to the untreated subjects, there was a marked discrepancy between those examined within 2 months and those examined more than 2 months post onset. "Time elapsed from onset is a very important prognostic factor in aphasia. . . . The end of the second month represents a turning point in the course of the disturbance. Indeed, it appears as if any degree of spontaneous restitution could occur in subjects examined for the first time within 2 months from onset, no matter how severely affected they were."

Schuell (1965), on the basis of her clinical experience, set a different limit to the period of spontaneous recovery. She stated, "The consensus is that most of the spontaneous recovery in aphasia occurs during the first 3 months. This is an arbitrary limit, and exceptions occur in both directions, but most investigators agree that significant changes do not often occur of themselves after this period and that one cannot be sure of obtaining a reliable test much earlier. . . . After patients are neurologically stable, performance is consistent and prediction tends to be highly reliable."

These opinions were arrived at retrospectively. Culton (1969) set out to develop more exact information about the period of spontaneous recovery in a prospective study. He studied 11 patients (Group I), whose onset of aphasia was not more than 30 days before initial testing, and another 10 patients (Group II), whose aphasia dated from 11 to 48 months before initial testing (mean, 27 months). The groups were comparable in age and etiology of aphasia (for the most part vascular). All Group II subjects and no Group I subjects had received speech therapy, and therapy was withheld from all subjects during the study. Both groups were administered a battery of eight language tests (recognizing pictured objects by name, following directions, matching printed words to pictures, reading sentences for comprehension, oral naming of pictures, answering simple questions, writing letters and numbers to dictation, and writing words to dictation) and the Raven Standard Progressive Matrices Test. The language battery was administered four times at 2-week intervals and the Raven test twice 6 weeks apart.

The results revealed spontaneous recovery during the 2-month period in the Group I patients. They showed a significant increase in mean scores on all eight language tests and on the Raven test, but the subjects in Group II demonstrated no significant improvement. "Rapid spontaneous recovery of language function was noted in the first month following the onset of aphasia. Although an increase in mean scores was noted, further significant improvement was not evident during the second month. This is somewhat incompatible with the predominant notion that significant spontaneous recovery of language function continues to occur 3 to 6 months after the onset of aphasia."

Further prospective data are supplied by Sarno and Levita (1971), who evaluated the language of 28 patients with severe aphasia due to stroke within 2 days of their cerebrovascular accidents (mean age, 66.5 years). The Functional Communication Profile was used for the language measure. Three months later, 18 of the patients were reevaluated, and 3 months after that, 14 were again evaluated. (The death of several subjects precluded serial evaluation of all 28 subjects.) None of the subjects received language therapy during the 6-month period. The investigators reported: "Greater change occurred within a 3- rather than 6-month period post stroke in the absence of formal speech therapy. . . . The present results would warrant the conculsion that in the natural course of recovery the most dramatic language improvement takes place during the first 3 months after a cerebrovascular accident."

Other prospective data are supplied by Hagen (1973). He studied two groups of 10 subjects each, male aphasic patients ranging in age from 49 to 57 years (mean age, 52.5 years), all of whom had had a single thromboembolic episode involving the left middle cerebral artery and all of whom were originally right-handed and English-speaking, without dysarthria, and available for study 3 months post onset. Ten patients received aphasia therapy for 1 year; the other 10 patients received all hospital services except aphasia therapy for 1 year. The patients in both groups were tested with the Minnesota Test for Differential Diagnosis of Aphasia (MTDDA) four times: (1) at 3 months post onset; (2) at 6 months post onset (after physical rehabilitation had been accomplished and at the time that aphasia therapy was to start); (3) 6 months later (12 months post onset); and (4) another 6 months later (18 months post onset). Scores on the various parts of the MTDDA were translated into severity scores; both at the time of admission into the program and at 6 months post onset, the two groups had comparable severity scores.

Hagen reported that both groups demonstrated some spontaneous recovery in the period from admission until the treated group began therapy (between 3 and 6 months post onset). This recovery was evident with regard to three dimensions of language: auditory retention span, visual comprehension (matching forms, letters, and words to pictures), and visual motor abilities (writing). Later comparison of the two groups indicated no differences between the treated and nontreated groups on these three dimensions and also on auditory comprehension. Hagen drew the following conclusions concerning spontaneous recovery: (1) Spontaneous recovery accounts for slight changes in all communication processes during the first 6 months post onset. (2) Spontaneous recovery accounts for the return of visual comprehension, visual motor abilities, auditory comprehension, and auditory retention span. (3) Visually mediated abilities spontaneously recover to a functional level within 6 months post onset. (4) Aurally mediated abilities spontaneously return to a functional level within 9 months post onset. (5) Speech production and reading comprehension abilities spontaneously improve during the first 6 months but not to a functional level. (6) Language formulation, spelling ability, and arithmetic ability spontaneously improve up to 9 months post onset but not to a functional level. Hagen demonstrated that further improvement in speech production, reading comprehension, language formulation, spelling, and arithmetic resulted from treatment.

Kertesz and McCabe (1977) have reported on the recovery of a group of 36 aphasic patients whose conditions were of vascular etiology, all of whom were initially examined within 45 days of onset. The Western Aphasia Battery (WAB) was administered initially 0 to 6 weeks post onset; the second test was administered 3 months later, a third test 6 months later, and further testing insofar as possible at yearly intervals up to 5 years. The results of the following language tests are reported: spontaneous speech, measured in terms of fluency and information content; comprehension, measured by responses to yes/no questions of graded complexity, pointing to objects, pictures, body parts, colors, letters, numbers, and shapes, and performing sequentially ordered auditory commands with three objects; repetition of words, numbers, and increasingly complex sentences; and naming tested by identifying 20 objects, finding names for an object category, sentence completion, and answering questions with single-word responses. "The subscores, which were scaled for equal difficulty level, are added and this provides the aphasia quotient (AQ) (maximum score = 100), which is used to follow progress in our patients."

These investigators took the differences between the AQs of the first test and the test 3 months later as the rate for the first interval; the 3- to 6-months test differences as the second; and the differences between the 6-month test and the last test (which might be anywhere up to 5 years) as the third interval recovery rate. They found that "the degree of improvement was by far the greatest in the first interval, that is, between the first test within a month and a half from onset and 3 months later [mean AQ differential = 16.64], but some recovery was noted in all subsequent intervals [3 to 6 month interval, mean AQ differential = 1.52; 6 to 12 or more months interval, mean AQ differential = 7.34]. That the improvement was greater in the third interval than in the second is probably the result of including some long-term patients in this group."

Kertesz and McCabe also studied a group of 22 patients who were not tested early enough for inclusion in the main study but who had tests and retests more than 1 year post onset. These patients, designated "chronic," displayed little or no improvement over the period of time tested, which extended as far as 17 years in one patient. It was concluded that little recovery takes place beyond 1 year. This conclusion "was fully supported by the very high test-retest reliability (r = 0.992, P <0.01), and the very low mean difference between tests-retests (a negligible value of 0.9)."

Lomas and Kertesz (1978) have reported on the recovery of 31 aphasic stroke patients in the first 3 months post onset (age range, 31 to 82 years). All patients had an initial language test (WAB) within 30 days post onset and a retest at or around 3 months post onset, with no intervening aphasia therapy. Test and retest information was reported on eight language tasks. Results indicated that during the 3-month period post onset the group as a whole showed recovery scores that were significantly different from zero.

Changes over time in the performance of aphasia patients have also been studied by Koura and associates (1978). In order to "measure language abilities as they changed during 3 years following onset in the absence of any specific language retraining," they studied three groups totalling 78 patients, all with aphasia of vascular etiology. Twenty-seven of these were first tested less than 30 days post onset and were designated "recent aphasics" (mean age, 51.23 years). A second group of 34 patients had been aphasic for more than 1 month (range, 1 to 6 months, mean 3.25 months) and were designated "delayed aphasics" (mean age, 56.8 years). A third group of 17 patients had been aphasic for more than 6 months (range, 6 months to 3 years; mean, 21 months) and were designated "stable aphasics" (mean age, 54.3 years). Language evaluations (an eight-task battery, 10 items per task) were administered to all patients four times at 4-week intervals.

Serial evaluations of the "recent aphasics" revealed "fair increase in mean scores on each task," an increase over the 16-week period that was statistically significant. The "delayed aphasics" showed lesser degrees of improvement on all the language tasks, but the increase was statistically significant. The improvement shown by the "stable aphasics" was not statistically significant, but there was some improvement. The investigators concluded: "Spontaneous recovery of language function is observed, within the time dimensions of this study, in aphasics [with disability of] up to 3 years' duration. However, recent aphasics reflected higher significant spontaneous recovery by increases in the overall scores of the subjects and by increases in mean scores on each of the eight different language tasks. . . . Moreover, despite the statistical insignificance of improvement in the stable aphasics, . . . the general clinical impression as well as the general configuration of the graph scoring indicates that some spontaneous recovery still occurs."

Basso and co-workers (1979) studied the effect of therapy on the language skills of 162 aphasic patients in their rehabilitation program. They also studied language changes in a group of 119 adult patients with aphasia, predominantly vascular in origin, who were unable to take advantage of treatment because of family or transportation problems but who were able to return 6 months or more later so that changes in their communication might be measured. These untreated patients, like those treated, were classified as having severe or moderate disability in terms of their degree of communication deficit in the two modalities of spoken language (oral expression and auditory verbal comprehension) measured on a scale from 0 to 4, where 0 represented no communication and 4 represented very good communication; patients rated 0 to 1 on oral expression and 0 to 2 on comprehension were designated as having severe aphasia; those rated 2 to 3 on oral expression and 3 to 4 on comprehension were designated as having moderate aphasia. The patients were also classified as fluent or nonfluent in terms of the quality of speech outflow in contextual speech, including rate of speech, phrase length, and articulatory difficulties.

Table 3–1 shows the percentage of untreated patients who improved in each of four language modalities — auditory verbal comprehension, reading, oral expression, and writing — between their initial evaluation (which varied from less than 2 months to more than 6 months post onset) and the second examination, administered in all cases at least 6 months later. It can be seen that some patients in all categories demonstrated spontaneous recovery in all modalities during the early months post onset.

In summary, studies of change in the language behavior of aphasic

Table 3–1. Percentages of Untreated Aphasic Patients (N = 119) Who Improved Spontaneously in Four Language Modalities Between First and Second Examinations*

	SEVERE		MODERATE	
	NF	*F*	*NF*	*F*
Auditory Verbal Comprehension	29	28	75	68
Reading	12	28	62	72
Oral Expression	3	12	37	34
Writing	3	8	42	20

*NF, Nonfluent; F, fluent.
From Basso, A., Capitani, E., and Vignolo, L. A.: Influence of rehabilitation on language skills in aphasic patients. Arch. Neurol., *36*:190–196, 1979.

patients who do not receive therapy are in agreement that spontaneous improvement is a reasonable expectation in the natural history of aphasia, although patients do not display equal degrees of it. The spontaneous recovery curve is generally a decelerating curve, steepest during the first month post onset, flattening out during the second and third months, but still rising at 6 and at 9 months and even longer. Perhaps it is fair to say that the aphasic patient has a continuing capacity for improvement and that no time limit imposes itself upon his potential. This potential is most evident in the first 3 months post onset and manifests itself less prominently and with lesser degrees of significance in the months that follow. An investigator of the effects of intervention on recovery from aphasia might be tempted to discount the less significant degrees of improvement that occur after the first month post onset; but for a more rigorous analysis of improvement attributable to treatment, a period of 6 months would appear to constitute a fairer definition of the stage of spontaneous recovery.

CHANGING PROFILES OF RECOVERY

Modality Shifts. During recovery, most patients display some improvement in all the language modalities, whether they are receiving therapy or not. But data indicate that the degrees of improvement in the various modalities are not equivalent.

Butfield and Zangwill (1946) treated a group of 70 aphasic patients for variable amounts of time; formal therapy was terminated when the patient had improved to the point at which little or no practical disability remained or, in the less responsive cases, when the language condition appeared to have become more or less stationary despite prolonged treatment. Language functions were rated on a three-point scale ("much improved," "improved," "unchanged"); ratings were relative, not absolute, as they were based on different degrees of original impairment. These investigators found that over the course of treatment, 82 per cent of their patients were much improved or improved in speech; 77 per cent were much improved or improved in reading; 72 per cent were much improved or improved in writing. Unfortunately, no information is provided concerning gains in auditory comprehension by these patients.

Wepman (1951) reported on the modality changes made during language rehabilitation by 68 patients with traumatically incurred aphasia: "The order of improvement in the four language areas, taught formally, is ... (1) reading, (2) mathematics, (3) writing, and (4) spelling. A significant improvement is noted in the area of speech performance." He reported a "general tendency of the language areas to improve to almost the same degree."

Vignolo (1964) reported on the "evolution of aphasia" in 27 aphasic patients who received no therapy and 42 patients who received a minimum of 20 therapy sessions over a course of not less than 40 days with a minimum frequency of one session a week. A standard aphasia examination was administered twice, with a minimum interval of 40 days between the first and second examinations. Vignolo reported that patients who on first examination had a severe impairment of both expression and comprehension, on second examination showed severe impairment limited to the expressive side. He stated, "This suggests that the receptive side clears up more than the expressive side during spontaneous evolution. In fact, a very definite trend seems to exist in the spontaneous evolution of aphasia in that the receptive side remains all the way along superior to the expressive. . . . On first examination, comprehension is preserved in more subjects than is expression; about 50 per cent of patients are able to communicate on the receptive side, while all of them fall below communication level in expression. On second examination, overall recovery of communication appears to be more frequent on the receptive than on the expressive side." With further regard to the untreated patients' expressive abilities, he found that their ability to name was consistently better than their ability to describe (male patients described what they do when they shave, female patients described what they do in cooking spaghetti); this pattern held true for every subject.

Vignolo found the patterns of change in treated and untreated patients to be quite similar. However, therapy tended to reduce the gap between expression and comprehension, which in the untreated patients was maintained throughout their spontaneous recovery.

Kreindler and Fradis (1968) tested aphasic patients in the early pretherapy stages of recovery from a vascular episode and retested them at the conclusion of therapy. They divided their battery of tests into three groups according to the frequency of improvement shown on them by the patients. The performances that showed the most frequent change were matching identical objects, matching dissimilar objects, oral imitation, auditory comprehension of nouns, and naming objects with visual, auditory, or tactile input. Lesser degrees of improvement were observed in repetition of syllables and words, reading aloud, copying and writing to dictation, executing one- and two-step spoken commands, and oral response to short questions. Performances which improved the least included repetition of sentences, executing a three-step spoken command, arranging letters into words, gesture-imitating tasks, and executing written orders.

Information about changing patterns of test response similar to that reported by Kreindler and Fradis was obtained by Kenin and Swisher (1972), who tested 15 aphasic patients once at the time of initial evaluation and a second time within 6 weeks to three months later. Patients (mean age, 58 years) were all receiving intensive aphasia therapy. The investigators administered 17 of the 20 subtests that compose the Neurosensory Center Comprehensive Examination for Aphasia.

Test-retest information indicated that tests of copying, sentence repetition, auditory and visual recognition of nouns and sentences, and visual naming improved in the majority of the patients. The test on which the largest number of patients improved was the writing test involving copying sentences. The tests on which the fewest patients showed improvement were the tests of visual graphic naming (writing the names of objects) and sentence construction (orally producing self-generated sentences containing two or three specific words). Concerning the amount of change shown in the various subtests, performance on the copying test showed the greatest amount of change, performance on the sentence construction test the least. Essentially imitative tasks (copying, repeating sentences) showed the greatest amount of improvement for the majority of the patients; tasks involving expressive language processes (describing the use of objects, sentence construction) showed the least improvement. The general conclusion was that "improvement in the comprehension of language was greater than the improvement in expressive language. . . . In addition, tests requiring the reception or spontaneous production of single words reflected more improvement than those requiring the comprehension or expression of longer verbal units."

On the basis of his study of 240 patients (61 per cent of 394 cases of left hemispheric lesions studied) who showed "signs of speech impairment in the early period," Luria (1970) emphasized the variability of patterns of change demonstrated by different patients:

> Such language disorders took various forms. Most often during the first days, and even weeks, they were characterized by total disruption of all forms of speech activity. Patients who had re-

ceived injuries of the left hemisphere a few hours before examination not only lacked the ability to speak spontaneously or to answer questions, but they could not understand what was said to them. That unity of the meaning and sound of a word which constitutes the special characteristic of any normal speech process was destroyed, and the patient was in no position either to recall the words which designate various objects or to recognize the significance of words spoken to him. Therefore, in the initial period of traumatic aphasia it most often turns out that even the simplest forms of language activity were severely disturbed, so that any communication with the patient became quite difficult. . . . Usually the recovery of speech function was quite gradual: at first the total block of expressive speech or comprehension and the unity of word and meaning which is basic to language function was reestablished. Difficulties of articulation, word finding, and slight disturbances of phonetic discrimination lasted considerably longer.

Earlier in this chapter, Hagen's (1973) study of spontaneous recovery was reviewed. It was his observation that visually mediated abilities spontaneously recovered earlier than aurally mediated abilities. The abilities that showed some spontaneous recovery but required treatment to return to a functional level were reading comprehension, spelling, speech production, language formulation, and arithmetic.

It was also noted earlier that Lomas and Kertesz (1978) studied changes over time (initial testing within 30 days post onset, retesting around 3 months post onset) on eight language tasks selected from the WAB: two comprehension tasks (yes/no questions and sequential commands); repetition of words, phrases, and sentences; and five expressive tasks (word fluency in producing as many animal names as possible in 1 minute; oral object naming; information content rated on a 10-point scale applied to spontaneous speech in the form of patients' responses to simple questions and their description of a picture; sentence completion; and responsive speech involving single-noun responses to simple questions). The recovery scores on these eight tests are shown in Figure 3–1. Yes/no comprehension recovered significantly more than all other tasks. Word fluency recovered significantly less than all other tasks; the investigators believed that the results suggested the isolation of this aspect of language from the normal recovery process.

Having developed the Porch Index of Communicative Ability (PICA) and administered it to large numbers of aphasic patients, Porch (1971a) reported a hierarchical pattern of test responses. "A large, random sample of aphasic patients has mean gestural, verbal, and graphic levels of about 12.00, 10.00, and 8.00, respectively." (The gestural score represents reading comprehension and various gestural responses to oral and written instructions.) In several public statements, Porch reported a consistent finding concerning modality sparing from least to most impaired: tactile, visual, auditory on the input

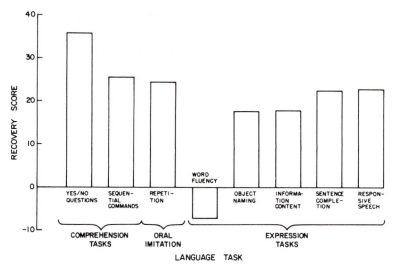

Figure 3–1. Recovery scores of 31 aphasic patients on eight language tasks over a 2 month period, as reported by Lomas and Kertesz. (From Lomas, J., and Kertesz, A.: Patterns of spontaneous recovery in aphasic groups: a study of adult stroke patients. Brain and Language, 5:388–401, 1978.)

side; gestural, verbal, graphic on the output side. Thus auditory input is more frequently and more severely impaired than visual or tactile input; patients are able to gesture more efficiently than they speak and speak more efficiently than they write. Porch says that this general pattern of modality ranking holds true during the course of recovery in patients who are receiving therapy. He has also stated that "the simpler subtest skills of matching, imitating, and copying improve more quickly or are lost later than the other subtest skills."

Using the PICA as the instrument for measuring language change, Hanson and Cicciarelli (1978) have further described the amount of change during therapy and also variations in modality change. They studied 13 patients (mean age, 56 years) with aphasia of vascular etiology, administering the PICA initially within a period ranging from eight to 64 days (mean, 33 days). Individual treatment was provided to the patients for a period ranging from 4 to 15 months (mean, 9 months), 3 hours per week. Retesting with the PICA was done approximately every 6 weeks, with between three and nine retests being administered (mean number of tests, 6). Analysis of the results of this serial PICA testing indicated that all 13 subjects made significant positive change in Overall score; the mean initial score was 9.48 (indicating marked difficulty with most communication skills), whereas the mean peak score was 12.72 (indicating that patients can handle most basic communication tasks without requiring much assistance). The difference was statistically significant. The average time from onset of aphasia to peak overall score was 8.94 months (range, 3.64 to 15.88

months). With regard to individual subtests, on most subtests patients reached their peak recovery between the fifth and the seventh month post onset. A high correlation ($r = 0.84$) was found between the order of the tasks in terms of time required to reach peak recovery and the order of tasks in terms of amount of change attained; that is, tasks requiring the most time to improve tended to reflect the most actual change; however, they did not reach as high a level of improvement on these tasks as on those that required less time for recovery. The mean Gestural score (reflecting performance in reading, visual matching, and matching in response to spoken instructions) reached a peak in the fourth month; the mean Graphic score reached a peak in the sixth month; the mean Verbal score reached a peak in the seventh month. Receptive language processes thus generally improved before expressive processes. Improvement peaks on the various subtests were noted in the first, second, fourth, fifth, sixth, seventh, and eighth months post onset, but 15 of the 18 subtests reached peak improvement after the fifth month post onset.

Earlier in this chapter, data provided by Koura and co-workers (1978) were reviewed. The three groups of aphasic patients — "recent," "delayed," and "stable" — were evaluated four times at 4-week intervals with a test battery involving eight tasks: visual naming, identification by name, description of use, identification by sentences, reading sentences for meaning, articulation, repetition of sentences, and writing to dictation. The group of "recent aphasics" displayed a significant increase in performance on all eight tasks; the configuration or profile of mean scores on these eight tasks remained the same over the four administrations of the test. In the group of "stable aphasics," however, the profiles changed irregularly, but "the final scores on all but one task were slightly higher than initial scores."

A comparison of improvement in spontaneous speech and improvement in language comprehension during a period of recovery was made by Prins and associates (1978). They studied 74 patients (mean age, 60.45 years) with aphasia of vascular etiology, all of them at least 3 months post onset. Patients were classified into four groups on the basis of the fluency of their spontaneous speech (speech tempo plus mean length of utterance) in the initial session: fluent (15), nonfluent (22), severely nonfluent (20), and mixed (17). (The 20 patients in the severely nonfluent group could not be scored on spontaneous speech because they produced only a few words, incomprehensible muttering, or verbal stereotypies). Patients were tested three times at 6-month intervals, during which time they received therapy. Two minutes of informal conversation by the subjects were elicited on three conversational topics with as little intervention by the clinician as possible. Spontaneous speech was scored on 28 variables, including such things as speech tempo (number of words produced in 6 minutes), a judgment of communicative capacity, melody, articulation, mean length of utterance, number of complex utterances, number of seconds of incomprehensible speech, paraphasias, and so forth. Two tests of comprehension were administered: a Morphosyntactic Comprehension Test consisting of 60 items, four for each of 15 morphosyntactic structures being tested, the sentence being read aloud to the patient, who was then asked to point to the picture that went with it; and an Ambiguity Comprehension Test consisting of eight items, each comprising one sentence and four pictures, in which each sentence was read aloud and the patient asked to point to the two pictures that were accurately described by it.

Results indicated that of the 28 variables used in analysis of spontaneous speech, five showed improvement: speech tempo, utterances shorter than five words, mean length of utterance, number of substitutions of function words, and unclassified mistakes. The three fluency indicators, (speech tempo, utterances shorter than five words, and mean length of utterance) all showed the greatest improvement between times I and II, with a slight deterioration between times II and III. Deterioration was observed on number of complex utterances, ratio of pronouns to number of content words, literal and verbal perseverations, and number of deletions of function words. None of the variables that changed significantly involved very large changes except literal perseverations; the amount of shift was, in all cases except literal perseverations, smaller than one standard deviation in either direction from the mean of the scores earned by a control group of 18 nonaphasic subjects. *Communicative capacity*, which reflected a clinical judgment of the patient's severity of aphasia, was one of the variables that showed no change over time. The investigators concluded that the changes in spontaneous speech over 1 year failed to show a clear pattern of either improvement or deterioration, and no changes were of great magnitude. This held true for all groups, including the severely nonfluent group, who at the end of the year still produced very few understandable words or only verbal stereotypies.

On the Morphosyntactic Comprehension Test, all four aphasic groups showed significant improvement from time I to time III and from time II to time III. All groups except the mixed group also improved significantly between time I and time II. On the Ambiguity Comprehension Test, significant improvement was shown by the nonfluent and the mixed groups from time I to time II and for the fluent group from time II to time III.

In summary, older patients with aphasia of vascular etiology over the course of 1 year showed no clear improvement as a group in spontaneous speech but did show considerable improvement in comprehension ability. "Our findings suggest that aphasic deficits in spontaneous speech production and in sentence comprehension are to some extent distinct, [and have] their own recovery histories. The pattern of change over the course of one year was essentially the same for all four patient groups studied."

Tonkovich (1980) used the same analysis of spontaneous speech used by Prins and colleagues as reported previously. He obtained speech samples at three 6-month intervals from a single subject. During the course of her recovery, she demonstrated increases in speech tempo, in communicative capacity, in number of nouns, and in number of self-corrections. She showed decreases in number of utterances shorter than six words, number of seconds during which speech was incomprehensible, ratio of personal pronouns to number of nouns, and number of automatisms, verbal paraphasias, neologisms, imitations of the examiner, verbal perseverations, substitutions of function words, and content word deletions.

Detailed information about improvement over time in the different language modalities has been provided by Basso and co-workers (1979). Table 3–2 shows percentages of patients who improved, classified according to the severity of their aphasia, whether they were fluent or nonfluent, and whether they were treated or untreated. The hierarchy of modalities with regard to percentages of patients showing improvement, from most to least, is highly consistent: auditory verbal comprehension, reading, oral expression, and writing. They summarized their findings as follows: "The relative improvement of the four modalities follows a consistent trend not only across aphasic syndromes but also across re-educated and nonre-educated groups: within both spoken and written language, comprehension improves more (that is, in a larger percentage of patients) than expression. A

Table 3–2. Percentages of Treated (N = 162) and Untreated (N = 119) Patients Who Improved in Four Language Modalities Between First and Second Examinations*

	SEVERE				MODERATE			
	NF		F		NF		F	
	R−	R+	R−	R+	R−	R+	R−	R+
Auditory Verbal Compression (N = 193 improved)	29	48	28	86	75	75	68	71
Reading (N = 228 improved)	12	43	28	69	62	66	72	68
Oral expression (N = 281 improved)	3	13	12	42	37	59	34	52
Writing (N = 279 improved)	3	9	8	37	42	43	20	61

*NF, Nonfluent; F, fluent; R−, untreated; R+, treated.
From Basso, A., Capitani, E., and Vignolo, L. A.: Influence of rehabilitation on language skills in aphasic patients. Arch. Neurol., 36:190–196, 1979.

weaker and less consistent trend disclosed . . . is that oral language modalities tend to improve more than the corresponding aspects of written language."

Smith (1972), observing the improvement in language functions of 80 treated aphasic patients, reported moderate or marked improvement in comprehension in 67 per cent, in reading in 61 per cent, in speech in 55 per cent, and in writing in 54 per cent. This hierarchy is identical to that reported by Basso and associates (1979).

Golper (1980) also studied the characteristics of spontaneous speech of 10 patients with aphasia of vascular etiology, comparing them with seven nonaphasic right hemisphere–damaged patients and three left hemisphere–damaged patients without aphasia. Picture-elicited contextual speech samples were analyzed for syllable rate, content units per minute, and number of grammatical strings within the sample. In order to characterize communicative recovery further, a ratio of number of content units to grammatical strings was computed, thus measuring the number of statements required to convey information. Speech samples were obtained from the patients at 1 week and at 1 month post onset. Over the period studied, all subjects demonstrated significant improvement in verbal fluency and in the use of content words. The aphasic patients (and also the left hemisphere–damaged nonaphasic patients) demonstrated an increase in the number of content units within a phrase or sentence, thus appearing to become more efficient communicators as they recovered. In contrast, the speech samples from the right hemisphere–damaged patients contained more redundant statements and noncontentive remarks, indicating that their recovery was characterized by a less efficient use of language for communication of content information than the left hemisphere–damaged patients.

In summary, studies are in substantial agreement that improvement in comprehension generally exceeds improvement in expression (Vignolo, 1964; Kreindler and Fradis, 1968; Porch, 1971a; Kenin and Swisher, 1972; Smith, 1972; Lomas and Kertesz, 1978; Prins et al., 1978; Hanson and Cicciarelli, 1978; Basso et al., 1979). Throughout their period of recovery, patients tend to understand what they hear better than what they read; understand what they hear and read better than they speak; speak better than they write; and read better than they write (Butfield and Zangwill, 1946; Porch, 1971a; Kenin and Swisher, 1972; Smith, 1972; Lomas and Kertesz, 1978; Prins et al., 1978; Hanson and Cicciarelli, 1978; Basso et al., 1979). They show earlier recovery of ability to perform imitative tasks (repeating, copying) than language generation tasks (Kreindler and Fradis, 1968; Porch, 1971a; Kenin and Swisher, 1972; Hagen, 1973; Lomas and Kertesz, 1978; Hanson and Cicciarelli, 1978). They progress farther and more quickly on tasks involving shorter input and output verbal units (repeating words, executing short spoken and written commands, naming, recognizing nouns) than longer verbal units (repeating sentences, executing complex commands, describing pictures, generating lists of categorical words) (Vignolo, 1964; Kreindler and Fradis, 1968; Porch, 1971a; Kenin and Swisher, 1972; Hagen, 1973; Lomas and Kertesz, 1978).

Changes in "Type" of Aphasia. Longitudinal studies of aphasic patients show that as their modality performances change, so do the gestalts of performance, to which various labels have been applied (Wernicke's, Broca's, conduction, anomic, and so forth). A number of studies confirm that in the course of recovery, seemingly dissimilar "types" of aphasia move together to display more commonalities than differences.

In a widely quoted report, Goodglass and co-workers (1964) described the use of the phrase-length ratio (five or more word groups divided by one-word and two-word groups) and several other highly correlated scales (speech melodic line, articulatory agility, variety of grammatical forms, and so forth). They presented the rationale and procedure for differentiating Wernicke's, Broca's, and amnesic "types" of aphasia on the basis of "productive speech defects." They made an important observation: "Severity of aphasia must be taken into account, since the profile offers no differentiation among patients who have recovered to a level of mild or slight residual aphasia."

Leischner (1960) reported on the "changeability of the aphasic syndromes" or what he called "the shifting of the disease" in a group of 46 patients classified as having motor aphasia (2), mixed aphasia (18), total aphasia (7), central aphasia (2), sensory aphasia (5), amnestic aphasia (5), motor-amnestic aphasia (2), sensory-amnestic aphasia (2), and amnestic-sensory aphasia (3). He made the following observations:

> There is still another reason to exercise caution in linking the individual aphasic syndrome with the localization of the cerebral lesions, namely, the observation that the aphasic syndromes often change during the course of the disease. . . . Originally, the great majority of the aphasics were displaying mixed aphasias. But in the course of improvement of the speech defects their number decreased visibly (from 18 to 12). On the other hand, the number of motor aphasias increased clearly during the course of rehabilitation (from two to 14). The sensory aphasias, too, showed a distinct decline (from five to two). A reverse trend appeared also in the total aphasias (from six to four) and in the central aphasias (from two to one). . . . There takes place a shift tendency from the mixed and total, as well as the sensory forms of aphasia, to the motor forms. From it can be deduced the important fact that the *symptomatological structures of the aphasias are often subject to a change during the course of recovery.* To the extent to which a small number of cases allow such a deduction, one gets the impression that the mixed, or total, or the central aphasias constitute the actual aphasic syndrome, which shows from case to case a variably pronounced recovery trend. Of the individual symptoms of this total syndrome,

the disturbances of the expressive speech, or, in other words, the motor-aphasic syndrome, is the most resistant. This may indicate that the motor aphasia is largely the recovery residue of an originally mixed aphasia. It is especially striking that the motor-aphasia syndrome is the only one which in a large number of observed aphasias increases in frequency within the course of the disease. This observation contradicts the classical concept about aphasia to the extent that it points out the fact that the individual *aphasic syndromes don't represent something stable, but something dynamic*, and that in most instances one does not do them justice by assuming a *direct relationship between a syndrome and a lesion site.*

In a study of recovery from aphasia due to various disorders of cerebral circulation, Kohlmeyer (1976) made similar observations concerning alteration of "type" of aphasia: "Nineteen per cent [56 cases] of all aphasias due to occlusion of left-sided cerebral arteries [303 cases] recovered completely during the first two weeks after the onset of the stroke. . . . In 68 per cent [207 cases] the type of aphasia did not change during the first two weeks post stroke. In 13 per cent [40 cases] the type of aphasia did change, most of the time turning to a milder form, for instance, from a global aphasia to a predominantly motor aphasia or a nominal aphasia, or from a conduction aphasia to a nominal aphasia."

Kertesz and McCabe (1977) present data about the evolution of aphasic syndromes resembling those provided by Leischner. Table 3–3 is taken from their report and summarizes the changes observed among their 93 patients. They reported as follows: "It appeared that anomic aphasia is a common end-stage of evolution in addition to being a common aphasic syndrome *de novo.* Four of 13 Wernicke's, four of eight transcortical and isolation, four of 17 Broca's, two of eight conduction, and one of 22 global aphasias evolved into anomic aphasia" [described as "the mildest language impairment"]. Twenty-one per cent of the patients attained a complete recovery, defined as a cutoff Aphasia Quotient of 93.8, which was the mean of the standardization group of brain-damaged patients clinically judged to be non-aphasic.

Similar findings were reported by Kertesz and associates (1979). They observed that global aphasia shows evolution toward Broca's aphasia in the chronic state, that acute Wernicke's aphasia patients recover most often as anomic aphasics and occasionally emerge in the conduction category, and that patients with an initially nonfluent aphasia (Broca's or transcortical motor types) often become anomic as time passes.

It is of interest that the patient studied for 1 year by Tonkovich (1980) on the basis of his performance on the WAB was initially identified as a "Wernicke's aphasic"; as he improved, it seemed appropriate to classify him as an "anomic aphasic"; ultimately his most appropriate classification was "alexia with agraphia."

Table 3–3. Evolution of Aphasia from Initial to End-stage Classification in 93 Patients (Percentages of Complete Recovery Are Shown on the Right)

CLASSIFICATION		PER CENT RECOVERED COMPLETELY
Initial	*Endstage*	
Global (22) ⟶	2 Broca's	
	1 Transcortical motor	
	1 Conduction	
	1 Anomic	
Broca's (17) ⟶	1 Transcortical motor	
	3 Anomic	
Conduction (8) ⟶	2 Anomic	
	5 Nonaphasic - - - - - - - - - - - - -(62.5)	
Wernicke's (13) ⟶	1 Global	
	1 Transcortical sensory	
	4 Anomic	
Isolation (2) ⟶	1 Anomic	
Transcortical motor 3 ⟶	2 Anomic	
(6)	1 Nonaphasic	
Transcortical sensory 3 ⟶	2 Nonaphasic - - - - - - - - - - (50.0)	
	1 Anomic	
Anomic (25) ⟶	12 Nonaphasic - - - - - - - - - - - - -(48.0)	
	Total 93	21.0

From Kertesz, A., and McCabe, P.: Recovery patterns and prognosis in aphasia. Brain, *100*:1–18, 1977.

It is evident that patients change in their performance on individual modalities and that their total profile can change so radically as to render their initial classification academic. The data reported above indicate that differential classification as to "type," which may appear justified in an acute stage, must be altered as the person improves and moves into less severe and finally mild degrees of aphasia. Rather than change labels, it seems more appropriate to recognize that the patient has moved from one pattern of multimodality dysfunction to a different pattern, with differential rates of improvement in the several modalities.

PROGNOSTIC FACTORS RELATED TO RECOVERY

Data reviewed in Chapter 2 showed that the initial severity of the aphasia is an important determinant of degree of recovery. Several studies confirmed the fact that the lower the level of performance at onset, the more limited the recovery and the more dismal the prognosis for the reacquisition of functional language. Other variables have been found to be likewise related to degree of recovery.

Etiology of Aphasia. From studies cited in Chapter 4 we will conclude that the amount of recovery resulting from programs of aphasia therapy is probably related to etiology. Other reports not concerned specifically with the effects of treatment will be reviewed here.

Alajouanine and co-workers (1957) studied 43 patients with traumatic aphasia and an undesignated number of patients with other causes of aphasia. They concluded that the prognosis for aphasic patients with closed head injuries was favorable, in contrast to a poorer prognosis for patients with aphasia due to open brain injuries and cerebrovascular accidents.

Leischner (1960), in discussing the outcome for 46 patients with aphasia, indicated that "the kind of aphasia is not necessarily decisive as to the course" but that "on the other hand, the kind of disease does affect the outcome. . . . In this respect, [patients with] closed cerebral injuries of long-standing were clearly in a better position than [those with] vascular diseases and the open brain damages."

Luria (1963) reported differential improvement between cases due to penetrating wounds of the brain (in a large percentage of which severe aphasia persists in the patient) and cases due to nonpenetrating wounds (in which persistent aphasia is exceptional). He reported that twice as many patients with nonpenetrating wounds recovered completely within 4 months as recovered in the group with penetrating wounds.

In Eisenson's (1964) experience, patients with single vascular episodes make better language recovery than those with recurrent vascular episodes. He observed that patients with traumatically incurred aphasia improved more than patients with neoplasms or cerebrovascular lesions.

Thomsen (1975) also reported favorable outcome of traumatically incurred aphasia. He studied 12 patients with severe closed head injuries (mean age, 25.5 years). Their communication was "observed" during the first 2 or 3 weeks post injury; then they were tested by a speech pathologist on the average of 4 months after injury, and a follow-up examination was performed another 12 to 50 months (mean, 33 months) after injury. Four of the 12 patients had no symptoms of aphasia on final testing, although spontaneous speech was aberrant in one. The remaining eight still had symptoms of aphasia, but in only one was the aphasia severe.

A less sanguine report of outcome was made by Heilman and co-workers (1971) concerning a group of 13 aphasic patients with closed head injuries. "In our cases recovery varied greatly and we could find no constant relationship that would help . . . to prognosticate."

On the basis of serial administrations of the PICA, Porch (1971b) has reported that patients with aphasia of thrombotic vascular etiology demonstrate a different recovery profile from those with aphasia of traumatic etiology. Those with vascular aphasia show an ascending recovery curve that plateaus at about 6 months post onset; patients with aphasia of traumatic etiology display a stair-step recovery that continues to improve beyond 6 months.

With further regard to vascular etiology, Anderson and colleagues (1970) studied predictors of recovery in completed stroke, including the outcome of aphasia. They concluded that hemorrhagic stroke results in the lowest recovery potential.

But Rubens (1977) has offered a less gloomy picture of the ultimate outcome of aphasia due to hemorrhage. "A circumscribed intracerebral hemorrhage often produces a potentially reversible though initially severe deficit. In our experience, the period of spontaneous recovery may not begin for weeks or sometimes months following deep cerebral hemorrhages. Several of our patients have left the hospital in three to four weeks post onset with a flaccid hemiplegia and a severe global aphasia, only to begin their spontaneous language recovery as late as the third, fourth, or sixth month post onset. This delayed improvement probably coincides with the late absorption of the hemorrhagic mass with concomitant reduction of pressure on and distortion of the language zone."

Kohlmeyer (1976) reported on aphasic impairments that result from cerebrovascular accidents and the spontaneous recovery demonstrated in two kinds of patients: those with occlusions of left-sided cerebral arteries and those with diminished local cerebral blood flow without evidence of arterial occlusion. He reported that rates of spontaneous recovery from aphasia due to diminished blood flow are much higher than in cases due to arterial occlusion. For example, 100 per cent of the 20 patients with Broca's aphasia due to diminished blood supply "recovered completely, or almost completely, within 14 days, eight of them within the first two or three days," whereas only 33 per cent of the Broca's aphasic patients with arterial occlusion recovered completely within 14 days. Similar discrepancies were observed in "sensory," "conduction," and "nominal" aphasic patients with and without arterial occlusion. Only in the case of "global" aphasia was no difference observed in rate of recovery between the two types of vascular disorder.

Kertesz and McCabe (1977), it will be recalled, followed a group of patients from initial testing done 0 to 6 weeks post onset, retesting them at 3 month, 6 month, and yearly intervals thereafter. Their total of 93 patients included 74 with infarcts and intracerebral hemorrhages, 12 with subarachnoid hemorrhage, and 7 with history of trauma. Excluding 22 "chronic aphasia" patients who had tests and retests more than a year post onset, they analyzed the course of recovery as related to etiology. "Aphasics after a subarachnoid hemorrhage showed wide variations in their recovery rates, presumably related to the variable extent of their hemorrhage and presence of infarcts or tissue destruction. . . . Some of the worst jargon and global [aphasic] patients were seen following ruptured middle cerebral aneurysms. Traumatic aphasia had a better overall prognosis than that of vascular disease. Many of these patients were younger, although the scatter of age factor was considerable. The extent and severity of lesions [were] quite variable in our motor vehicle accident population, most of them closed head injuries, a few with subdural or intracerebral hemorrhage or contusion. Younger patients with milder injuries showed excellent spontaneous recovery." They further stated, "It was demonstrated that the prognosis and recovery [were] significantly different according to etiological varieties, such as cerebral infarcts, intracerebral and subarachnoid hemorrhage and trauma. Although this is also evident from the literature, various etiologies are still often lumped together. Post-traumatic aphasia seemed to have a more benign course and sometimes surprisingly dramatic spontaneous recovery was witnessed. One of our young patients was considered global aphasic, but recovered to a mild anomic state, a phenomenon not seen in infarcts or other vascular lesions with this extent of initial language impairment. Complete recovery was seen in more than half of our traumatic cases."

The data indicate, then, that traumatically incurred aphasias generally have a more favorable prognosis than those of vascular origin, especially if the injury is a closed head injury rather than a penetrating wound. Of all the vascular etiologies, hemorrhage appears to carry the poorest prognosis, and multiple vascular episodes make the ultimate outcome of aphasia less favorable than if only a single episode is responsible. Recovery from aphasia due to diminished cerebral blood supply is generally better than it is in cases due to vascular occlusion. Data are lacking concerning the prognosis for patients with aphasia of infectious, neoplastic, or surgical origin.

Site and Extent of Lesion. Russell and Espir (1961) studied 255 aphasic patients who had suffered penetrating wounds of the brain in World War II. They charted the "speech territory" in the left hemisphere, "the regions of the brain important for speech": "The surface marking of the speech territory . . . includes the lower half of the left pre-central and post-central gyrus, the supramarginal and angular gyrus, the inferior parietal gyrus, and a large part of the temporal lobe" but does not include any of the occipital lobe or the inferior temporal gyrus. "This surface marking is just as likely to indicate the importance of underlying tracts as of the cortical cell-layers themselves. This territory is a meeting-ground for cerebral mechanisms connected with the elaboration of the auditory and visual afferent systems, and with the sensorimotor organization for the muscles used for articulation and for writing." To clarify further the anatomic boundaries of the speech territory, they reviewed nine cases "in which the wound was near the margin of the speech area and in which there is a good record of the preservation of speech after wounding."

They then presented a series of 11 patients who suffered small wounds in the center of the speech territory; all showed catastrophic "disorganization of all aspects of speech. . . . Speech means nothing to the patient and if he can himself speak or write at all he talks or writes jargon. . . . The term global aphasia might . . . be used for this group . . . but we propose to refer to this group as the cases of *Central Aphasia.* . . ; the term *central* provides the important indication that the wound involves the center of the speech territory." "It is necessary to emphasize that these central wounds often cause motor aphasia, nominal aphasia, jargon, word deafness, alexia, agraphia, and loss of memory and capacity for thought. This global effect does not mean that all aspects of the mechanism, say for reading, are situated where the wound is, but rather that even if certain contributions to the speech mechanism are untouched, they are useless without the integrity of the central speech organization. This is important when considering the effects of wounds at the periphery of the speech territory in which the central mechanisms are relatively intact."

Russell and Espir then reviewed three groups of such cases of small wounds at the periphery of the speech territory: 30 patients with small wounds of the rolandic area ("motor aphasia," our apraxia of speech), "which not infrequently render the wounded man speechless, and yet the understanding of speech, whether spoken or written, remains good or even unimpaired," patients who typically showed "remarkable recovery"; seven cases with small posterior parietal wounds (region of angular gyrus), with agraphia much more severe than other dysphasic features; and 11 cases with small inferior parietal wounds with disproportionate alexia.

In addition to their presentation of the results of small wounds in various areas, they reviewed four cases with more extensive, "severely destructive wounds of the left cerebral hemisphere." One patient demonstrated severe global aphasia with fair recovery; a second had global aphasia with good recovery of speech, although reading remained difficult; a third demonstrated global aphasia and showed some recovery of speech and understanding, but reading and spelling recovered little, and writing consisted of only a few words; the fourth patient initially displayed severe aphasia, his speech returning satisfactorily but not his reading or writing.

Russell and Espir make only a few rather general allusions to the recovery patterns of their groups of cases. Their data suggest, in summary, that small lesions in the central portion of the "speech territory" cause severe aphasia with variable degrees of recovery; small lesions in the periphery of that territory cause disproportionate unimodality impairment associated with less severe or no aphasia, with many instances of excellent recovery; and extensive destructive lesions cause severe aphasia with limited recovery.

Luria (1963) also commented upon the disparity between the initial severity and eventual good outcome for aphasic patients with lesions occurring near but not in the classic language zone. Lesions directly involving the language areas appeared to him much less likely to resolve in significant spontaneous gains than lesions in the bordering areas.

Penfield and Roberts (1959) studied patients with seizures. They mapped the brain in terms of language function by electrical stimulation of the cerebral cortex and also reported on the effects of excision of affected areas of the brain in 273 operations. "It should be remembered that these patients were operated upon because they had brain functioning abnormally to the extent that it had been giving rise to seizures. There were at least seven patients who had dysphasia before operation; this number probably would have been higher had all patients been examined in detail from the standpoint of language." Five of these seven patients, following excision of part of the left hemisphere, "had increased difficulties in speech after operation, with the exception of one, who had no changes immediately and nine months later showed improvement."

Penfield and Roberts reported that aphasia occurred immediately after excision of areas in the left hemisphere 22 times in the 273 operations. They made the following conclusions concerning the size of the areas excised: "Limited excisions of any previously damaged part of the left hemisphere may be followed by only transient dysphasia, provided the remaining brain functions normally. Persistent dysphasia may occur during abnormal function or with extensive destruction of the left hemisphere."

Yarnell and associates (1976) related outcome of aphasia to size, location, and number of lesions in 14 patients with acute onset of thromboembolic cerebrovascular accidents who were available for long-term follow-up. In the acute stage, angiographic and radioisotopic findings were obtained, and the MTDDA and the PICA were administered within the first month of illness. These tests were readministered a second time over a period ranging from 8 months to 3½ years later, and the identity of the lesions at time of follow-up was determined by computed tomography (CT). In the interim, the patients received speech therapy of undescribed type and amount. Outcomes were graded as good (minimal to mild impairment), fair (moderate to moderately severe impairment), and poor (severe). Six of the 14 patients were rated as having good outcome at the time of the second test, three as fair, and five as poor.

The investigators reported their findings as follows: "Bilateral, in part temporal, or large single dominant-hemisphere lesions correlated with the acute severe global aphasic states. These patients had general-ly poorer aphasia recoveries. Alternately, relatively small-sized dominant-hemisphere CT lesions correlated with acute expressive much greater than receptive difficulties and a more benign aphasia resolution. . . . The long-term CT scan showing the size, location, and number of lesions had a good correlation with aphasia outcome. Most patients with large dominant-hemisphere inolvements, either one large or many smaller lesions, fared poorly, while those with lesser lesions did better. Bilateral lesions, at times evasive clinically, helped to account for significant aphasia residuals."

Gloning and co-workers (1976) also reported the deleterious effect of bilateral cerebral involvement. In a study of 19 variables they found that the existence of bilateral cerebral lesions (diagnosed via EEG, neurologic examination, and brain scans) had a statistically significant negative prognostic effect on recovery from aphasia in a group of 107 patients whose progress was followed for 18 months post onset.

Another study using computed tomography for determining lo-calization and size of lesion and relating these to prognosis in aphasia has been reported by Kertesz and colleagues (1979). Their findings were further summarized by Kertesz (1979). They obtained computed tomography scans on 23 aphasic patients within 35 days of onset and on 39 other patients 1 year post onset (designated chronic). Ten patients had scans in both the acute and chronic stages. Patients were administered the WAB and the results were correlated with the data obtained either in the acute phase or in the chronic phase; in those cases in which CT data were available in both acute and chronic stages, the correlation was determined between language recovery and lesion size.

Considering first the data on the total group of patients, the correlation coefficient between the largest area traced in each aphasic patient and the AQ (the summary score of the WAB) was -0.57, significant at $P \leq 0.01$. The negative correlation indicates that the larger the lesion, the more severe the aphasia.

Considering only the patients tested in the acute stage, "The larger the lesion, the poorer is the comprehension ($r = 0.595$, significant $P \leq 0.01$). Similar trends (negative correlations) were seen for naming (-0.357), repetition (-0.328), and overall severity (-0.367). . . . On the other hand, fluency did not correlate with lesion size (-0.1437)."

The chronic aphasic patients who were tested only after a year post onset showed significant negative correlations between lesion size and all language parameters: comprehension (-0.74), repetition (-0.679), naming (-0.702), fluency (-0.666), and overall severity as measured by AQ (-0.725).

Concerning patients with both early and late data: "The extent of language recovery was calculated as the difference in scores between the initial and the one-year follow-up examination in 32 patients. The positive correlation (+0.35) between recovery of comprehension and lesion size was the only one reaching statistical significance. A trend of negative correlation was observed for the other parameters (severity as measured by AQ, −0.253; fluency, −0.348; repetition, −0.300; naming, −0.255)." These negative correlations between the recovery rate and lesion size indicate that the larger the lesion, the less overall recovery occurs in the total language deficit (AQ) and in parameters other than comprehension.

Kohlmeyer (1976), as noted earlier, related aphasia and recovery from it to focal disorders of cerebral circulation. We have already reviewed his data concerning the better outlook for patients with diminished local cerebral blood flow as opposed to patients with demonstrated occlusions of left-sided cerebral arteries. He provides further information about the more specific site of lesion. Patients whose aphasia was due to an occlusion of the *posterior cerebral artery* recovered completely during the first 2 weeks post onset but, Kohlmeyer added, "unfortunately the latter site of cerebroarterial occlusion is very rare, only 4 per cent (14 cases out of 303)." Concerning occlusions of other vessels he reported as follows:

> Broca's aphasias due to occlusion of the *internal carotid artery* in the neck are marked by a favorable spontaneous course. Thirty-three per cent (35 cases) . . . recovered completely during the 14 days following the stroke. The remaining 65 cases continued to show a more or less severe motor aphasia.
> Only five per cent (four cases) of all aphasias due to occlusion of the *middle cerebral artery* recovered completely during the first 14 days; 43 per cent (36 cases) of all patients surviving the first 14 days retained a severe global aphasia [the remainder showing a change to milder forms].
> Aphasias due to occlusions in *branches of the middle cerebral artery* were remarkably stable. One could observe some recovery. But only 3 per cent (three cases) recovered completely during the first 14 days, 12 per cent (12 cases) changed the type of aphasia, 85 per cent (85 cases) remained unchanged.

Rubens (1975) supplements these comments with some observations on the results of large infarctions in the territory of the left *anterior cerebral artery*. He describes profound but transient disturbances of speech and language: "Despite the initially severe and profound motor aphasia, serviceable spontaneous speech returns within weeks. . . . The short duration of the major aphasic symptoms is probably due to the fact that these regions have extensive bilateral connections with subcortical structures and with each other, so that the function of one may be readily assumed by its remaining counterpart."

Mohr and co-workers (1975) have reported on the language consequences of hemorrhage in the thalamus of the left hemisphere. These patients are described as logorrheic, paraphasic, and echolalic. One patient who survived is described as having a very severe early deficit but recovering language to complete normalcy by the second month post onset.

In summary, even small lesions of the central core of the dominant-hemisphere language area, the area served by the middle cerebral artery, result in severe aphasia. The more extensive the lesion, the more lasting the effect on language functions and the poorer the ultimate outcome. The prognosis is also poorer if contralateral hemisphere areas are implicated and if there are several, even small lesions in the dominant hemisphere. More peripheral single lesions, including infarctions related to posterior cerebral artery, anterior cerebral artery, and internal carotid artery occlusions, may result in initially severe aphasia, but the course of recovery is more rapid and the outcome is generally more favorable.

Review of case data presented by Russell and Espir and by others indicates that in *individual* cases it is difficult to predict outcome of aphasia even though it is possible to draw certain group generalizations about outcome. Despite the fact that in general the larger the dominant-hemisphere lesion, the poorer the outcome, many investigators have reported individual patients who apparently had large lesions yet recovered well. Rubens (1977) has highlighted the wide differences that exist among individual brains: "It is quite possible that many variations in the rapidity and degree of recovery seen in patients with lesions of similar size and location reflect this underlying inborn variability of the cortical speech apparatus."

General Health and Associated Sensory and Motor Deficits. There are some indications that the patient's good general health and his freedom from motor and sensory deficits may provide a more favorable prognosis for his recovery from aphasia. Eisenson (1949), on the basis of clinical experience, reached the conclusion that the better the patient's physical condition, the better his chances of language improvement, largely because of his greater mobility and opportunity for environmental stimulation. Elsewhere, Eisenson (1964) stated his conviction that "patients who do not incur, or who did not previously have, a hearing or visual defect do better than those with such sensory impairments. . . . Patients with few somatic complaints do better than those with many such complaints."

Leischner and Linck (1967) tried to account for the relative lack of progress shown by some of their treated patients. They listed as probably the second most frequent contributor to negligible progress (after unfavorable personality characteristics) the existence of associated "bodily or psychic diseases, which necessitated a temporary interruption of the treatment and thus brought about an essential slowdown of the latter. In this category belong paroxysms of angina pectoris, cardiac and circulatory failure, alcoholism, depressed state of mind, frequent cerebral cramps, or an organic change of disposition."

Anderson and colleagues (1970), in a study of rehabilitation predictors in completed stroke, concluded that prognosis is better if there are no coexisting sensory deficits. They confirmed a finding made earlier by Van Buskirk (1955) and subsequently supported by Smith (1972). Smith reported on the effects of therapy with a group of 18 aphasic patients with normal sensory functions as contrasted with a group of 21 patients who had sensory problems demonstrated on double simultaneous testing. The patients without sensory loss showed higher gains in comprehension, reading, and writing; however, their gains were lower than those of patients with sensory loss in speech, digit span, oral substitutions, and visual retention. Despite sensory problems, Smith concluded that aphasic stroke patients with marked sensory defects but with no dementia can benefit significantly from therapy.

Keenan and Brassell (1974) studied the clinical records of 39 aphasic patients in order to identify and correlate factors noted in their initial examination with their subsequent progress in communicative performance. Three nonlanguage variables and, as reviewed in Chapter 2, five language variables were studied. A clinical scale of speech performance based on the patient's most characteristic conversational responses was used to classify the patient's ultimate communicative performance as "good," "fair," or "poor." General health of the patient before onset of aphasia was one of the nonlanguage variables related to scaled language outcome. It was rated on the basis of information in the medical history; those with no report of prior serious disease or general debilitating condition were rated as in "good health"; "fair health" meant that the patient had been functioning in a somewhat restricted manner, usually under sustained medication; a rating of "poor health" was assigned to patients who for more than a month before the onset of aphasia had been severely restricted in activity or were under continual medical care. Outcome data revealed little difference in the general health of the three groups of patients divided according to their terminal level of speech performance. "Whatever their terminal speech performance levels, most patients tended to be healthy. Put another way, patients who had been in good health were well distributed among those dismissed in each speech performance category. Thus, we found insufficient predictive value in ratings of general health before the onset of aphasia."

Contradictory statements have been made about the relationship of hemiplegia to outcome of aphasia in stroke patients. In an early report, Bateman (1890) indicated that whereas the nonhemiplegic aphasic patient may benefit from treatment, little can be done to improve language function in aphasic patients with hemiplegia. Smith (1972) compared the outcomes of therapy with 42 hemiplegic and 25 non-hemiplegic aphasic patients. The hemiplegics as a group tended to be more impaired in communication skills before therapy began than the nonhemiplegic group, but the gains of the two groups after therapy were almost identical except for higher gains by the hemiplegic group in digit span, oral substitutions, and visual retention. The findings of Gloning and co-workers (1976) are in agreement; in their statistical study of the influence of 19 variables on the recovery of 107 aphasic patients, they found that presence of mono- or hemiplegia did not negatively affect outcome. Kertesz and McCabe (1977) do not indicate how they arrived at the conclusion, but they report, in contrast, "In our experience. . .persisting hemiplegia. . .is a poor prognostic sign."

Age. There are many expressions of opinion in the aphasia literature that age at onset of aphasia is an important determinant of degree of recovery. Goldstein (1948) concluded that patients under 50 years of age have a better chance for language recovery than those over 50 years old. Eisenson (1949) observed that progress was favorable in a group of 13 patients in an army hospital with a mean age of 24 years (range, 20 to 32 years), whereas progress was poor in a group of eight other army personnel with a mean age of 31 years (range, 22 to 47 years).

Sands and associates (1969) reported on language progress made by 30 patients (mean age, 56.5 years) who were followed from 4 to 12 months after termination of variable periods of aphasia therapy; Functional Communication Profile scores were obtained pretreatment, at discharge, and on follow-up. Age was found to be "the most potent variable influencing recovery." The one sixth of their group which improved most had an average age of 47 years, whereas the one sixth which recovered least averaged 61 years.

Schuell (1965) also acknowledged the influence of age in recovery from aphasia but suggested that it is only indirect. In her clinical experience, she encountered young patients with persisting severe aphasia and other patients over 60 years old who made good recovery. She felt that a generalization concerning age as a single prognostic factor was unwarranted.

Kertesz and McCabe (1977) included age as a parameter to be investigated in the study alluded to previously in which patients, some treated, some untreated, were initially tested with the WAB in the period 0 to 6 weeks post onset and subsequently retested at 3-month, 6-month, and yearly intervals thereafter. They found that the age of the patients was negatively correlated with recovery rates in the first 3-month interval ($r = -0.240$). But this correlation, indicating that the younger the patient, the higher the initial recovery rate, did not reach statistical significance. The investigators suggest that it did not because of certain marked exceptions in the group, such as two older patients who recovered remarkably well and two young patients who made a poor recovery.

One of the nonlanguage variables studied by Keenan and Brassell (1974) was age. The 39 subjects were divided into 10-year age groups to compare age at onset of aphasia with level of terminal speech performance (good, fair, or poor). The subject distribution was marked by dispersion rather than by any central tendency. "When the seven subjects from 29 to 39 years of age completed therapy, three had good speech, two had fair speech, and two had poor speech. There was little difference for the seven subjects from 60 to 69 years of age, for when they completed therapy, three had good speech and four had poor speech. While advanced age may complicate recovery from aphasia, for the patients of this study, it was not a reliable factor for predicting speech return."

Further information about the effect of age on recovery in patients who receive treatment for aphasia is given in Chapter 4. It will be seen from those data that studies of the effect of treatment on older and younger groups of aphasic patients are again in some conflict, but most of the recent studies indicate that age appears to be neither an important deterrent to nor a facilitator of recovery.

Sex. The differential outcome of aphasia in male and female patients has scarcely been studied. Kertesz and McCabe (1977) compared the initial 3-month recovery rates of groups of 23 male and 23 female aphasic patients. The difference in the recovery rates of the two groups was not statistically significant. Similarly, Gloning and co-workers (1976) found that the sex of the patients was not significantly related to degree of recovery in a group of 107 patients with aphasia of traumatic or vascular etiology.

Psychosocial Factors. Eisenson (1947) and others have suggested that the more highly educated the aphasic patient, the less favorable his recovery, but no firm data support this notion. Wepman (1951) in his study of the recovery of a group of 68 patients with traumatically incurred aphasia provides some information about the relationship between educational level and recovery from aphasia. He reported: "One highly consistent factor. . .is the low positive correlation between the subjects' educational achievement rank order at the three stages. The tendency seemed to remain constant for the group to maintain to a slight degree their relative rank order in terms of language ability. Low positive correlation coefficients were found between (1) the pretraumatic and the posttraumatic stages [0.36], (2) the pretraining and post-training stages [0.31], and (3) even the preinjury and posttraining stages [0.28]. The fact that the better educated students tended to remain at somewhat higher educational levels after injury and that the subjects who were highest in rank order of educational achievement after injury were also highest after training would indicate that, to the degree of significance that the statistics have, it would be possible to predict the amount of loss and amount of gain a particular individual would have were he to suffer a brain injury. It should be pointed out, however, that the actual correlations are so slight as to make this prediction hazardous at best."

Sarno and colleagues (1970a) studied the same 31 severely aphasic patients whose lack of progress in therapy was reported by Sarno and co-workers (1970b). They found that educational level and premorbid language proficiency were not related to the degrees of negligible improvement shown by these severely aphasic patients.

Smith (1972) compared improvement during therapy of 18 patients with less than 12 years of formal education with that of 29 patients with 18 or more years of education. The better educated group made greater gains than the others in four areas — reading, writing, digit span, and oral substitutions; both groups showed comparable gains in all other areas of performance appraised by means of a comprehensive battery of language and nonlanguage tests. Smith concluded that limited education is not a significant obstacle in language rehabilitation of aphasic patients.

Similarly, Gloning and associates (1976) found that educational level did not significantly influence recovery from aphasia. In their follow-up of 107 treated and untreated patients (mean age, 39 years) with aphasia of traumatic or vascular etiology, they found that patients with eight or more years of schooling did not recover to a greater or lesser degree than those with less than eight years of schooling.

Data about the effect of level of intelligence on recovery are scanty. Wepman (1951) reported a positive correlation between pretraumatic IQ and posttraining IQ, and another positive correlation between gain in IQ and gain in educational achievement in his group of 68 treated aphasic soldiers. It seems reasonable to conclude that the higher the original IQ, the greater the gains in therapy. In their multiple linear regression analysis of the relationship of 19 variables to recovery, Gloning and co-workers (1976) found that "feeblemindedness before onset of illness" (based on school reports and family estimates that IQ was 70 or lower) was one of four prognostic factors significantly affecting recovery negatively. Messerli and colleagues (1976) found a significant positive relationship between "operational" intelligence level (measured by the Piaget Conservation of Physical Quantities Test) and the level of communication reached by the 53 patients they studied (age range, 17 to 74 years) with aphasia of vascular and traumatic etiology.

Personality characteristics of aphasic patients, as Wepman (1953) has pointed out, constitute a convenient but possibly irrelevant explanation for failures encountered in therapy; "personality" is a peculiarly handy scapegoat because it is difficult to specify and quantify. Nevertheless, some clinical workers have been convinced that certain personality characteristics may inhibit whereas others may facilitate recovery. Eisenson (1947) has suggested that "there is a psychological overlay which influences the presence and nature of aphasic disturbances. Subjectively, I am inclined to believe that those of our aphasic patients who showed severe expressive disturbances were for the most part withdrawn individuals prior to their head injury. . . . Withdrawn individuals made slow progress and needed constant psychological support in the course of their training. On the other hand, persons whose histories revealed so-called extrovertive tendencies appeared to make rapid improvement. They 'took chances' more often than did the introvertive type of patient and were less embarrassed by errors in their speech. . . . Several of the patients were involved in accidents about which they felt guilty. . . .In these instances, little spontaneous improvement took place and the aphasic disturbances tended to persist despite early efforts at training.'' Eisenson (1949) also has considered euphoria, too high a level of aspiration, and excessive dependency as negative prognostic characteristics.

Leischner and Linck (1967) felt that the primary reason why several of 70 patients receiving therapy did not improve was "the personality of the patient." They referred to lack of interest, actual resistance to participation, lack of realization of being sick, and lack of motivation. Anderson and co-workers (1970) emphasized motivation and high level of aspiration as favorable prognostic signs in aphasia.

Although Stoicheff (1960) has shown that the attitudes surrounding the patient and characterizing the stimulation that he receives can importantly influence his level of language function, few data are available concerning the effect of the social milieu of the patient on his recovery from aphasia. Sarno and collaborators (1970a) found that current living environments (whether at home or in a nursing home, hospital, or rehabilitation center) had no significant effect on degree of improvement in their 31 elderly, severely aphasic patients.

Keenan and Brassell (1974) studied the relationship of prior employment to the ultimate communicative performance of their 39 subjects. Their findings were that patients were unemployed, employed part time, or employed full time in about equal proportions in all three terminal speech performance categories (good, fair, poor).

Sarno and co-workers (1970a) placed their 31 elderly, severely aphasic patients in two groups with respect to occupational status. The group of subjects involved in unskilled and skilled labor was compared with the group of businessmen, professionals, and housewives. No significant difference in level of recovery was found between the two groups.

This review of possible prognostic variables leads to the conclusion that in addition to the initial severity of the aphasia (more severe deficits eventuating in less complete recovery), the etiology of the aphasia and the extent and site(s) of the lesion are the most important determinants of outcome. Traumatically incurred aphasia improves more than aphasia of vascular etiology. Additional hazard for recovery is contributed by multiplicity of lesions, bilateral involvement, and (possibly) hemorrhagic etiology. The greater the extent of damaged brain tissue, the poorer the prognosis. Long-term gains are poorest in patients whose lesion involves the central portion of the dominant-hemisphere language area, the area served by the middle cerebral artery, aphasias resulting from more peripheral lesions showing faster and more complete recovery.

Variables of apparently lesser negative influence in general are poor general health, coexisting sensory and motor deficits, advanced age, low intelligence, and emotional maladjustment (depression, introversion, lack of motivation). In individual cases these may exert more potent influence, and the generally more powerful prognostic variables may exert less influence than expected because of individual variability with regard to brain structure and plasticity.

REFERENCES

Alajouanine, T., Castaigne, P., Lhermitte, F., Escourolle, R., and DeRibaucourt, B.: Etude de 43 cas d'aphasie post-traumatique. Encephale, 46:1–45, 1957.

Anderson, T. P., Bourestom, N., and Greenberg, F. R.: Rehabilitation Predictors in Completed Stroke: Final Report. Minneapolis, American Rehabilitation Foundation, 1970.

Basso, A., Capitani, E., and Vignolo, L. A.: Influence of rehabilitation on language skills in aphasic patients. Arch. Neurol., 36:190–196, 1979.

Bateman, F.: On Aphasia or Loss of Speech and the Localization of the Faculty of Articulate Language. London, Churchill, 1890.

Butfield, E., and Zangwill, O. L.: Re-education in aphasia: a review of 70 cases. J. Neurol. Neurosurg. Psychiatry, 9:75–79, 1946.

Culton, G. L.: Spontaneous recovery from aphasia. J. Speech Hearing Res., 12:825–832, 1969.

Eisenson, J.: Aphasics: observations and tentative conclusions. J. Speech Dis., 12:290–292, 1947.

Eisenson, J.: Prognostic factors related to language rehabilitation in aphasic patients. J. Speech Hearing Disord., 14:262–264, 1949.

Eisenson, J.: Aphasia: a point of view as to the nature of the disorder and factors that determine prognosis for recovery. Int. J. Neurol., 4:287–295, 1964.

Gloning, K., Trappl, R., Heiss, W. D., and Quatember, R.: Prognosis and speech therapy in aphasia. In Lebrun, Y., and Hoops, R. (Eds.): Recovery in Aphasics. Atlantic Highlands, New Jersey, Humanities Press, 1976.

Goldstein, K.: Language and Language Disturbances. New York, Grune & Stratton, 1948.

Golper, L. C.: A study of verbal behavior in recovery of aphasic and non-aphasic persons. In Clinical Aphasiology Conference Proceedings 1980. Minneapolis, BRK Publishers, 1980, pp. 28–37.

Goodglass, H., Quadfasel, F. A., and Timberlake, W. H.: Phrase length and the type and severity of aphasia. Cortex, 1:133–153, 1964.

Hagen, C.: Communication abilities in hemiplegia: effect of speech therapy. Arch. Phys. Med. Rehabil., 54:454–463, 1973.

Hanson, W. R., and Cicciarelli, A. W.: The time, amount, and pattern of language improvement in adult aphasics. Br. J. Disord. Commun., 13:59–63, 1978.

Heilman, K. M., Safran, A., and Geschwind, N.: Closed head trauma and aphasia. J. Neurol. Neurosurg. Psychiatry, 34:265–269, 1971.

Keenan, J. S., and Brassell, E. G.: A study of factors related to prognosis for individual aphasic patients. J. Speech Hearing Disord., 39:257–269, 1974.

Kenin, M., and Swisher, L.: A study of pattern of recovery in aphasia. Cortex, 8:56–68, 1972.

Kertesz, A.: Aphasia and Associated Disorders: Taxonomy, Localization, and Recovery. New York, Grune & Stratton, 1979.

Kertesz, A., Harlock, W., and Coates, R.: Computer tomographic localization, lesion size, and prognosis in aphasia and nonverbal impairment. Brain Lang., 8:34–50, 1979.

Kertesz, A., and McCabe, P.: Recovery patterns and prognosis in aphasia. Brain, 100:1–18, 1977.

Kohlmeyer, K.: Aphasia due to focal disorders of cerebral circulation: some aspects of localization and of spontaneous recovery. In Lebrun, Y., and Hoops, R. (Eds.): Recovery in Aphasics. Atlantic Highlands, New Jersey, Humanities Press, 1976, pp. 79–85.

Koura, F., Taher, Y., Barrada, O., and Mostafa, M.: Effect of temporal factor in the prognosis of aphasia due to vascular stroke. In Multinational Conference on Rehabilitation Research in Disorders of Central Language Processing. Cairo, Egypt, S.O.P. Press, 1978, pp. 77–86.

Kreindler, A., and Fradis, A.: Performances in Aphasia. A Neurodynamical, Diagnostic and Psychological Study. Paris, Gauthier-Villars, 1968.

Leischner, A.: Zur Symptomatologie und Therapie der Aphasien. Nervenarzt, 31:60–67, 1960.

Leischner, A., and Linck, H. A.: Neuere Erfahrungen mit der Behandlung von Aphasien. Nervenarzt, 38:199–205, 1967.

Lomas, J., and Kertesz, A.: Patterns of spontaneous recovery in aphasic groups: a study of adult stroke patients. Brain Lang., 5:388–401, 1978.

Luria, A. R.: Restoration of Function After Brain Injury. New York, Macmillan, 1963.

Luria, A. R.: Traumatic Aphasia. The Hague, Netherlands, Uitgeverij Mouton, 1970.

Messerli, P., Tissot, A., and Rodriguez, J.: Recovery from aphasia: some factors of prognosis. In Lebrun, Y., and Hoops, R. (Eds.): Recovery in Aphasics. Atlantic Highlands, New Jersey, Humanities Press, 1976.

Mohr, J. P., Watters, W. C., and Duncan, G. W.: Thalamic hemorrhage and aphasia. Brain Lang., 2:3–17, 1975.

Penfield, W., and Roberts, L.: Speech and Brain Mechanisms. Princeton, New Jersey, Princeton University Press, 1959.

Porch, B. E.: Porch Index of Communicative Ability. Manual, Vol. 2, Revised Ed. Palo Alto, California, Consulting Psychologists Press, 1971a.

Porch, B. E.: A comparison of unilateral and bilateral PICA profiles on brain-damaged adults. Paper presented at 47th Annual Convention, American Speech and Hearing Association, Chicago, 1971b.

Prins, R. S., Snow, C. E., and Wagenaar, E.: Recovery from aphasia: spontaneous speech versus language comprehension. Brain Lang., 6:192–211, 1978.

Rubens, A. B.: Aphasia with infarction in the territory of the anterior cerebral artery. Cortex, 11:239–250, 1975.

Rubens, A. B.: The role of changes within the central nervous system during recovery from aphasia. In Sullivan, M., and Kommers, M. S. (Eds.): Rationale for Adult Aphasia Therapy. Lincoln, Nebraska, University of Nebraska Press, 1977, pp. 28–43.

Russell, W. R., and Espir, M. L. E.: Traumatic Aphasia: A Study of Aphasia in War Wounds of the Brain. London, Oxford University Press, 1961.

Sands, E., Sarno, M. T., and Shankweiler, D.: Long-term assessment of language function in aphasia due to stroke. Arch. Phys. Med. Rehabil., 50:202–206, 222, 1969.

Sarno, M. T., and Levita, E.: Natural course of recovery in severe aphasia. Arch. Phys. Med. Rehabil., 52:175–178, 1971.

Sarno, M. T., Silverman, M., and Levita, E.: Psychosocial factors and recovery in geriatric patients with severe aphasia. J. Am. Geriatr. Soc., 18:405–409, 1970a.

Sarno, M. T., Silverman, M., and Sands, E.: Speech therapy and language recovery in severe aphasia, J. Speech Hearing Res., 13:607–623, 1970b.

Schuell, H.: Differential Diagnosis of Aphasia with the Minnesota Test. Minneapolis, University of Minnesota Press, 1965.

Smith, A.: Diagnosis, Intelligence, and Rehabilitation of Chronic Aphasics. Final Report. Ann Arbor, Michigan, University of Michigan Press, 1972.

Stoicheff, M. L.: Motivating instructions and language performance of dysphasic subjects. J. Speech Hearing Res., 3:75–85, 1960.

Thomsen, I. V.: Evaluation and outcome of aphasia in patients with severe closed head trauma. J. Neurol. Neurosurg. Psychiatry, 38:713–718, 1975.

Tonkovich, J. D.: A longitudinal case study of expressive language changes in aphasia resulting from herpes encephalitis. Clinical Aphasiology Conference Proceedings 1980. Minneapolis, BRK Publishers, 1980, pp. 331–337.

Van Buskirk, C.: Prognostic value of sensory defect in rehabilitation of hemiplegics. Neurology, 6:407–411, 1955.

Vignolo, L. A.: Evolution of aphasia and language rehabilitation: a retrospective exploratory study. Cortex, 1:344–367, 1964.

Wepman, J. M.: Recovery from Aphasia. New York, Ronald Press, 1951.

Wepman, J. M.: A conceptual model for the processes involved in recovery from aphasia. J. Speech Hearing Disord., 18:4–13, 1953.

Yarnell, P., Monroe, P., and Sobel, L.: Aphasia outcome in stroke: A clinical neuroradiological correlation. Stroke, 7:516–522, 1976.

4 • THE EFFECT OF TREATMENT

Studies without No-Treatment Control
  Groups
Studies Using No-Treatment Control
  Groups
Individual Case Studies
Additional Testimony
Conclusions
References

>"What is very sure is that aphasia in most cases needs to be at-
>tacked."
>
>JOSEPH M. WEPMAN

It is evident that the language status of aphasic patients seldom remains static. A reasonable expectation is that even if left relatively to themselves, most aphasic patients spontaneously demonstrate some increments in their ability to process incoming language and to respond to it in some meaningful way. Weisenburg and McBride (1935) point out, "As a matter of fact, most intelligent patients begin to train themselves very soon" and benefit from "incidental training from daily experience." Persons around them inevitably provide input for the patients' brains to react to, and they establish an environment which facilitates (or inhibits) language processing.

Beyond these influences, can the course of recovery from aphasia be influenced by deliberate intervention in the form of language treatment? What evidence is there that a program of language rehabilitation accomplishes measurable gains in language function beyond what can be expected as a result of spontaneous recovery and incidental influences? Does language-specific intervention significantly influence recovery of language processing skills? These important questions have long been asked by neurologists, physiatrists, and other physicians responsible for the management and rehabilitation of brain-injured patients; by the patients and their families, who may potentially invest significant amounts of time, effort, and money; by speech pathologists, who are expected to provide treatment and counsel; and by agencies whose financial support of rehabilitation programs requires getting a dollar's worth of gain from a dollar's worth of investment.

Answers to these questions should emerge from studies designed to document degree of improvement rather than from opinions founded only on intuition and bias. The inquirer finds published declarations that the effectiveness of treatment "remains a subject of considerable doubt" because changes due to therapy have "proved almost impossible to measure" (Benson, 1979). A *Lancet* editorial (1977) pronounces

144

that "assessment of the value of therapy is virtually impossible." A group of discussants, ignoring most published data, report "Definitive answers to questions about the degree of recovery possible after an aphasia and the role that the therapy may play in augmenting such recovery do not, at the moment, exist" (Marshall et al., 1975). Counter to these expressions of skepticism, studies have been designed and completed that provide a reasonable answer to the questions. Objective tests have been developed and applied that provide accurate, repeatable measurement of language performance. Rational therapy regimens have been described. Individual patients and groups of patients have been selected for controlled study. We will consider these studies and the data they provide, and we will abstract from them such conclusions as we can about whether treatment is efficacious; whether the timing of intervention, its nature, and its intensity make a difference; and for what patients it seems to be most helpful.

Data are of several types, varying in scientific merit, reliability, and the provision of a basis for generalization. We will first consider data provided by studies of appreciable numbers of subjects meeting specified criteria, in which baseline and end-point performance have been measured, but which have not included a control group of subjects who received no treatment; second, data coming from studies including control groups of subjects given no formal treatment; third, data from single-case studies and reports; and fourth, expert testimony from aphasiologists who, without providing documentation, have generalized from their experience. We will consider these studies individually and chronologically, reporting whenever possible the number of patients involved in the treatment group; their characteristics in terms of etiology of aphasia, severity of aphasia, age, and length of time post onset before treatment began; how the language status and changes in it were measured; and the intensity of the treatment, its duration, and by whom it was administered. In this way we may be able to make some generalizations about the effect of treatment, although from the outset it must be acknowledged that so many interacting factors influence recovery from aphasia that it is probably not reasonable to reach a single all-inclusive conclusion about the effect of treatment.

STUDIES WITHOUT NO-TREATMENT CONTROL GROUPS

In a study of 200 military personnel who suffered gunshot wounds of the head in World War I, Frazier and Ingham (1920) reported on the treatment of 16 patients of unspecified ages who demonstrated a residual aphasia 6 months or more after they were wounded. "Of these, ten were of the motor or dysarthric type, three of the sensory type with alexia as the most prominent symptom, and three were of the mixed type, manifesting disturbances both in the expression and in the interpretation of language. In none of the patients were the residual aphasic symptoms of severe degree, and all were able to carry on simple conversations fairly well. . . . Trained teachers gave the members of this group daily individual instruction and exercise in conversation, reading, and writing adapted to the needs of the patient and the character of his language disturbance. . . . The improvement has been marked in every patient in this group, the aphasic symptoms of some of whom had previously remained stationary for several months. . . . The patients with alexia were ultimately able to recognize letters and many words, but did not regain the ability to read understandingly to any practical extent."

Franz (1924) reported intensive work with three patients with the goal of reeducating them in object naming, color naming, naming of forms, reading letters and words, and matching printed words to objects. He concluded that "the relearning process is at first slow, but . . . as the period of training continues, learning becomes easier and things are acquired more rapidly. . . . It seems certain that patients with obvious similar speech defects must be reeducated individually, because obvious differences are to be detected."

Weisenburg and McBride (1935) conducted a 4-year study of 60 aphasic patients, all below the age of 60 years. In detailed testing (average duration, 19 hours) they determined the nature and the extent of their language impairments, correlated these with data concerning localization of lesion, and charted improvement in language facility. In one part of their book, they describe the multimodality training methods used as being adapted to the individual patient's needs. They provide a lengthy report of one case (summarized later in this chapter) and briefly describe the results of treatment of four other subjects given somewhat more therapy (1 to 3 hours per week for periods of 5 to 30 months) than others (numbers unspecified) in the study. With regard to the effects of treatment, they drew the following conclusion:

> Reeducation increases the rate of improvement and aids in overcoming specific difficulties and also in helping the patient to find new ways of achieving the results which he can no longer achieve in a normal manner. In none of the cases where training was given did the patient regain what might have been expected to be his former ability, but in all he made considerable progress and was significantly encouraged by his progress to have a different attitude toward the disorder. Thus, the training was of value directly for the improvement in speaking and other specific performances, and it was of tremendous value indirectly for its effect on the patient's morale.

Objective data in support of their conclusions are not presented.

As an introduction to a report of their own treatment study, Butfield and Zangwill (1946) referred to an unpublished report by

Isserlin concerning work at the Brain Injuries Institute in Munich. "Of 178 cases of aphasia given reeducational treatment at this Centre, complete recovery was reported in 10.1 per cent, marked improvement in 23.3 per cent, some improvement (partial recovery) in 55.6 per cent, and no significant change in 9 per cent."

Butfield and Zangwill (1946) reported on the results of treatment of aphasia in the Brain Injuries Unit, Edinburgh, Scotland, of 70 aphasic patients, 59 of whom were under the age of 45 years and 11 over age 45 years. Of these, the etiology in about half was traumatic, in about one third it was vascular, and in the rest neoplastic. The patients were divided into two groups, about two thirds composing one group whose treatment began less than 6 months post onset, the rest beginning treatment more than 6 months post onset. Clinicians rated the patients' impairments in speech, reading, writing, and calculation as severe, moderate, or mild. Aphasia treatment was presented by speech thera- pists in 2 half-hour sessions daily, the number of treatments varying for the group from a minimum of five to a maximum of 290 sessions. Treatment was terminated "when the patient had improved to a point at which little or no practical disability remained or, in the less responsive cases, when the language condition appeared to have become more or less stationary despite prolonged reeducation." At the conclusion of treatment, the patient's language functions were rated by the senior member of the clinical staff as "much improved," "im- proved," or "unchanged."

Concerning the total group, the following ratings are reported: speaking: 48 per cent much improved, 33 per cent improved, 19 per cent unimproved; reading: 36 per cent much improved, 41 per cent improved, 22 per cent unimproved; writing: 38 per cent much im- proved, 34 per cent improved, 28 per cent unimproved. For half the patients whose treatment began less than 6 months post onset and nearly one third of those whose treatment began more than 6 months post onset, the speech "was judged to be much improved after reeducation." With regard to speaking performance alone, 40 per cent of the severe cases, 56 per cent of the moderate cases, and 58 per cent of the mild cases showed much improvement. Again with regard to speaking performance, 21 of 35 traumatic cases were much improved; speech was improved to some degree in two thirds of the cases with vascular and neoplastic etiology. Two thirds of the patients former- ly employed were resettled in gainful employment following their treatment.

Wepman (1951) studied the language rehabilitation of 68 young soldiers (age range, 19 to 38 years) with traumatic head injuries incurred during World War II. None of the patients received formal language treatment for aphasia until 6 months post onset. One group of 36 patients began treatment within the first posttrauma year (6 to 12 months post onset), and a second group of 32 began treatment more than 1 year post onset. The two groups were equated within three tenths of a grade level at the beginning of treatment.

All subjects were given formal training in four language areas: reading, writing, spelling, and mathematics; speech training was given whenever indicated, at the beginning of the training process, by developing recognition of verbal language symbols, and throughout the process by provision of speech correction for errors in articulation and rhythm. Training was provided by skilled teachers of the subject matter areas, not by trained speech pathologists. Half the subjects were taught by a single instructor who covered all subject matter areas, whereas the other half were taught by teams of instructors. Language retraining was conducted for approximately 18 months in each of two Army hospitals, classes meeting 6 hours a day, 5 days a week, with planned extracurricular activities in the evenings and on weekends.

Wepman reported that after this treatment was completed, using the Butfield and Zangwill scale of change, 51 per cent of his patients were much improved, 35 per cent improved, and 14 per cent unimproved. Results of Progressive Achievement Tests showed that as a group these patients' injuries had caused them to lose approximately six school grades of achievement in reading, writing, spelling, and arithmetic. Retesting showed that language rehabilitation led to a mean gain of better than five school grades, the greatest gain being made in reading, followed by arithmetic, writing, and spelling. Speech improvement amounted to two steps on a five-point scale used by clinicians in judging speaking performance. The mean grade level after training was more than one grade better in those whose treatment began during the first year post onset than in those whose treatment began after a full year had elapsed. The group taught by a single instructor and the group taught by a team of instructors made comparable gains in language; after training, a mean of only two tenths of a grade separated the attainments of the two groups, a nonsignificant difference.

Marks and co-workers (1957) reported on the changes in language function of 159 patients treated in a rehabilitation setting during a 3-year period. In 94 per cent of these patients "disease processes," mostly cerebrovascular accidents, were considered the primary cause of the aphasia; the rest of the cases were of traumatic etiology. The patients ranged in age from 3 to 80 years; 7 per cent were under 30 years old, 29 per cent were between 30 and 50 years old, and 64 per cent were over 50 years of age. Individual stimulation therapy was provided to these patients in highly variable amounts, ranging from only one session to more than 110 sessions and in duration from less than 1 month to more than 12 months; 48 per cent received therapy for no more than 2 months. Therapy was terminated "when it was considered that the patient had reached his maximum level of language functioning"; other causes of termination were "disinterest of the patient in continuing therapy" or inability to finance further treatment. Three speech pathologists judged improvement in language function using a four-point scale, with the following distribution of results: excellent, 7 per cent; good, 22 per cent; fair, 21 per cent; and poor, 50 per cent.

Although it is often quoted, a report by Godfrey and Douglass (1959) of the course of aphasia in patients provided group socialization opportunities can scarcely be considered a "study" of the effects of the *treatment* of aphasia. They describe a rehabilitation program carried on for 1 year, ultimately involving 38 patients with aphasia of vascular etiology ranging in age from 33 to 83 years (mean age, 68 years). Thirty-four of the patients had fairly recently become aphasic (mean time post onset, 3.5 weeks); the aphasia of the remaining four patients was of longer duration (8 months to 2 years). These patients were gathered into groups of no more than six and provided with socialization experiences described as follows: "The mechanics of speech retraining were not emphasized in this group rehabilitation program, . . . a typical physically oriented rehabilitation regimen . . . including physiotherapy, exercises, gymnasium, walking, and pool activities. Included, however, as a part of the day's rehabilitation activities were 'social-speech' group therapy sessions utilizing two occupational therapists who had only the most elementary knowledge of speech therapy techniques. Although these therapists offered so-called 'direct' language therapy, this of necessity was of a primitive nature owing not only to lack of specialized knowledge of the subject, but also to lack of technical aids in the way of equipment designed for language reeducation."

Patients were included in the program for periods of undesignated length. Language was reassessed every 3 months through the use of a "standard aphasia protocol," the scoring of which was done by group discussion of observations made by those working with the patients. It was reported that 37 per cent of the patients demonstrated "good results" (language ability and psychosocial adjustment improved); 42 per cent showed "fair results" (language showed no improvement but adjustment was better in several respects); and 21 per cent were unchanged both in language ability and psychosocial adjustment. "There were obvious signs of markedly reduced anxiety, lowering of defensive attitudes, less withdrawal from human relationships, and lifting of depression." Four of the patients with "long-standing aphasic conditions" made "fair" progress, comparable to that of patients with aphasia of more recent onset.

Schuell and associates (1964) presented information on 155 patients studied and treated at the Minneapolis Veterans Administration Hospital. They included the percentages of patients in each of five classifications who returned to gainful employment or to vocational training. Although it is impossible to recapture specific data from their report, one would conclude that a large number of patients were substantially helped by the rehabilitation program. Only in the case of their Group 4 and Group 5 patients, whose aphasia was most severe, was there no return to vocational training or employment on the part of the patients.

Beyn and Shokhor-Trotskaya (1966) reported the effect of one specific therapy program. They endeavored to "*prevent* the appearance of some of the speech defects of aphasic patients which up to now seemed to be inevitable," specifically "telegraphic style of responses." With 25 patients whose aphasia had resulted from cerebrovascular disease, they avoided teaching nominative words, teaching at first only simple words that can function as a sentence — words like "no," "there," "here," "give," "tomorrow," and "thanks." Only when words appeared spontaneously in a patient's speech were nouns introduced, and then never in the nominative case but only in one of the other five cases in the Russian language involving inflection. The investigators report that the results of the rehabilitation of active speech varied: 12 per cent attained a level of spontaneous conversation consisting of single-word responses; 42 per cent became able to speak in single sentences; 36 per cent became able to discourse more extensively, though "with elements of agrammatism." "But the most important fact is that telegraphic style, which is *inevitable* with other methods of rehabilitation, did not emerge in any of our patients." Sixty-four per cent showed some "incompleteness of utterances" and "pronounced agrammatism in the agreement of parts of the sentences;" the remaining 36 per cent displayed only "difficulties in the use of prepositions."

Leischner and Linck (1967) reported the results of treatment of two groups of aphasic patients. One was a group of 46 patients originally described in 1960 by Leischner; they ranged in age from 14 to 62 years. Of these cases of aphasia 17 were of traumatic, 25 of vascular, three of neoplastic, and one of infectious etiology. A second group of 70 patients ranged in age from roughly 20 to 70 years (mean age, 46.1 years); ten cases were of traumatic, 53 of vascular, and six of neoplastic etiology, and one was a case of early childhood brain damage. Both individual and group treatment were provided (duration of therapy not reported), geared to the individual needs of the patients, supplemented with activities other than language-centered. A six-point scale was used to judge the outcome of therapy: linguistic recovery (best results), 2 per cent; practical recovery (speech improved to a point sufficient for daily use), 9 per cent; pronounced improvement, 45 per cent; moderate improvement, 29 per cent; slight but noticeable improvement, 11 per cent; no improvement or worsening, 5 per cent. The level of practical recovery was achieved only by patients who began treatment not later than half a year post onset; patients treated after 3 years or more post onset, on the other hand, attained only moderate to slight improvement.

Sands and co-workers (1969) reported on the results of treatment of 30 patients, with a median age of 56.5 years, who had had a cerebrovascular accident. These patients received therapy daily for periods ranging widely from 2 weeks to 32 months, the median duration of therapy being 7.5 months. Therapy was initiated between 2 weeks and 48 months post onset. The Functional Communication Profile (FCP) was used to measure status initially, at the conclusion of treatment, and on subsequent follow-up (median, 13 months later). Twenty-seven patients showed measured improvement while three remained the same or regressed. "The median overall gain in language function for the whole group as measured by the FCP was ten percentage points. In the interval between the discharge from treatment and reevaluation, the group gained an average of five per cent. Thus, from the time of beginning treatment to the follow-up reevaluation, there was a gain of 15 per cent, modest, but surely significant. Examining the upper and lower sixth of the total group, we find that those who improved most achieved an average gain of 36 per cent, whereas those who experienced the least change gained an average of four per cent on the FCP."

Sarno and associates (1970) reported the results of treatment of 31 stroke patients, all described as having a severe expressive-receptive aphasia. They ranged in age from 46 to 83 years old. The period post onset before treatment began ranged from 3 to 144 months. "Severe aphasia was operationally defined as an Overall Functional Communication Profile score of below 31 per cent." At the outset, these patients had essentially no speech and little understanding of it; some were able to say a few words and understand some simple commands. They were assigned to one of three treatment groups: programmed instruction, nonprogrammed instruction, and no treatment. The groups were comparable with respect to age, sex distribution, and education, less comparable with regard to duration of symptoms (median, 19.5, 18, and 45 months, respectively). The treated patients were given 13 to 91 half-hour sessions (mean, 56) over a period of 3 to 36 weeks (mean, 17). A battery of 10 tests of terminal language behaviors toward which both programmed and nonprogrammed instruction were directed was administered before treatment, at termination of treatment, and 1 month later. Test results revealed no significant differences among the three treatment conditions. The investigators concluded:

> Results strongly suggest that current speech therapy does not modify verbal behavior in this population. . . . Although gains were small and similar for all groups, many of the study patients showed at least minimal gains. What is surprising is that this was true for the untreated patients as well. . . . The fact that speech therapy, of either type, did not affect language recovery in this study is no doubt related to the severity of their aphasia.

Perry (1972) used an experimental design that permits comparison of the relative effects of spontaneous recovery and formal language training on the language performance of adult aphasic patients without using an untreated control group. The design compares the rate of improvement shown by treated patients with an empirically validated theoretic rate associated with spontaneous recovery. As reported in Chapter 3, Culton (1969) plotted successive test score levels over a 2-month period for a group of recently aphasic patients without therapy. He showed *decreasing* difference scores from one test date to another. Perry reasoned that if one could show that language therapy resulted in *equal* or *increasing* difference scores over two or more successive therapy periods, the null hypothesis of no effect produced by language therapy on aphasic language performance could be reject-ed. He tested the null hypothesis by comparing difference scores on the Peabody Picture Vocabulary Test for successive treatment periods, usually 20 to 30 days each, during which therapy was administered at least three times a week. Of the 50 patients at the Cleveland Veterans Administration Hospital who participated, more than half displayed patterns of successive difference scores that led to rejection of the null hypothesis. Perry concluded that there was reason to believe that language training had a unique influence on the spoken language comprehension of the patients beyond that which could be attributed to spontaneous recovery.

Messerli and co-workers (1976) reported a study not dealing specifically with the effects of language therapy for aphasia but investigating the relationship between certain prognostic factors and improvement shown in speech therapy. The report concerned only aphasic patients "who have *benefited* from speech therapy or those who have been subjected to neuro-psychological treatment" at the University Neurological Clinic in Geneva, Switzerland. Data are pre-sented on 53 subjects ranging in age from 17 to 74 years; aphasia was due to vascular accident in 36, subdural hematoma or aneurysm in ten, and trauma in seven. The length of time the patients spent in speech therapy, the levels of communication they had attained at the conclu-sion of therapy, and the amount of their recovery (differences between initial and posttreatment language status, measured in a manner not described) were related to type of aphasia, severity of aphasia, exis-tence of apraxias, age, socio-professional level, and intellectual level. A significant relationship was found between the severity of the aphasia and the level of communication ultimately attained. "The severity of aphasia influences to a large extent the amount of residual disorders of language. The severe aphasic patients rarely recover their previous verbal capacities completely, even though it is among these patients that we find the longest periods of therapy." Another significant relationship was found between the severity of aphasia and the duration of therapy, which the investigators state indicated simply that therapy had been continued until no further progress could be expect-ed. Type and severity of aphasia were significantly related, and both were significantly related to the level of communication ultimately attained. Detailed analysis of the results led the investigators to conclude that "among all aphasic patients of equal severity, Broca's aphasics and Wernicke's mixed aphasics [both phonemic and semantic problems] have a greater probability to attain a relatively good level of communication at the end of the period" than globally aphasic patients, Wernicke's aphasic patients with predominantly phonemic disorders, and Wernicke's aphasic patients with predominantly semantic disorders. "Nevertheless, all types of aphasics are able to recover, at least to some degree." "We can conclude from all of our work that the clinical picture with the most favourable prognosis is the following: a not too severe Broca's or mixed Wernicke's aphasic without apraxia but with a good operational intelligence level." "The age of our patients. . .has nothing to do (contrary to what we would have thought) with the severity of aphasia, the judged importance of recovery [in terms of degree of recovery from initial status], the level attained at the end of the therapy period, or the duration of therapy."

Broida (1977) reported the results of intensive work with 14 aphasic patients long post onset, all with aphasia of vascular etiology (one cerebral hemorrhage, 13 thrombotic cerebrovascular accidents), ranging in age from 43 to 79 years (mean, 55 years). The Porch Index of Communicative Ability (PICA) was administered before therapy began and readministered every 2 months. Individual 50-minute therapy sessions were provided from three to five times a week over periods ranging from 2 to 21 months (mean treatment time, 9 months). At the conclusion of treatment, all subjects had improved on some measures, and 11 made notable improvement on all aspects measured (PICA overall score and three modality scores). Whereas only 43 per cent of the group earned a PICA overall score above the 60th percentile at the beginning, 89 per cent scored above the 60th percentile at the conclusion of treatment. In the group were four patients who had earlier had treatment which was interrupted for from 6 to 18 months; when their treatment was resumed, all improved significantly on several measures. The effect of spontaneous recovery for all 14 patients was obviated since all were between 1 and 6 years post onset. The investigator concluded: "The results of this study support the contention that language therapy can be effective in improving the communicative abilities of some aphasic patients, even if they are from 1 to 6 years post onset."

A carefully designed study of the effect of two types of treatment has been reported by Wertz and co-workers (1978). The patient groups in this study were defined in careful detail: all patients were 4 weeks post onset; had had one left hemisphere embolic or thrombotic episode; were between 40 and 80 years of age; were male; were natively English speaking; had no worse than 20/100 vision; had hearing no poorer than 45 dB SRT in the poorer ear; and scored between the 15th and 75th percentiles on the PICA. These Veterans Administration investigators reported on four cohorts of patients: 11 weeks (N = 58), 22 weeks (N = 45), 33 weeks (N = 39), and 44 weeks (N = 34). Patients were evaluated every 11 weeks by means of a neurologic examination; screening of auditory, visual, and tactile acuity; administration of the PICA, the Token Test, a word fluency measure, and the Ravens Colored Progressive Matrices; a motor speech evaluation; a rating of conversational ability; and a rating by some family informant of the patient's functional language use.

Patients were divided into two treatment groups. Both received 4 hours a week of prescribed therapy, with 4 additional hours of supplementary activity. One group received intensive traditional individual, stimulus-response aphasia therapy; the other received nonspecific socialization in small-group activities (discussion, role-playing, guest speakers and discussions, hobby activities, excursions, puzzles). Results indicated that both groups improved significantly on several measures, especially during the early weeks of treatment but continuing beyond the 6 months which some have considered to be the limit of spontaneous recovery. Few significant differences were found between individual and group treatments; those that did occur, all confined to performance on the PICA, favored individual treatment.

David and colleagues (1979) have reported a feasibility trial of a larger study of the efficacy of aphasia therapy in progress. They reported observations made of two groups of aphasic patients all with aphasia of vascular etiology, ranging in age from 51 to 80 years, none of whom had had previous treatment for their aphasia. Treatment was started from 3 to 30 weeks post onset. A group of seven patients received 40 hours of "conventional individual therapy from a speech therapist" during a period of 12 weeks, "unless they recovered in that time, in which case treatment was discontinued." Members of a second group of six patients each received 40 hours of stimulation during a 12-week period from a volunteer; the volunteers were given no training, but were simply "asked to encourage their patients to communicate." (There is regrettably no way to determine how structured and language-centered the "encouragement" was that the volunteers provided.) The Functional Communication Profile (FCP) was used to plot changes in language function over a 52-week period following initial assessment. Results indicated that the two groups were comparable in the shape of their recovery curves; a plot of results obtained with the Minnesota Test for Differential Diagnosis of Aphasia (MTDDA) was similar. "Almost all the recovery appeared to have taken place in the first month of treatment, irrespective of the length of time between onset and initial assessment. . . . It was interesting that the first month of treatment was crucial even for those patients with long-standing dysphasia, and the rapid improvement during this period could not, therefore, be assigned to spontaneous recovery." Although the difference between the two treatment groups was not judged to be significant, the patients who received conventional aphasia therapy performed on the FCP at a higher level than those who received stimulation from volunteers.

Studies of More Limited Scope

The studies cited have reported in most cases the results of comprehensive multimodality treatment programs on the full spectrum of language functions of groups of aphasic patients. Many other studies can be mentioned that have investigated either the effects of multimodality treatment on some specific input or output function, or the effects of therapy techniques confined to specific modes of input or output in modifying some selected language behavior(s). The scope of generalization possible from such studies is more limited, but they can provide specificity in witnessing to the power of treatment regimens described. A sampling of four such studies will be presented.

Improvement in auditory comprehension of words as a result of aphasia treatment was studied by Schuell and associates (1961). Their group of 48 aphasic patients had a mean age of 47 years; in etiology, 36 cases were vascular, six traumatic, three infectious, two neoplastic, and one undetermined. The Ammons Full-Range Picture Vocabulary Test, Form A, was administered twice, once before treatment and again after treatment. Treatment was the intensive stimulation therapy described by Schuell and co-workers (1964), the range of treatment times extending from 1 to 12 months (mean, $3\frac{1}{2}$ months). Of a total of 83 words tested, the initial mean number of errors for the group was 29.58, and the final mean number of errors was 21.81, a significant difference. Forty-one of the patients improved, five became worse, and two did not change. The investigators concluded, "Comprehension of words tends to improve during the course of treatment . . . in an orderly and predictable manner."

The effect of language stimulation on the ability to evoke specific words was tested by Weigel-Crump and Koenigsknecht (1973). Four adult aphasic patients with "predominant word retrieval deficits characterizing amnesic aphasia," all of them at least 3 months post onset, all of whom had had a minimum of previous treatment, were given an intensive stimulation program of the type described by Schuell (1964). A pool of 150 frequently occurring picturable words was selected for study; after initial testing with these words, examples from each subject's errors were selected randomly either to be drilled on or not to be drilled on. Eighteen 1-hour therapy sessions were held, two or three a week. During these sessions, the words selected for drill were presented ten times in isolation, then in five simple sentences, and then ten more times in isolation. The sentences used in the word presentations were short, and they were presented at a slow rate. Following such stimulation, the patients were asked to say the words in response to the pictures; facilitatory techniques were used to elicit the words, including gestures, associated words, synonyms, carrier phrases, and prompting initial phonemes or syllables. At six-session intervals the subjects were tested with 40 items, 20 of which had been drilled on, 20 of which had not been. After six sessions, the patients' naming scores rose from 0 to 61 per cent correct; after six more sessions they rose to 74 per cent correct; after all 18 sessions scores had risen to 84 per cent correct; the latencies of response were also decreased. The mean latency of response for drilled items dropped from 24.4 seconds in the pretreatment testing to 3.3 seconds following 18 therapy sessions; the mean latency of response for nondrilled items decreased from 23.6 to 9.3 seconds during the same period. "The reduction of latency of response to drilled items is 25.8 per cent greater than the reduction in latency of response to nondrilled items, again pointing up the value of concentrated drill in reducing latency of response on word-retrieval tasks." A similar degree of improvement was evidenced in all five categories of words (clothes, household items, living things, action verbs, foods). "This equivalence of progress across superordinate categories reflects the rapid generalization of progress from categories drilled on in therapy to other categories, as was demonstrated by the generalization to the category receiving no treatment (foods) and indicated that the amnesic component is symptomatic of disturbance of lexical retrieval and does not represent an absolute loss of information from the lexical store."

The relative effects of treatment confined to the modality of writing versus multimodality language treatment were investigated by Schwartz and co-workers (1974). Two groups of aphasic male adults were matched on PICA scores (mean score of about 12), age (53 versus 52 years), education level (about 12 years), and months post onset of left cerebrovascular accidents (19 versus 21 months). The experimental group of eight subjects received 20 half-hour sessions of writing therapy (writing the alphabet from memory, writing the names of monosyllabic pictured objects, writing monosyllabic words to dictation, writing such words to dictation after each was said three times by a clinician, and writing monosyllabic words to dictation after each was put into a sentence by a clinician). The control group of six subjects received 20 sessions of multimodality language therapy related to word-level auditory comprehension, reading, naming, repeating, and writing the names of pictured objects. Subjects were retested on the PICA following treatment. Results indicated that the groups did not significantly differ on their post-treatment tests, although the 0.05 level of significance was approached. The experimental group that received writing therapy obtained a significantly greater degree of improvement from pretreatment to posttreatment tests than did the control group;

three lower-level subjects accounted for the significance of the difference of scores; the higher-level subjects did not make as great gains as the lower-level subjects.

Sparks and colleagues (1974) describe the results of a program of Melodic Intonation Therapy (MIT) with eight patients with severe (but not global) aphasia of vascular etiology. In all patients "verbal output was severely impaired, with better preservation of auditory comprehension and other language modalities"; all had had previous treatment, but no improvement in verbal output in any of the patients had occurred for at least 6 months.

All patients completed the MIT program of daily individual and group therapy (duration of program not specified). The nine-step graduated "program involves sung intonation of propositional sentences in such a way that the intoned pattern is similar to the natural prosodic pattern of the sentence when it is spoken." Pre- and post-MIT scores on the Boston Diagnostic Aphasia Examination showed significant gains on each of three verbal subtests: responsive naming, confrontation naming, and phrase length. "Recovery of some appropriate propositional language occurred for six of the eight patients as a result of Melodic Intonation Therapy."

STUDIES USING NO-TREATMENT CONTROL GROUPS

Studies that permit comparison between the results of the treatment of a group of aphasic subjects and the course of recovery in a comparable group of untreated subjects are difficult to plan and execute. And even though one might not be persuaded of the efficacy of treatment, concern arises about the ethics of deliberately excluding from treatment patients who might conceivably benefit from it. Eight studies which have used no-treatment control groups have been reported.

Eisenson (1949) briefly reported on what he called "a somewhat informal experiment" conducted at an Army hospital. He initiated treatment with (supposedly all) aphasic patients in the hospital, only to discover 8 months later 12 additional patients. They had been in the hospital for as long as the patients with whom the staff had been working, but their limited spontaneous language recovery compared unfavorably with the improvement shown by the patients who had been receiving training. "Many of the new group of patients presented evidence of psychological obstacles which had to be overcome before direct language training was possible. Several were convinced that their cases were hopeless and that language learning for them was an impossible task."

Smith (1972) reported on the progress made by a group of 80 treated aphasic patients ranging in age from 18 to 60 years (mean, 51.3

years). The 67 patients with aphasia of vascular etiology had been aphasic an average of 21.6 months (range, 3 to 114 months) prior to the initiation of treatment; the 13 patients with aphasia of traumatic etiology, an average of 26 months (range, 7 to 72 months). All 80 patients received no less than 5 hours of individual and group therapy of unspecified type daily for at least 5 weeks; the amount of therapy ranged from 125 to 1000 hours over a period ranging from 5 to 40 weeks. Therapy was administered by graduate students under the supervision of experienced clinicians. The language progress of the group was contrasted with that of a group of 15 patients who received no formal treatment: five because of poor health, dementia, or evidence of severe diffuse bilateral cerebral damage; ten because of various personal or financial reasons. They did not constitute what could be considered a matched control group because of higher mean age, lower mean education, and more severe impairment of language and non-language functions than the treated group.

The efficacy of intensive language therapy was reflected by a marked contrast between negligible changes in the mean language test scores of the untreated patients over a mean period of 22.6 months and marked improvement in all language functions of the 80 patients who received therapy, as measured by a series of objective tests, including the MTDDA. Among the treated patients, there was moderate or marked improvement in speech in 55 per cent, in comprehension in 67 per cent, in reading in 61 per cent, and in writing in 54 per cent. Some of the patients with very severe language impairment showed significant improvement after therapy.

Gloning and co-workers (1976) studied the language changes of 107 patients with aphasia of traumatic and vascular etiology who were examined, reexamined after 7 days, and again reexamined after approximately 18 months. Patients ranged in age from 2 to 78 years (mean age, 39 years). The relationship of each of 19 different factors to measured changes in language function was studied.

Some patients (number not designated) received no aphasia treatment because they lived where none was available or for "other bureaucratic reasons." The treated subjects (number not designated) received at least 6 months of therapy (intensity of treatment not stated).

At the conclusion of the study, two variables were found that had a significant positive influence upon improvement in language functions. One of these was treatment of the aphasia. Indeed, 46 of the total of 107 patients were reported to have recovered completely. "The usefulness of language therapy has been experimentally confirmed." The other variable found to be significantly related positively to outcome was improvement of aphasia within 1 week. Variables found to have a significant negative effect upon outcome were age (being 51 years old or older), "feeblemindedness before onset of illness," severe aphasia ("verbal communication between examiner and patient was completely lacking"), and severe dysarthria (patient anarthric or at least half of the utterances being unintelligible). Type of aphasia and duration of aphasia for 1 year or more prior to initial examination of the patient were found not to be significantly related (either positively or negatively) to outcome of language recovery.

Three studies of language change in treated and untreated aphasic patients have been reported by the personnel of the Milan Neurological Clinic. In all three, the control groups were chosen not by design but as the result of "unintentional selection due to extraneous factors"; personal, family, or transportation problems prevented certain patients from participating in a language rehabilitation program. In the first study, Vignolo (1964) studied a group of 69 patients, in all but a few of whom aphasia was of vascular etiology, representing a broad range of severity. All patients were tested twice with a "standard examination for aphasia" with a minimum time interval of 40 days between the first and the second examination. Twenty-seven patients received no treatment; the remaining 42 patients were treated with a minimum of 20 therapy sessions over not less than 40 days, with a frequency of at least one session per week. Difference scores (initial test versus final test) for the two groups were found not to be significantly different.

Appreciating the fact that some of the treated patients were probably not treated long enough, Vignolo further analyzed the results and concluded that patients who were treated for more than 6 months improved significantly more than patients treated for less than 6 months. The percentage of patients who improved decreased as the time interval from onset increased; the longer the delay in receiving treatment, the more prolonged the treatment needed. Improvement was less frequent in older than in younger patients; over 70 per cent of younger patients (under 40 years old) improved, whereas only 22 per cent of older patients (over 60 years old) improved. Those patients over 60 years old who improved began their aphasia treatment less than 2 months post onset. Vignolo found that the majority of treated subjects who were seen before 2 months had elapsed improved, but so did the majority of nontreated patients; subjects who came for help 2 or 3 months post onset did not improve unless they were treated; and subjects who came more than 6 months post onset did not improve unless they were treated for more than 6 months. Vignolo concluded that treatment has a beneficial effect provided it lasts for more than 6 months and, further, that during the period from 2 to 6 months post onset the potentiality for recovery can be significantly enhanced by formal treatment.

In a second study, Basso and co-workers (1975) reported on the change in language function in 185 aphasic patients described as having a mean age of 48 years, the etiology of aphasia being nonprogressive lesions (70 per cent cerebrovascular accidents). Ninety-one subjects received intensive treatment, three to four sessions per week for a period of more than 6 months; 94 patients were not treated. All patients were tested twice with the standard aphasia battery, once at some variable period post onset and a second time no less than 6 months later. Differences between initial and final tests for the two groups indicated that "language rehabilitation has a positive effect on the improvement of oral expression." Age, educational level, etiology of the aphasia, and clinical type of aphasia were found not to be related to the outcome, but, as in the former study, delay of initiation of treatment did have a significant negative effect on improvement; the incidence of improvement decreased significantly with increase of time post onset.

In the third study, Basso and colleagues (1979) investigated the influence of language rehabilitation on language skills in 162 aphasic patients who received intensive treatment, comparing the results of treatment with changes in language performance in 119 untreated aphasic patients. In the total group, the etiology of the aphasia in 85 per cent of the patients was vascular, in 11 per cent traumatic, in 3 per cent neoplastic (ablation of a benign tumor), and in 1 per cent other nonprogressive focal lesions. The interval between onset and first examination was less than 2 months in 137 cases, from 2 to 6 months in 86 cases, and more than 6 months in 58 cases. All patients were tested by means of the standard language examination employed in the two earlier studies. Patients were classified as fluent or nonfluent, and the severity of their defect in each of four language modalities (oral expression, auditory verbal comprehension, reading, and writing) was rated on a scale ranging from 0 (no communication) to 4 (very good communication). All patients were tested a second time after an interval of no less than 6 months. Only patients who received treatment for no less than 5 consecutive months and at a rate of at least three individual sessions per week were included in the treatment group; some of these had four sessions per week and a few as many as five. "In order to be considered improved in any given modality, patients had to progress at least two points on the second examination with respect to their score on the first examination. In clinical terms, this gain reflects a remarkable progress. . . . Patients who progressed zero or one point only were considered 'unchanged.' "

Statistical tests of the differences between the initial and final tests indicated that treatment significantly influenced language function; the investigators concluded: "The main finding of this study is the demonstration that formal language rehabilitation in aphasics does have a positive effect on the improvement of the ability to communicate through speaking, listening, writing, and reading, provided that it is carried out during at least 6 months and at a rate of no less than three individual sessions per week. The gains in these specific language modalities are significantly more frequent in treated than in nontreated patients." It was also found that time post onset has a significant negative effect; delay in initiating treatment resulted in significantly less improvement than when treatment was started early. Overall severity of aphasia was also found to be significantly related to outcome, those with severe aphasia showing less improvement than those with more mild aphasia. Type of aphasia was found not to have a significant effect upon outcome: "There is no evidence that, other things being equal, the outcome of global aphasics is worse than that of the severe Wernicke's aphasics, nor that Broca's aphasics improve less than the moderate forms of fluent aphasia. The fact that the influence of rehabilitation is not significantly different in the several groups indicates that all aphasics, if treated, increase their chances of improvement by about the same proportion, in comparison with their expected 'spontaneous improvement.' This means, on the one hand, that all types of aphasics are equally good candidates for treatment; but, on the other hand, it means that patients with severe and long-standing deficits on first examination are still those with the worst prognosis even among the treated group." Only a weak relationship between improvement and age of patients was found, too weak to be judged to interfere significantly with the effects of treatment. The investigators further indicated that their results can be generalized beyond simply the language tests used, for their tests measured symptoms of consequence to the patient in his personal and working life. The improvement measured in the study appears to reflect functional communication rather faithfully and tells us about their language recovery in real life.

Hagen (1973) made a deliberate selection of his control group of nontreated patients in a study conducted at a rehabilitation hospital (Rancho Los Amigos Hospital, Downey, California). He first established criteria for inclusion of aphasic subjects in his study: all were to be classified as Class III on the Minnesota Test for Differential Diagnosis of Aphasia (aphasia with sensorimotor impairment), with a single neurologic lesion that is embolic or thrombotic in origin, involving left middle cerebral artery only, originally right-handed, originally English speaking, without dysarthria, with no history of mental deterioration or psychiatric disturbance, at least 3 months post onset. The first 10 subjects who met these criteria were designated the treatment group, and the second 10 subjects who met the criteria were designated the untreated control group. (Hagen explains that there was a high patient-to-therapist ratio in the hospital at the time; patients were not arbitrarily denied therapy for the purposes of the investigation: "the use of a control group reflects the fact that at the time, we could treat a small number of patients and only conduct a diagnostic workup on the remainder.") His 20 subjects ranged in age from 49 to 57 years (mean age, 52.5 years.) For a period of 1 year the patients in the treatment group received aphasia therapy, whereas those in the no-treatment group received all hospital services except aphasia therapy. Those treated received 4 hours of individual therapy, 8 hours of group therapy, and 6 hours of programmed therapy (visual discrimination work, matching, reading, spelling) for a total of 18 hours of therapy weekly. The Minnesota Test for Differential Diagnosis of Aphasia was administered to both groups four times: at 3 months post onset, 6 months post onset (after physical rehabilitation had been accomplished and when aphasia therapy was to be instituted), 12 months post onset, and 18 months post onset. Scores on the various parts of the MTDDA were translated into severity scores ranging from 0 (no impairment) to 3.5 (extremely severe impairment). The two groups were comparable on the various language measures on hospital admission and at the beginning of therapy.

Hagen found that spontaneous recovery accounted for slight changes in all communicative processes during the first 6 months post onset. During the year that followed, the two groups did not show significant differences in their gains in auditory comprehension, auditory retention span, visual comprehension (matching forms, letters, and words to pictures), and visual motor abilities (writing). However, significantly greater improvement was shown by the treated than by the untreated group in reading comprehension, language formulation, speech production, spelling, and arithmetic. Improvement in these areas was shown to be a function of treatment, not of the passage of time. Hagen concluded, "For this type of patient, recovery of communication abilities is a function of therapy rather than spontaneous recovery."

Deal and Deal (1978) studied four groups of patients (ages not reported) with aphasia of vascular etiology who received treatment, comparing them with one group who received no treatment. The four treatment groups were divided as follows: Group 1: 17 patients, therapy initiated during the first month post onset; Group 2: 9 patients, therapy initiated during the second month post onset; Group 3: 9 patients, therapy initiated during the third month post onset; and Group 4: 10 patients, therapy initiated during the fourth to seventh months post onset. All 45 patients in the four groups had 24 therapy sessions over a 2-month interval, averaging three sessions per week. The 10 members of the untreated control group (Group 5) were evaluated during the first month post onset but were discharged without treatment to a facility or to their home, where no treatment was available. The initial language status and language changes were measured with the PICA administered initially and 12 months post onset.

Results indicated that although all five groups initially had comparable performance levels (there were no significant differences among the five initial PICAs), and in all five groups the final PICA scores were significantly higher than the initial PICA scores, within-group change scores were quite different. The differences between the change scores of Group 1 and Groups 4 and 5, those between Group 2 and Groups 4 and 5, and those between Group 3 and Groups 4 and 5 were all significant, but the differences between the change scores of Group 4 and those of Group 5 were not. To the question as to whether treated patients improved more than untreated, the answer that emerged was positive, if patients are treated early. Patients treated during the first 3 months post onset changed significantly more than those treated later and those untreated. The late treatment group was not different in its gains from the untreated group. Furthermore, achievement of a level of so-called "functional" communication (defined as achieving an overall PICA score at the 50th percentile or higher) was found to be more likely if treatment was started early than if it was started later or not at all. Age was not found to be a significant factor in the occurrence of change; there was no correlation between age and amount of change, and dividing the patients into groups under 55 years old and over 55 produced no significant differences between the two.

Finally, a study using a somewhat different kind of control group has been reported by Holland (1980). In connection with her development of the measure of functional communication entitled Communicative Ability in Daily Living (CADL), she administered 68 test items twice to 28 aphasic patients, the times between administrations ranging from 8 to 15 months. Seventeen of the patients showed improved scores, eight scored lower on the second test, and three remained the same. Analysis of the characteristics of the "improvers" and the "non-improvers" failed to show that age, months post onset, type of aphasia, severity of aphasia, or institutionalization accounted for the improvement; almost accidentally it was learned that certain of those who had improved had continued in therapy for at least 6 months. Further investigation revealed that of the 28 patients involved, 15 had not continued in therapy for at least 6 months in the interim between tests, whereas 13 had. Twelve of these 13 were among the 17 "improvers." These patients could appropriately be called "chronic" aphasia patients, all being at least 1 year post onset; they were provided a variety of treatments rather than any particular type of treatment; and they represented a range of severity and "types" of aphasia. Whatever the possible reasons why therapy was discontinued with 15 of the patients, it appeared that a high percentage of the 13 who continued in therapy showed greater improvement than the rest in terms of more language output and more efficiency in producing that output.

INDIVIDUAL CASE STUDIES

Useful data bearing on the issue of the effect of treatment can be derived from single-case studies and reports. Studies of groups of subjects are generally considered preferable since they allow generalization to the population from which they are drawn, permit the control of certain variables, and allow evaluation of the reliability of results. However, group studies involve the assumption that the subjects are similar and respond in a similar manner to the experimental condition being studied, but this assumption may not be appropriate. Furthermore, group studies allow generalization to the "typical" behavior of the mean or median group member, an entity that may not correspond to any individual member of the group. Therefore, group studies often have limited applicability to individual clinical cases. Individual case studies obviously permit more limited generalization, but generalization is possible if the subject being studied is described completely, clearly, and longitudinally, providing the opportunity for replication, which allows a demonstration of generalization across subjects and across behaviors. The picture of "typical" behavior derived from a single case study relates to a given, living individual and can allow generalization to the population from which the subject was drawn. Single-case studies provide useful information about what procedures work in treatment, how well, over what period of time, with what kinds of patients. Single-subject time series (subject-as-his-own-control) studies provide information about the results of treatment on specific tasks, including baseline, status after stopping therapy, status after resuming therapy, and task performance in contrast to tasks not treated.

Weisenburg and McBride (1935) present detailed information about one of their patients, "the most satisfactory case for the purpose of a controlled study of the effect of reeducation." This 45 year old patient with six grades of schooling suffered an embolism of the left middle cerebral artery with a residual aphasia described as "a case of predominantly expressive disorder with marked difficulty in articulation and word-formation and a tendency to leave out the less important words in speaking and in writing."

Detailed examination of the patient 2 weeks post onset revealed a severe disorder of the type that we would designate an apraxia of speech. In addition, her writing was "disturbed by spelling errors, abbreviated structure, and some serious confusions." Her understanding of spoken language "was fairly satisfactory in ordinary conversation. At the same time, she often failed to grasp more complex questions and her execution of twofold or threefold commands was poor." Her comprehension of reading was "to be classed among the poorest of the performances of literate normal subjects." In writing, the patient formed letters poorly, "sometimes actually misformed them," reversed letters, omitted letters, and used an abbreviated form of expression.

The patient returned home and for the next 7 months had no treatment for her aphasia. "Seven months after her discharge, the patient sent for the examiner through the Social Service Department of the University Hospital, and asked to be taught to speak better. She was discouraged and depressed because she did not think she had made any progress since leaving the hospital. . . . She was anxious for further training." Reexamination revealed that she could now speak somewhat more easily and attempted to speak more, but the clarity of her rapid speech showed little improvement. Her understanding of spoken language had improved considerably: "She no longer made errors in following two- or threefold directions. She had no difficulty understanding conversation, even when several people were talking with her. Her only limitations now appeared in grasping complex statements such as those of the Absurdities Test." Her reading comprehension was somewhat improved but still defective. She was now writing with her left hand, still making letter and spelling errors, and producing simplified and abbreviated sentences.

A treatment program was instituted immediately (7 months post onset). The treatment program provided was meager, only 1 or 2 hours a week. This was supplemented by assigned homework performed faithfully, including copying of sentences, saying sentences aloud, practicing the production of polysyllabic words, reading newspaper reports or magazine articles and writing accounts of what she had read, and writing or telling about what she heard on the radio or had been doing. Treatment continued for 17 months.

Considerable progress was reported in the patient's language functions as a result of this program. Her articulation improved considerably; she learned to slow down her speech so that it was more intelligible. "The structure of both spoken and written expression is far more complete and the vocabulary more extensive." Data on a wide range of language tests were presented graphically, representing status 2 weeks post onset, 7 months post onset, 13 months post onset, and 19 months post onset. "There was great improvement in the first 6 months of training in reading comprehension, oral spelling, arithmetic, the performances required by the Sentence Completion and the Absurdities Test, and in vocabulary. As was to be expected, with the more satisfactory speech production, the quality and speed of oral reading also improved, but the extent of the improvement does not show in the graph because the patient's performance was still far below the normal range. In the next 6 months of training, although the progress in speaking continued, there was much less change in other performances. . . . The only marked improvement during the second 6 months, aside from that in spontaneous speaking and writing, was in oral reading and reading comprehension. This condition was interesting, for these were performances which were being trained."

Weisenburg and McBride present more sketchy information about the effects of treatment of other individual patients. Another of their patients, a professor of Romance languages, began treatment 2 months post onset, receiving 3 hours per week of treatment for a period of 9 months. "Since he was not examined immediately after the attack, there is no means of estimating his improvement in the first 2 months. His family's reports indicate that there had been progress, and psychological examinations made in the fifth and ninth months after the attack show that the progress continued. The question as to how much of this progress resulted from the training cannot be answered definitely, but there is this significant fact: a comparison of the patient's condition just after the onset with the findings of the first psychological examination [done 3 months post onset] indicates less change than that which was manifested between the first and second examinations [second examination, fifth month post onset]. In other words, it seems that the rate of improvement increased around the third and fourth months, a condition which is undoubtedly to be attributed to the training." Then improvement slowed down, in spite of treatment, but was still apparent on examination about a year post onset. Greatest improvement occurred in those areas of language performance in which treatment was administered. "However, . . . there was some improvement in almost all performances."

The investigators present evidence on a few other cases and then conclude: "The evidence in all the cases . . . goes to show that speech can be improved by training, both in respect to articulation and in the more complex processes of language expression."

The differential effects of two treatment procedures upon a selected language performance (naming) in a single patient were described by Helmick and Wipplinger (1975). Following a stroke, their 54 year old patient presented a mild aphasia with primary deficit in naming skills and less impairment in auditory and visual comprehension skills. From among the words that he was unable to name on the Peabody Picture Vocabulary Test, three groups of 15 words were selected: 15 for a maximum stimulation, 15 for a minimum stimulation, and 15 for a nontreatment condition. Starting 8 weeks post onset, therapy was conducted for four weeks. On odd-numbered days the patient was presented with 24 stimulations of each of the 15 words, the stimulations involving several different types of activities, including identification, contextual cuing, differentiation, tracing, and copying. On even-numbered days, the patient was presented with only six stimulations of the second group of 15 words. After 4 weeks of such stimulation, it was found that correct naming was greater for both the maximum and minimum stimulation condition words than it was for the nontreatment condition words. The number of correct naming responses was essentially the same for the two treatment conditions, at the beginning of therapy and throughout the therapy period. The fact that the patient improved in naming the 15 words not used in treatment indicated generalization from words stimulated to words not stimulated. The investigators concluded that large amounts of stimulus repetition do not enhance naming skills more than small amounts, but the application of a systematic stimulation program of either kind enhances naming skills.

Concentration on Auditory Comprehension

Kushner (1975) and Kushner and Winitz (1977) have reported on the effect of extended practice in listening comprehension on language functions in a single case. The patient, a 47 year old male with a traumatically incurred aphasia, was tested 1 month post onset and at monthly intervals during a 4-month period during which treatment was provided. Treatment was confined to programmed practice in the comprehension of single words, using the comprehension approach to the learning of foreign languages developed by Winitz and Reeds (1975). At the beginning of treatment, the patient scored overall at the 24th percentile on the PICA, indicating marked impairment in communication. He scored only 10 words correct on the Peabody Picture Vocabulary Test; performed only 12 items correctly on the Token Test; scored 67 per cent on the Discrimination Between Paired Words subtest of the MTDDA; and got only 40 per cent of the items correct on the Auditory Comprehension Test, which measures comprehension of sentences presented orally. His verbal production was characterized by both intelligible and unintelligible perseverations, difficulty in imitating words, difficulty in verbalizing names of objects and people, and numerous refusals to engage in verbal output tasks. He was able to name none of the 19 items used in the training program.

The patient was treated for 1 month, beginning 1 month post onset. A no-treatment period occurred at 2 months post onset when he left the hospital. He returned at 3 months post onset and treatment was conducted until 4 months post onset.

Over a period of 5 months, the patient showed steady improvement in listening comprehension. Although oral production of the words being worked on in listening comprehension training was never practiced, after 11 sessions the patient correctly produced 63 per cent of the words. There was a drop in performance to 42 per cent following the no-treatment period, but at the conclusion of training he was able to produce all 19 items correctly; this performance was maintained during subsequent periods of no treatment. The patient advanced to an overall PICA percentile of 72 per cent; to a 100 per cent correct score on the Discrimination Between Paired Words subtest; to a score of 98 correct on the Peabody Picture Vocabulary Test; to 71 per cent correct on the Auditory Comprehension Test, and to a score of 31 of 61 items correct on the Token Test. "Of particular interest is the fact that on the three comprehension tests (Peabody, Auditory Comprehension Test, Token Test), the patient continued to improve during the no-treatment periods. This finding suggests that training in the comprehension of specific single lexical items generalized to the comprehension of other words and to complex structures as well. Although no formal assessment was made, it was observed that at the end of treatment the patient, on occasion, spontaneously produced short sentences. However, word recall was still impaired."

Wertz (1978) reviews the case of a 56-year-old man who suffered a left hemisphere subdural hematoma from a fall; the hematoma was not evacuated. After 1 month in the hospital he returned home for 5 months, after which time his language performance was evaluated and treatment instituted. "Speech and language evaluation results indicated marked aphasia in all communicative modalities, including auditory comprehension, reading, speaking, and writing deficits. . . . PICA performance was at the 32nd percentile, overall. . . . His functional language was fluent but contained essentially no nouns and only a few verbs. . . .He gave a total of seven correct answers on the 61-item Token Test, produced no words on the Word Fluency Measure." By the time therapy was instituted, his overall performance had advanced to the 37th percentile on the PICA.

The treatment program consisted of speech and language therapy, 4 hours a day, 5 days a week, 1 hour of physical therapy, and evening assignments using the Language Master along with written work. After 1 month of therapy he returned home for 1 month. Although his PICA overall performance at that time was at the 45th percentile, no overt changes were seen on the other measures. The patient believe he had improved during the month's treatment, but he continued to feel that he "didn't know nothin'." He was given a home program that included reading and writing exercises and verbal practice using the Language Master.

He returned for an additional month of in-patient therapy, his PICA overall performance at the time being at the 50th percentile; his Word Fluency Measure performance showed four words produced compared with zero on previous tests; his Token Test performance had improved to 16 correct items. At the conclusion of the second month's treatment, his overall PICA score was at the 60th percentile. His performances on the Boston Diagnostic Aphasia Examination and the MTDDA had improved. His Word Fluency Measure performance now showed eight words produced; his Token Test total was 13. When he was discharged with a new home program, he reported, "Now, I know something." The review of his progress indicated that the patient's performance improved most on those aspects that had been treated or that had been focused on in treatment. Graphic presentations of PICA performance showed gains in auditory comprehension, reading comprehension, speaking ability, and writing.

Base-10 Measurement of Gains

In connection with his presentation of the Base-10 programmed stimulation approach to aphasia therapy, LaPointe (1978) presents illustrative information about several individual cases. The procedure suggested by LaPointe involves selection of a specific task, measurement of baseline behavior, defining an acceptable criterion level of performance, specifying 10 stimulus items to be used in repeated evaluation, and graphic display of performance levels on these items in terms of percentage over 10 sessions. The patient's base rate performance is measured pretreatment, therapy judged to be relevant to the specific task is designed and carried out, and the 10-item probe is administered at the conclusion of work on that task during each session. The PICA multidimensional scoring system or any other quantitative system can be used.

One patient described by LaPointe was a 28 year old man with war-incurred traumatic aphasia. Fourteen months post onset his language impairment was mild (PICA overall score at the 86th percentile) and included difficulty in spelling verbs during writing and impairment in retrieving and producing connective and functional words. Therapy devoted to improving his writing of verbs to dictation was successful, as shown by the fact that on the Base-10 record he reached the criterion (100 per cent) performance in five sessions. Another plot indicated that on the task of generating and uttering sentences using selected prepositions, he reached criterion level after eight sessions of therapy. Retested 6 weeks later, he performed on this task at the 90 per cent level.

A second, 61 year old patient displayed a moderate to severe aphasia (PICA overall 47th percentile) of thromboembolic etiology, incurred 6 years before treatment. On a task requiring oral reading of printed commands without omitting, adding, or substituting words, baseline performance was 47 per cent. Therapy consisted of isolating the error words in each sentence and repeating them five times with the clinician, saying the complete sentence after the clinician, and then rereading the sentence without being prompted. Criterion performance level (100 per cent) was reached after eight sessions. After 5 months the patient was retested; he had maintained performance on the task at the 90 per cent level. Two months later his performance was at the 80 per cent level. "Since it had been approximately 6 years since the onset of this patient's illness, it is reasonable to assume that his progress was not the result of spontaneous recovery. Further, since he demonstrated no progress on several very similar language tasks, on which performance was measured over the same time span but without a concentrated effort to correct error performance, this progress probably did not reflect ... improvement merely because the patient received the attention of a clinician." On another task requiring spoken sentence responses to a series of questions, baseline performance was 59 per cent. Following therapy consisting of verbal reinforcement of complete sentence responses with neutral or no response from the clinician when sentences were incomplete, the patient achieved criterion level after seven sessions. When he was retested 5 and then 10 months later, his performance had decreased to 73 per cent and 87 per cent, respectively.

Recovery in Bilingual Patients

Watamori and Sasanuma (1976, 1978) have reported on the effect of language treatment on the relative degree of recovery of function in two languages in two bilingual aphasic patients. The first patient, a 65-year-old, university-educated Japanese-American brought up in a bilingual environment, was equally proficient in English and Japanese. He became aphasic as a result of cerebral thrombosis and was diagnosed 2 months post onset as having severe Broca's aphasia with oral and verbal apraxias. Initial evaluation using parallel English and Japanese subtests from the MTDDA indicated that the patterns of impairment in English and Japanese were almost equal in all language modalities, with English slightly less impaired. The patient early felt that he could not improve in Japanese, so treatment thereafter was conducted exclusively in English. One-hour therapy sessions in English were given four times a week until 18 months post onset; then, because the patient exhibited increasing interest in the Japanese language, therapy was modified to incorporate Japanese as well as English. Beginning at 18 months post onset, language therapy in two languages was provided, each once a week until 30 months post onset. Therapy consisted of intensive multimodality stimulation of the type described by Schuell and co-workers (1964). Parallel tests in the two languages were administered at 14, 26, and 49 months post onset. Whereas initial tests revealed essentially identical patterns of impairment in the two languages, treatment in English for a year had produced a considerable gap between the patterns as well as in the degree of impairment between the two languages; improvement in English was clearly greater than that in Japanese across all modalities and particularly in writing, which apparently benefited most from therapy. The results of therapy in both languages between 18 and 26 months post onset indicated that the writing modality in Japanese had improved considerably; the gap between the two languages in the oral production modality did not narrow even after therapy in Japanese was initiated.

Therapy in English terminated at 30 months but was continued in Japanese twice weekly. Evaluation of language status in both languages at 49 months indicated that the degrees and patterns of impairment of the two languages had again become almost identical, with English still being somewhat less impaired than Japanese. Only negligible regression had occurred in English after 19 months of nontreatment.

The second patient, a 52-year-old Japanese, prior to a stroke spoke and understook both English and Japanese competently; although he had a functional knowledge of written Japanese, he wrote primarily in English. Initial evaluation 3 months post onset resulted in a diagnosis of severe Wernicke's aphasia. Parallel English and Japanese subtests from the MTDDA indicated that the degrees and patterns of impairment of the two languages were almost identical across all language modalities, with English slightly less impaired. Intensive stimulation therapy in English was provided for a period of 6 months, with two 1-hour sessions per week. Comparison of evaluations pre- and posttreatment indicated that the gap between the two languages had widened, English being more improved than Japanese; however, the patient's ability in Japanese had also improved slightly. Discrepancies between the two languages were most apparent in the reading and writing modalities.

Watamori and Sasanuma concluded that "systematic, controlled language therapy is one decisive variable affecting the relative degree of recovery in a bilingual aphasic's two languages. In either of the patients reported in this study, all the language modalities recovered, by and large, for the language under therapy. Improvement in the nontreated language, on the other hand, was confined to certain modalities predicted from the specific types of aphasia, and the amount of improvement even in these modalities tended to be less than that for the treated language." Auditory comprehension was the modality in which similar improvement was observed in the treated and the nontreated languages, regardless of type of aphasia. Writing ability seemed to improve as a function of language therapy in both languages. With regard to reading, while the Broca's aphasic patient showed a similar recovery rate for both the treated and the nontreated language, the Wernicke's aphasic patient showed a selective recovery only for the treated language. In the oral production modality, differential recovery patterns were observed between the two types of aphasias: the Wernicke's aphasic patient showed improvement not only in the treated but in the nontreated language as well, though to a lesser degree; the Broca's aphasic patient showed improvement only in the treated language until therapy in the other language was initiated.

Cases from the Milan Study

Following presentation of their group data concerning the effects of intensive treatment of 162 aphasic patients, Basso and colleagues (1979) supplement their findings as follows: "Further evidence of the effectiveness of rehabilitation is provided by the study of single cases, in whom treatment was initiated more than six months after onset . . . when spontaneous restitution had reached a plateau. In a sense, these patients serve as their own controls. It is difficult to attribute to chance the dramatic improvement of language (up to complete recovery in one case) that occurred following the prescribed period of formal treatment."

The first case reviewed is that of a 49 year old teacher with aphasia of vascular etiology. For 11 years following her stroke she received no language rehabilitation because it was unavailable where she lived. When she learned of the aphasia program in Milan, she moved there to participate. The language diagnosis arrived at was severe Broca's aphasia. Using the five-point scale described earlier in which 0 represents "no communication" and 4 represents "very good communication," the patient had an expression score of 0 and a comprehension score of 3; on the Token Test she got 18 of 39 right. Reading comprehension was reported to be good. She could not write, even her name. Language therapy was provided in five sessions per week for 8 months. On second examination, her oral expression, while still somewhat slow and paraphasic, was flawless so far as grammar and meaning were concerned; she was given an expression score of 3. Writing improved dramatically; she was able to write a letter consisting of seven well-constructed, meaningful sentences, although with some literal paraphasias, hesitations, and rewritings. Auditory-verbal comprehension had improved to a score of 4; she got 23 of 39 right on the Token Test. Reading comprehension was reported to be good. "In summary, this patient, while well integrated in a helpful and motivated family, was still a severe Broca's aphasic 11 years after her stroke. Eight months of systematic language retraining were sufficient to bring about a dramatic improvement."

The second case was that of a 17 year old boy with a traumatically incurred aphasia and right hemiparesis. Seven months later, his motor problem had subsided but his language difficulties remained quite severe. He did not seek language rehabilitation because he was employed and because he believed that his communication would improve spontaneously, as had the strength of the right arm and leg; language rehabilitation was not available in his hometown. When he found that spontaneous improvement was not occurring, he moved to Milan 26 months post onset. On first examination, he earned scores of 0 on both expression and writing. He earned a comprehension score of 4 (Token Test, 33 of 39 correct), and his reading comprehension was also good. The diagnosis was moderate fluent aphasia with prominent word-finding difficulties and severe agraphia. He was treated in three to four sessions per week and was judged to be recovered after 5 months; on examination at that time, he earned expression and writing scores of 4. "In summary, language in this patient progressed little if at all during the first 2 years and 2 months, although he was a young person, had resumed regular work, and had been leading a life that provided him with a variety of language stimuli. Intensive formal rehabilitation brought him to virtually complete recovery in 5 months."

The third case was a 60 year old nurse who following a stroke developed aphasia with conspicuous difficulties in reading and writing, right visual field defect, and hemiparesis. During the following 6 months she underwent intensive physical rehabilitation in her hometown but received no language therapy because it was unavailable. Seven and a half months post onset she moved to Milan to receive language therapy. On first examination her expression score was 0; writing was limited to her signature; comprehension score was 2, but on the Token Test she got only 11 of 39 right; reading was possible but so slow as to be nonfunctional. Diagnosis was fluent aphasia with marked anomia, agraphia, and alexia.

The patient underwent language rehabilitation for 6 months, three sessions per week. On final examination she earned expression and comprehension scores of 4 (Token Test, 21 of 39 right). "The most striking progress, however, concerned reading and writing, which were now virtually perfect, while the right visual field defect remained unchanged. . . . In summary, language in this patient was still severely defective seven and a half months after stroke, in spite of the fact that she had undergone continuing and intensive physical therapy, a type of activity that implies close personal contacts and much verbal stimulation. Progress was brought about only by formal language rehabilitation."

Personal Accounts

Detailed case reports are also available in biographic or autobiographic accounts of recovery from aphasia and the role of aphasia treatment in it. These present a broad spectrum of reactions to aphasia and efforts made to reduce it through language therapy.

In *Stroke: A Study of Recovery*, Douglas Ritchie (1961) recounts his slow recovery of language functions and the contributions made to it by the staff of a British medical rehabilitation center; his contempt for his initial speech therapist and her seemingly unorganized and inappropriate approach, as though to a child; his debt to his later speech therapist, Miss B., and some of her student therapists who "played a considerable part in my recovery. . . . Much as I used to grumble, inwardly and outwardly, I heeded her advice and usually profited by it. . . . Yet I hated those half-hour sessions. . . . Miss B.'s influence was not confined to speech, or language reeducation as one might better call it. Victims of aphasia did want to regain the power of language but, above that, nearly all of them unconsciously craved for some emotional balance of which they had been robbed by the stroke. Ability to help in this need was Miss B.'s real quality. . . . Miss B. summoned up an emotional equilibrium for me, and from then on she had a clear course with me."

In *Silent Victory*, Carmen McBride (1969) reveals the sorrow and frustrations experienced by her and her severely aphasic husband, whose impairment of language function was never significantly reduced by language treatment. She documents their development of "ability to communicate in other ways."

Barry Farrell's *Pat and Roald* (1969) recounts the incredibly intensive and pressure-filled program of language work which helped return the eminent actress Patricia Neal to professional work in cinema and television.

The psychologist C. Scott Moss tells his story in *Recovery With Aphasia: The Aftermath of My Stroke* (1972). A "high-level" aphasic patient, he describes his skepticism about language therapy and the challenge which he presented his clinicians, who were used to dealing with more severe problems and less daunting personalities and intellects. The speech pathologist in charge, Robert K. Simpson, summarizes the role of language treatment: "The goals of therapy were to obtain appropriate stimulation for Dr. Moss and to decrease his fears of venturing into his professional activities, which he had to reexplore. . . . The goal was to help Dr. Moss reach the point where he could assume the major responsibility for this therapy, in essence, to become his own clinician. . . . Therapy from my point of view has been successful. . . . The success is aptly demonstrated in part by his present social and professional activities, in part by his continued professional growth, and in part by his proposed book on his personal encounter with aphasia."

Helen Wulf in her personal narrative, *Aphasia, My World Alone* (1973), describes the supporting, galvanizing effect on her of her speech pathologist (Josephine Simonson) and the benefits that resulted from being instantly understood by that insightful person even without the vehicle of verbal communication. Her testimonies to the importance of language treatment are eloquent: "I have a sickish feeling that speech therapy, and everything it stands for, tends to be shoved aside as a minor key in rehabilitation. It should be the most important factor if the patient's needs are to be met intelligently." "My experience has been that the speech therapist was the only person . . . on whom I could pin my hope for understanding what made me tick. Patients quickly know that the speech therapist is someone to whom they can relate because he has already related to them; that they can count on his interest and his willingness and ability to accept them as part of the human race despite aphasia." "The teaching techniques of speech therapy I don't pretend to know anything about — what their results were are tangible. Speech therapy for me was effective in helping me regain the following facilities in communication: talking, reading, writing, arithmetic, thinking, post-stroke activities." "Bless all therapists whose forte is aphasia. . . . Theirs is a healing art used deftly with a disorder whose implications are only now beginning to be understood. . . . The interaction between a therapist and the aphasic is vital in the patient's success in areas where he wishes to achieve. The aphasic may never be able to make much progress in speaking, but a sanguine attitude toward the total picture means progress in his revival as an adjusted, functioning person — progress sparked and nurtured by the techniques and perception of the therapist."

ADDITIONAL TESTIMONY

Some aphasiologists, without providing complete documentation, have generalized from their experience in the rehabilitation of aphasic patients. Hillbom (1965) described the rehabilitation of brain-injured war veterans in Finland and stated, "Extremely good results were obtained in the treatment of aphasia, where training could in many cases be continued for several years."

Fenelon and co-workers (1969) described a program of aphasia treatment and stated, "There has been neither a sufficient follow-up period nor enough experience to indicate percentages of improvement or failure, but it seems that reeducation of the patient's speech helps his recovery, removes stumbling blocks, and makes a definite contribution to rehabilitation in aphasia."

The late eminent Russian neurophysiologist Luria devoted a major part of his book *Traumatic Aphasia* (1970) to the subject of rehabilitating patients with aphasia of traumatic etiology. He stated: "We have shown that in some, though by no means all, cases the function disturbed may be restored in its original form." "A consciously directed, systematic course of retraining is the only method of compensating for a defect arising from primary brain damage. By reorganizing the disturbed function, it is possible to restore activities which once appeared hopelessly lost."

CONCLUSIONS

No single study reviewed has proved to be so comprehensive and so creatively and rigorously designed and executed as to provide by itself the unequivocal answer to questions about the efficacy of aphasia treatment. But the foregoing collage of studies of groups and individuals collectively provides a series of answers and together lays our doubts about efficacy to rest. The studies are uneven in their scientific merit, and the generalizations that we can draw from each of them are limited. Nevertheless, in many of these studies are seen careful efforts to describe in detail the patients studied; to measure objectively and quantitatively their language status and changes in it over time or in connection with a course of treatment; to specify the nature of the therapy, its intensity, and its duration; and to tease out the influence of variables related to the observed outcomes.

The answers to our questions about the efficacy of aphasia treatment, as we had anticipated, are multiple. There is no single yes-or-no statement that can be offered without qualification. But the following statements are clearly supported by the data compiled during more than 60 years of research:

1. Language treatment leads to significant improvement in the majority of cases of aphasia. Percentages are sometimes reported of treated cases who improved significantly: 100 per cent (Frazier and Ingham, 1920); 33 per cent total or marked, 56 per cent partial (Isserlin, in Butfield and Zangwill, 1946); 81 per cent much improved or improved in speaking, 77 per cent in reading, 86 per cent in writing (Butfield and Zangwill, 1946); 86 per cent much improved or improved (Wepman, 1951); 29 per cent excellent or good, 21 per cent fair (Marks et al., 1957); 56 per cent practical recovery or pronounced improvement, 29 per cent moderate improvement (Leischner and Linck, 1967); and 55 per cent moderately or markedly improved in speech, 67 per cent in comprehension, 61 per cent in reading, 54 per cent in writing (Smith, 1972).

Other studies report significant gains in language functions as measured quantitatively by designated test instruments: on Progressive Achievement Tests (Wepman, 1951); on the Functional Communication Profile (Sands et al., 1969; David et al., 1979); on the Peabody Picture Vocabulary Test (Perry, 1972; Kushner and Winitz, 1977); on the Ammons Full-Range Picture Vocabulary Test (Schuell et al., 1961); on the PICA (Schwartz et al., 1974; Broida, 1977; Wertz et al., 1978; Deal and Deal, 1978; Wertz, 1978); on the MTDDA (Smith, 1972; Hagen, 1973; Kushner and Winitz, 1977; Wertz, 1978; Watamori and Sasanuma, 1976, 1978; David et al., 1979); on the Boston Diagnostic Aphasia Examination (Sparks et al., 1974; Wertz, 1978); on the Token Test (Kushner and Winitz, 1977); on the CADL (Holland, 1980); and on other standardized test batteries (Weisenburg and McBride, 1935; Vignolo, 1964; Basso et al., 1975, 1979.)

Significantly greater language gains using a variety of measures in groups of treated patients in contrast to untreated patients are reported by Eisenson (1949); Smith (1972); Hagen (1973); Gloning et al. (1976); Basso and co-workers (1975); Deal and Deal (1978); and Basso and associates (1979).

Data of these three types together strongly support the general conclusion that aphasia treatment helps the majority of patients.

2. Improvement in language functions is clearly attributable to treatment and cannot be assumed to be the result solely of spontaneous recovery. Significant language gains have been reported in groups of aphasic patients treated after intervals post onset that in almost all cases exceed the 6 months commonly (though probably overgenerously) defined as the period of spontaneous recovery: Butfield and Zangwill (1946), 6 months post onset; Wepman (1951), one group 6 months, one group at least 12 months post onset; Smith (1972), mean of over 22 months post onset (range, 3 to 114 months); Weigel-Crump and Koenigsknecht (1973), at least 3 months post onset; Hagen (1973), 6 months post onset; Schwartz and co-workers (1974), mean of 19 months post onset; Sparks and colleagues (1974), no improvement in prior therapy for at least 6 months; Broida (1977), between 1 and 6 years post onset; Wertz and associates (1978), treatment continuing with benefit beyond 6 months post onset; Holland (1980), at least 1 year post onset. Similar gains are reported in individual cases reported by Weisenburg and McBride (1935), 7 months post onset; Watamori and Sasanuma (1976, 1978), treatment continuing with benefit until 49 months and 9 months post onset, respectively; Wertz (1978), 6 months post onset; LaPointe (1978), 14 months and 6 years post onset; and Basso and co-workers (1979), 11 years, 26 months, and 7½ months post onset.

3. The restoring effect of treatment extends beyond content specifically used as stimulus material to linguistic units and modalities not so used. Generalization is found to occur with regard to lexical units not drilled on (Weigel-Crump and Koenigsknecht, 1973; Helmick and Wipplinger, 1975; Kushner and Winitz, 1977); to modalities not concentrated on in treatment (Weisenburg and McBride, 1935, Case 4; Schwartz et al., 1974; Sparks et al., 1974; Kushner and Winitz, 1977; Wertz, 1978); even to some degree to impairment in use of another language in which bilingual patients had been proficient but which was not simultaneously treated (Watamori and Sasanuma, 1976, 1978). It becomes apparent that treatment is not an "educational" process for reteaching "lost" bits of language (words, rules) via rote memorization but a stimulating, reintegrating process that facilitates retrieval of temporarily unavailable language still in storage.

4. Gains in language function are enduring, for the most part irreversible. Continuing improved performance beyond the period of active treatment has been implied in the reports of most of the investigators quoted and has been specifically reported by Schuell and co-workers (1964); Sands and associates (1969); LaPointe (1978); and Watamori and Sasanuma (1976, 1978).

5. Early initiation of treatment results in significantly greater improvement than results when treatment is delayed. This contrast between the results of early and delayed treatment has been confirmed by Butfield and Zangwill (1946); Wepman (1951); Vignolo (1964);

Leischner and Linck (1967); Basso and colleagues (1975); Deal and Deal (1978); and Basso and co-workers (1979). Although these studies provide incontrovertible evidence concerning the importance of early treatment, no study has been reported that clarifies exactly how early "early treatment" should be. No available data clarify the relative merits of beginning treatment within days versus weeks following onset of aphasia. The closest answer is provided by Deal and Deal (1978), who showed that patients for whom treatment was initiated within the first month post onset (as well as for those for whom it was initiated within the second and third months) improved significantly more than those whose treatment began 4 months post onset or later.

Despite the considerable weight of evidence that early treatment is significantly related to recovery, it is also clear that a later start does not necessarily result in negligible or no gains. Several studies have reported significant improvement in language functions despite prolonged intervals of no treatment post onset: Frazier and Ingham (1920), "The aphasic symptoms of some . . . had previously remained stationary for several months"; Weisenburg and McBride (1935), one patient improved with treatment begun 7 months post onset; Godfrey and Douglass (1959), four patients with "long-standing aphasic conditions" made "fair" progress; Smith (1972), patients who benefited from treatment represented a wide range of periods from the onset of aphasia, up to 9½ years; Sparks and co-workers (1974), eight patients helped by Melodic Intonation Therapy had shown no prior improvement in verbal output for at least 6 months; Gloning and associates (1976), two patients who benefited from treatment were treated 2 and 6 years post onset; Broida (1977), 14 patients were treated 1 to 6 years post onset; Wertz (1978), the patient's treatment begun 6 months post onset was beneficial; LaPointe (1978), two patients benefited from treatment started 14 months and 2 years post onset; and Basso and co-workers (1979), highly beneficial treatment began in three patients 11 years, 26 months, and 7½ months post onset.

6. For maximum gains, treatment must often be continued for several months. Prolonged treatment with beneficial results has been described by Weisenburg and McBride (1935), up to 30 months; Wepman (1951), approximately 18 months; Marks and associates (1957), more than 12 months in some cases, although 48 per cent of 159 patients received therapy for no more than 2 months; Schuell and colleagues (1961), 48 patients treated from 1 to 12 months (mean, 3½ months); Vignolo (1964), patients whose treatment began more than 6 months post onset improved only if treated for more than 6 months; Sands and co-workers (1969), median duration of treatment of 30 patients was 7½ months; Smith (1972), 80 patients treated from 5 to 40 weeks; Hagen (1973), 10 patients treated for 12 months; Basso and collaborators (1975), 91 subjects treated for more than 6 months; Gloning and others (1976), all treated patients were treated for at least 6

months; Messerli and associates (1976), a significant relationship was reported between severity of aphasia and duration of treatment; Watamori and Sasanuma (1976, 1978), two patients treated for 49 months and 6 months; Broida (1977), 14 patients receiving treatment over periods ranging from 2 to 21 months (mean, 9 months); Wertz and co-workers (1978), treatment given for up to 44 weeks; Basso and colleagues (1979), "formal language rehabilitation ... does have a positive effect ... provided that it is carried out during at least six months... "; Holland (1980), treatment lasted at least 6 months. Although some investigators whose work has been reviewed have reported significant and even total recovery within a relatively short period, the more usual expectation is a necessary prolongation of treatment for several months in order to attain maximum levels of language performance.

7. Treatment should be intensively administered. The reports of the greatest gains and the clearest contrasts in improvement between treated and untreated patients are based upon programs of individual sessions scheduled daily (sometimes multiple sessions daily) or no less often than three times per week: Frazier and Ingham (1920); Butfield and Zangwill (1946); Wepman (1951); Sands and co-workers (1969); Perry (1972); Smith (1972); Hagen (1973); Weigel-Crump and Koenigsknecht (1973); Sparks and associates (1974); Basso and colleagues (1975); Broida (1977); Watamori and Sasanuma (1976, 1978); Deal and Deal (1978); Wertz (1978); and Wertz and collaborators (1978). This evidence would motivate the development of intensive schedules of consistent treatment application and the abandonment of homeopathic dosage (occasionally or perhaps once a week).

8. The age of the patient is not necessarily either significantly limiting or facilitating in recovery from aphasia in response to treatment. Some studies suggest that younger patients can be expected to have a more favorable treatment outcome than older: most of Wepman's (1951) young aphasic soldiers (mean age, 26 years) made significant recovery of performance in all language areas (86 per cent judged improved or much improved); Vignolo (1964) found that over 70 per cent of patients under 40 years old improved in treatment, whereas only 22 per cent of patients over 60 years old improved; the severely aphasic patients studied by Sarno and co-workers (1970), who as a group did not improve with treatment, were older than patients studied by others, ranging in age from 46 to 83 years, with a mean age of about 65 years; and Gloning and associates (1976) reported that older age (51 years of age or older) had a significant negative effect upon the outcome. But other studies, in contrast, have found age not to be a significant determinant: Smith (1972) found relatively slight differences in the gains in all four modalities of a group of 19 patients who were 19 to 40 years of age and a group of 27 patients ranging in age from 51 to 56 years. Basso and colleagues (1975) found that age was not

related to outcome in their 185 patients, and in their later study of 281 patients with a mean age of 50 years, Basso and co-workers (1979) found only "a rather weak inverse relationship between age and improvement, which, however, does not significantly interfere with the effects of rehabilitation." Messerli and collaborators (1976) likewise found in their study of 53 patients ranging in age from 17 to 74 years that "age . . . has nothing to do . . . with the severity of aphasia, the judged importance of recovery [in terms of change from initial to final status], the level attained at the end of the therapy period, or the duration of therapy." Deal and Deal (1978) similarly found age not to be a significant determinant of change; patients under 55 years of age improved no more as a group than did patients over 55 years old. The first patient described by Watamori and Sasanuma (1976, 1978) was 65 years old; he made significant improvement in two languages as a result of prolonged intensive treatment.

9. The outcome of treatment does not appear to be importantly determined by the "type" of aphasia that patients are sometimes classified as displaying. Most studies reviewed have ignored such classification and have considered their patients to share a disorder of unitary nature. Some investigators have described their patients as falling within various clinical "types," but in analyzing the outcome of treatment have not bothered to relate type to outcome or have reported that all types improved (e.g., Frazier and Ingham, 1920). A few studies have provided more specific data on this issue: Wepman (1951) (see Table 4–1) reported that his 30 "expressive" patients (symptoms predominantly motor or productive in nature) showed the greatest improvement and the highest level of attainment of four groups; his 17 "expressive-receptive" patients (approximately equal disturbance of input and output modalities) started at the second lowest level and were next to highest in attainment; his 10 "global" patients ("all language forms seriously affected") started lowest and attained the lowest level of accomplishment; his 11 "receptive" patients ("symptoms predominantly sensory or receptive") started second highest and ended next to the lowest, gaining less than all the other groups. Godfrey and

Table 4–1. Amount of Gain Shown by Four Groups of Treated Aphasic Patients

PATIENT GROUPS	MEASURED ACHIEVEMENT LEVEL (IN GRADES)		MEAN DIFFERENCE
	Pretraining	Posttraining	
Expressive (N = 30)	4.1	9.9	5.8
Receptive (N = 11)	3.7	8.4	4.7
Expressive-receptive (N = 17)	3.5	8.7	5.1
Global (N = 10)	2.9	7.9	5.0

From Wepman, J. M.: Recovery from Aphasia. New York, Ronald Press, 1951.

Douglass (1959) reported best results with their "expressive" patients (13 "good results," seven "fair") and poorest results with three "global" patients ("unchanged"). Vignolo (1964), in the first of the three Milan studies, drew "a provisional conclusion" that "expressive disorders have poorer prognosis and much greater negative effect on overall recovery than do receptive disorders; moreover, the initial level of comprehension does not seem to influence the evolution of expressive disorders; in particular, poor auditory comprehension does not prevent improvement of oral expression . . . [from taking] place." Leischner and Linck (1967) classified 49 of their patients as "total" or "mixed" aphasics; the remaining 21 were divided into 10 other "types"; their analysis of outcomes showed that some of all types made "small," "slight," or no improvement, and they attribute these failures to personality factors, other illnesses, or late treatment. Messerli and co-workers (1976) found type and severity of aphasia to be jointly related to level of communication attained and concluded that Broca's aphasics and Wernicke's mixed aphasics (both phonemic and semantic paraphasic problems) are more likely to improve significantly than globally aphasic patients or Wernicke's aphasic patients with either predominantly phonemic or predominantly semantic disorders; "nevertheless, all types of aphasia [patients] are able to recover, at least to some degree." Gloning and co-workers (1976) in their study of 107 patients found that type of aphasia was not related either positively or negatively to the outcome of treatment or the degree of language recovery without treatment. Basso and associates (1975) found no relationship between clinical type of aphasia and outcome of treatment, a finding confirmed by Basso and colleagues' later study (1979); their conclusion was that "the influence of rehabilitation is not significantly different in the several groups. . . . All aphasics, if treated, increased their chances of improvement by about the same proportion." It appears that the influences of severity and clinical type of aphasia were not adequately separated in some studies, this contaminating effect preventing unequivocal statements about the effect of type alone. Data from studies that were designed to obviate this contamination attest that clinical type of aphasia is not a significant determinant of the outcome of treatment.

    10. The initial severity of the aphasia is an important determinant of the outcome of treatment, patients with less severe impairment generally attaining higher levels of achievement than those with more severe impairment. This generalization is supported by the findings of Frazier and Ingham (1920), none of whose 16 patients had "residual aphasic symptoms of severe degree"; those of Butfield and Zangwill (1946), 58 per cent of whose mild cases, 56 per cent of moderate cases, and only 40 per cent of severe cases showed marked improvement in speech; of Wepman (1951), whose "global" patients made the least gain of all; of Schuell and co-workers (1964), whose most impaired

Group IV and Group V patients made the poorest gains in treatment; of Sarno and associates (1970), all of whose patients were very severely aphasic and did not benefit from treatment; of Messerli and collaborators (1976), who found a significant relationship between severity and level of function attained and stated that "severe aphasic patients rarely recover their previous verbal capacities completely" despite even prolonged treatment; of Gloning and co-workers (1976); and of Basso and colleagues (1979), who found that overall severity of aphasia has a significant negative influence on "the subsequent course of nontreated as well as that of treated patients." Tempering this conclusion are findings by Smith (1972) and Sparks and associates (1974) and individual cases reported by Wertz (1978), Watamori and Sasanuma (1976, 1978), and Basso and co-workers (1979), which testify that at least some severely aphasic patients can be helped to improve significantly.

Associated impairments that complicate the language problem and recovery from it have been reported to have a negative influence, include personality factors (including lack of interest in or resistance to treatment, denial of disability, poor motivation) and additional "bodily or psychic diseases" (Leischner and Linck, 1967); and "feeblemindedness before onset of illness" and severe dysarthria (Gloning et al., 1976). Vignolo (1964) also reported that an associated speech deficit, "anarthria" (our apraxia of speech), probably constituted a negative influence on recovery of expressive functions, but the two later Milan studies did not confirm this conclusion.

11. The etiology of the aphasia appears to influence the outcome of treatment, inconclusive data suggesting that patients with traumatically incurred aphasia generally attain greater degrees of recovery than those whose aphasia is of vascular etiology. Especially good gains have been reported on the part of trauma cases by Frazier and Ingham (1920), Isserlin (quoted in Butfield and Zangwill, 1946), Butfield and Zangwill (1946), Wepman (1951), and Hillbom (1965). Studies that have included patients with aphasias of various etiologies (traumatic, vascular, neoplastic, infectious) have failed to provide data contrasting outcomes in the disorders of various etiologies, except that the study by Gloning and co-workers (1976) reported no significant differences in improvement between patients with aphasia of traumatic origin and those with aphasia of vascular etiology.

12. A cluster of several negative influences can so combine as to make treatment ineffective. For example, the patients treated without benefit by Sarno and associates (1970) were all globally aphasic, were older as a group than any other group studied, and in many cases were treated long post onset; their failure to improve is attributed by the investigators to the severity of their aphasia, but the additionally deleterious effects of age and delayed treatment would seem to help explain the uniformly poor outcomes with this group, which stands

unique among the studies reviewed. The bulk of the data from all the studies would compel one to believe that no *single* factor that negatively influences recovery appears to be so uniformly potent as to justify automatically excluding a patient from at least a trial of therapy on the basis of its existence.

13. The gains that result from treatment are not confined to language functions but are also noted in attitude, morale, appropriateness of affect, and maintenance of social contact. These values have been reported by Weisenburg and McBride (1935), every patient being "significantly encouraged by his progress to have a different attitude toward the disorder. Thus, the training . . . was of tremendous value indirectly for its effect on the patient's morale." Godfrey and Douglass (1959) spoke of reduced anxiety, defensiveness, withdrawal, and depression. Wepman (1951) concluded that the treatment program used "succeeded in obviating many common personality aberrations in the aphasic subject." Personal testimonials about gains in insight, a feeling of acceptance, optimism, and emotional stability are offered by Wulf (1973) and Ritchie (1961), and even by Moss (1972).

References

Basso, A., Capitani, E., and Vignolo, L. A.: Influence of rehabilitation on language skills in aphasic patients: a controlled study. Arch. Neurol., 36:190–196, 1979.

Basso, A., Faglioni, P., and Vignolo, L. A.: Etude controleé de la rééducation du language dans l'aphasie: comparaison entre aphasiques traités et non-traités. Rev. Neurol. (Paris), 131:607–614, 1975.

Benson, D. F.: Aphasia rehabilitation. Arch. Neurol. 36:187–189, 1979.

Beyn, E. S., and Shokhor-Trotskaya, M. K.: The preventive method of speech rehabilitation in aphasia. Cortex, 2:96–108, 1966.

Broida, H.: Language therapy effects in long term aphasia. Arch. Phys. Med. Rehabil., 58:248–253, 1977.

Butfield, E., and Zangwill, O. L.: Re-education in aphasia: a review of 70 cases. J. Neurol. Neurosurg. Psychiatry, 9:75–79, 1946.

Culton, G. L.: Spontaneous recovery from aphasia. J. Speech Hearing Res., 12:825–832, 1969.

David, R. M., Enderby, P., and Bainton, D.: Progress report on an evaluation of speech therapy for aphasia. Br. J. Disord Commun., 14:85–88, 1979.

Deal, J. L., and Deal, L. A.: Efficacy of aphasia rehabilitation: preliminary results. *In* Clinical Aphasiology Proceedings 1978. Minneapolis, BRK Publishers, 1978, pp. 66–76.

Editorial: Prognosis in aphasia. Lancet, 2:24, 1977.

Eisenson, J.: Prognostic factors related to language rehabilitation in aphasic patients. J. Speech Hearing Disord., 14:262–264, 1949.

Farrell, B.: Pat and Roald. New York, Random House, 1969.

Fenelon, J., Dissez, A., Crouigneau, C., and Arne, L.: Rééducation de l'aphasie. Experience d'un service de rééducation. Bordeaux Med., 2:2557–2570, 1969.

Franz, S. I.: Studies in re-education: the aphasias. J. Compar. Psychol., 4:349–429, 1924.

Frazier, C. H., and Ingham, S. D.: A review of the effects of gunshot wounds of the head: based on the observation of two hundred cases at U.S. General Hospital No. 11, Cape May, N.J. Arch. Neurol., 3:17–40, 1920.

Gloning, K., Trappl, R., Heiss, W. D., and Quatember, R.: Prognosis and speech therapy in aphasia. *In* Lebrun, Y., and Hoops, R. (Eds.): Recovery in Aphasics. Atlantic Highlands, N.J., Humanities Press, 1976, pp. 57–62.

Godfrey, C. M., and Douglass, E.: The recovery process in aphasia. Can. Med. Ass. J., 80:618–624, 1959.

Hagen, C.: Communication abilities in hemiplegia: effect of speech therapy. Arch. Phys. Med. Rehabil., 54:454–463, 1973.

Helmick, J. W., and Wipplinger, M.: Effects of stimulus repetition on the naming behavior of an aphasic adult. J. Commun. Disord., 8:23–29, 1975.

Hillbom, E.: Rehabilitation of brain-injured war veterans. Suom. Lääk, 20:1104–1110, 1965.

Holland, A. L.: The usefulness of treatment for aphasia: a serendipitous study. In Clinical Aphasiology Conference Proceedings 1980. Minneapolis, BRK Publishers, 1980, pp. 240–245.

Kushner, D.: Extended comprehension training leading to improved verbal production: a treatment program for the aphasic patient. In Clinical Aphasiology Conference Proceedings 1975. Minneapolis, BRK Publishers, 1975, pp. 79–88.

Kushner, D., and Winitz, H.: Extended comprehension practice applied to aphasic patients. J. Speech Hearing Disord., 42:296–306, 1977.

LaPointe, L. L.: Aphasia therapy: Some principles and strategies for treatment. In Johns, D. F. (Ed.): Clinical Management of Neurogenic Communicative Disorders. Boston, Little, Brown, 1978, pp. 129–190.

Leischner, A.: Zur Symptomatologie und Therapie der Aphasien, Nervenarzt, 31:60–67, 1960.

Leischner, A., and Linck, H. A.: Neure Erfahrungen mit der Behandlung von Aphasien. Nervenarzt, 38:199–205, 1967.

Luria, A. R.: Traumatic Aphasia. The Hague, Netherlands, Uitgeverij Mouton, 1970.

Marks, M., Taylor, M., and Rusk, H. A.: Rehabilitation of the aphasic patient: a summary of three years' experience in a rehabilitation setting. Arch. Phys. Med. Rehabil., 38:219–226, 1957.

Marshall, J. C., Holmes, J. M., and Newcombe, F.: Fact and theory in recovery from the aphasias. In Outcome of Severe Damage to the Central Nervous System. CIBA Foundation Symposium 34. New York, North-Holland Publishing Co., 1975, pp. 245–254.

McBride, C.: Silent Victory. Chicago, Nelson-Hall Co., 1969.

Messerli, P., Tissot, A., and Rodriguez, J.: Recovery from aphasia: some factors of prognosis. In Lebrun, Y., and Hoops, R. (Eds.): Recovery in Aphasics. Atlantic Highlands, New Jersey, Humanities Press, 1976, pp. 124–134.

Moss, C. S.: Recovery with Aphasia: The Aftermath of My Stroke. Urbana, Illinois, University of Illinois Press, 1972.

Perry, P.: The comparative effectiveness of language training and spontaneous recovery in improving the spoken language vocabulary comprehension of adult aphasics. Paper presented at 48th Annual Convention, American Speech and Hearing Association, San Francisco, 1972.

Ritchie, D.: Stroke: A Study of Recovery. Garden City, New York, Doubleday, 1961.

Sands, E., Sarno, M. T., and Shankweiler, D.: Long-term assessment of language function in aphasia due to stroke. Arch. Phys. Med. Rehabil., 50:202–206, 222, 1969.

Sarno, M. T., Silverman, M., and Sands, E.: Speech therapy and language recovery in severe aphasia. J. Speech Hearing Res., 13:607–623, 1970.

Schuell, H., Jenkins, J. J., and Jiménez-Pabón, E.: Aphasia in Adults: Diagnosis, Prognosis, and Treatment. New York, Harper & Row, 1964.

Schuell, H., Jenkins, J., and Landis, L.: Relationship between auditory comprehension and word frequency in aphasia. J. Speech Hearing Res., 4:30–36, 1961.

Schwartz, L., Nemeroff, S., and Reiss, M.: An investigation of writing therapy for the adult aphasic: the word level. Cortex, 10:278–283, 1974.

Smith, A.: Diagnosis, Intelligence, and Rehabilitation of Chronic Aphasia: Final Report. Ann Arbor, Michigan, University of Michigan, 1972.

Sparks, R., Helm, N., and Albert, M.: Aphasia rehabilitation resulting from Melodic Intonation Therapy. Cortex, 10:303–316, 1974.

Vignolo, L. A.: Evolution of aphasia and language rehabilitation: a retrospective exploratory study. Cortex, 1:344–367, 1964.

Watamori, T. S., and Sasanuma, S.: The recovery process of a bilingual aphasic. J. Commun. Disord., 9:157–166, 1976.

Watamori, T. S., and Sasanuma, S.: The recovery processes of two English-Japanese bilingual aphasics. Brain Lang., 6:127–140, 1978.

Weigel-Crump, C., and Koenigsknecht, R. A.: Tapping the lexical store of the adult aphasic: analysis of the improvement made in word retrieval skills. Cortex, 9:411–418, 1973.

Weisenburg, T., and McBride, K. E.: Aphasia: A Clinical and Psychological Study. New York, Commonwealth Fund, 1935.

Wepman, J. M.: Recovery from Aphasia. New York, Ronald Press, 1951.

Wertz, R. T.: Neuropathologies of speech and language: an introduction to patient management. In Johns, D. F. (Ed.): Clinical Management of Neurogenic Communicative Disorders. Boston, Little, Brown, 1978, pp. 1–101.

Wertz, R. T., Collins, M., Weiss, D., Brookshire, R. H., Friden, T., Kurtzke, J. F., and Pierce, J.: Veterans Administration Cooperative Study on Aphasia: preliminary report on a comparison of individual and group treatment. Paper presented at 54th Annual Convention, American Speech and Hearing Association, San Francisco, 1978.

Winitz, H., and Reeds, J.: Comprehension and Problem Solving as Strategies for Language Training. The Hague, Netherlands, Uitgeverij Mouton, 1975.

Wulf, H. H.: Aphasia, My World Alone. Detroit, Wayne State University Press, 1973.

5 • MAXIMIZING INPUT AND OUTPUT

The Arousal Power of the Stimulus
  Auditory input
  Visual input
The Role of Cues, Context, and
    Redundancy
Syntactic and Semantic Complexity
Avoiding Information Overload
Selection of Input Modality
Variations in the Time Dimension
  Rate of presentation
  Effect of internal pauses in sentence
    stimuli
  Imposed response delay
Scheduling of Stimuli Presentation
Situational Factors
The Content of Therapy
Other Facilitators of Output
The Importance of Attitude
References

"We must insure that the stimuli we use get into the brain."

HILDRED SCHUELL

Data make it clear that most aphasic patients demonstrate a degree of spontaneous recovery of their ability to process language input and produce language output (Chapter 3). Data also show that a program of intervention facilitates recovery of language functions and the attainment of higher levels of achievement than would be the case without formal treatment (Chapter 4). How does treatment accomplish this acceleration and maximization of recovery?

Evidence abounds that indicates that the aphasic patient has not lost his words nor forgotten the rules for putting words together into sentences nor any other specific bits of information. In the course of treatment, using given stimulus materials and a limited number of semantic items and syntactic forms, generalization is observed: other words and structures not worked on return to functional usage as well as the words and sentences that are concentrated on in therapy. As gains are demonstrated in a given modality of concentration, parallel gains in other modalities that have not been stressed are observed. If a bilingual patient has therapy in one language, he shows gains in his other language which may not have been worked on at all. It appears that "language" has not been lost. Rather, brain damage interferes with language function. As Schuell and co-workers (1964) stated, "The clinical evidence in aphasia indicates that the language storage system is at least relatively intact, but the integrity of previously stored patterns is not a sufficient condition for complex discriminatory and selective behavior." It is necessary to present to the brain some kind of stimulus that activates it to function better again. Wepman (1951) stated, "The recovery process must include a program leading to reintegration of the activity of the cortex and not to specific skills. . . . Recovery follows reintegration of the remaining cortical tissue into a functioning whole." He further stated, "The changed brain . . . must form new integrations in ways that require considerable training."

Schuell and associates (1964) expressed it clearly: "We regard aphasia primarily as an interference with language processes resulting from brain injury. . . . Converging evidence from many lines of research indicates . . . that repeated sensory stimulation is essential for organization, storage, and retrieval of patterns in the brain, and it would be strange if language patterns operated according to some other principle. . . . It would seem that sensory stimulation is the only method we have for making complex events happen in the brain. All the evidence suggests that auditory stimulation is crucial in control of language processes. However, since feedback from more than one sensory modality may contribute to behavior, there is no reason for using this mode exclusively. This suggests that the first principle of treatment for aphasia should be the use of intensive auditory stimulation, although not necessarily stimulation through auditory channels alone. . . . In aphasia, combined auditory and visual stimulation is effective in eliciting language on progressive levels of complexity. It should be continued until the patient can respond to each modality alone on any given level. Skills become functional if this procedure is followed."

A second principle follows, namely, that of "the adequate stimulus. . . . We must insure that the stimuli we use get into the brain." That is the crux of the matter: to stimulate the brain, to give it something to react to. How can we insure that the stimuli we use get into the brain?

This chapter is devoted to a scrutiny of ways in which we may proceed that will help to insure that the brain gets stimuli to react to. We will review many studies designed to reveal what works better and what works less well in stimulating the aphasic patient to respond. Most of the information is based on experimental studies; other material has been derived from interviews with patients about their problems and their treatment; still other material reflects what clinicians who have worked with aphasic patients have abstracted from their experience.

It should be stated that the following review is descriptive, not critical. The experimental investigations reported are not analyzed with regard to the nature or adequacy of the population samples studied, the reasonableness of the procedures employed, the rigor of the statistical analyses applied, or the justifiability of the conclusions reached. Rather, research reports, most of them taken from refereed journals, are summarized without critique. Practical considerations prevent doing otherwise, particularly since it is believed that a detailed analysis of each study would add relatively insignificant gains to our knowledge of the issues being considered.

There are many ways to present stimuli to patients, and there are also many ways to measure their success in responding. One can measure recognition; comprehension demonstrated by matching, pointing, or executing a task; naming; spelling; completing or producing a sentence; writing a response; repeating a stimulus; and so forth. This review is not confined to any particular type of stimulus material or mode of input or output but covers, insofar as is possible, every means that people have tried and reported on that is relevant to the issue of stimulating the brain so that the patient can react and perform. The outcomes of this search for ways to maximize input to and output from aphasic patients is organized into 11 parameters of stimulus control.

THE AROUSAL POWER OF THE STIMULUS

Stimuli vary in their capacity to arouse attention and interest, evoke associations, and elicit response. They can be said to vary in their arousal or activating power. Several dimensions of this capacity to arouse will be considered, first with regard to auditory input and then with regard to visual input.

Auditory Input

Saliency. Goodglass has proposed the concept of saliency, which grew out of his analysis of the grammar of aphasic patients. Saliency is defined by Goodglass (1973) as "the psychologic resultant of the stress, the informational significance, the phonological prominence, and the affective value of a word." The data indicate that patients' comprehension of language and especially their fluency in initiating language are influenced by the saliency of words. Aphasic patients appear to need a salient word in order to initiate speech. When asked to repeat phrases, some opening with nonsalient function words and some with salient substantive words, they have more trouble with the former than with the latter. It is easier for a patient to repeat a sentence like "Murder will out!" than one like "It seems likely that murder will out." The implication for therapy is clear: we can help patients initiate speech by making it easy for them to "get hold of" a salient word. Repetition or spontaneous production is easier if sentences are constructed or stimuli are presented so as to allow a quick clutching of salient words. Saliency, then, is a germinal notion that clarifies our consideration of several aspects of the stimulus.

Loudness of Stimuli. Is it possible that increasing the loudness of the stimulus will increase its power to elicit responses? McNeil (1977) studied the effect on auditory processing of diotic intensity increments, that is, equal increments in both ears, simply increasing the loudness of the message. He studied the effects of three different levels of intensity (70 dB, 85 dB, and 100 dB SPL) on the performance of 10 aphasic patients with normal hearing on four dependent variables, representing different levels of linguistic processing: (1) the P_1 and N_2 components of cortical auditory evoked responses (AER) for both the right and left hemispheres, (2) the patients' ability to sequence loud and soft bursts of speech noise, (3) their performance on a minimally varied initial phoneme word discrimination and sequencing task involving from one to four words, and (4) performance on portions of the Revised Token Test. The increased intensity levels did result in the predicted increased amplitude and decreased latency of the AER components, but these changes were not statistically significant. The increased intensity levels did not alter the performance of the patients either statistically or substantively on the other three tasks. McNeil concluded that simple diotic increase of stimulus intensity does not improve the comprehension abilities of aphasic patients. We do not help them understand better by simply presenting the message more loudly.

Binaural Intensity Variations. A second question posed by McNeil pertained to the effects of selective binaural intensity variations on the auditory processing performance of these patients. It is known that a unilateral cortical lesion leads to unilateral unresponsiveness to stimuli applied simultaneously and bilaterally, an effect called extinction; when the message is introduced bilaterally, the message travels faster to the intact hemisphere; the message is interfered with in the damaged hemisphere and arrives later at its destination. It has been determined that this extinction effect can be reduced by trading intensity for time in the central nervous system, including the auditory system. So McNeil asked, "Can the extinction-interference phenomenon be overcome in the auditory system of aphasic patients by selectively raising the intensity of signals to one ear?" He studied these combinations of intensities in decibels: left 70/right 85, left 70/right 100, left 85/right 70, and left 100/right 70. He measured the effects on the patients' performance on the same four dependent variables studied in the first experiment. He found that selective amplification of the left ear resulted in smaller interhemispheric differences in the latencies of both AER components as well as increased amplitudes in both hemispheres and smaller interhemispheric amplitude differences. With regard to the other tasks, he reported: "Speech intensity can be traded for time in quantities large enough to overcome the extinction-interference of auditory stimuli. Although meaningful trends toward improved performance were evident in the nonverbal and the discrimination and sequencing tasks, unilateral increase of stimulus intensity did not prove to be a very potent mechanism for improving auditory comprehension in the aphasic patients tested. Sentence length (Revised Token Test) was not affected in either direction by selective binaural amplification." The results, then, were in the hypothesized direction but were mostly nonsignificant. Although increasing loudness differentially in the ears proved not to be a potent tool for increasing patients' comprehension, the possibility of left ear/right hemisphere stimulation as a facilitator in the processing of linguistic and nonlinguistic material was suggested.

Masking Noise. For a while, research seemed to advocate influencing the expressive performance of aphasic patients by the use of an intense auditory masking noise during the presentation of stimulus materials. First Birch and Lee (1955), then Birch (1956) reported improved performance on the part of 10 of 14 aphasic patients when a 60 dB, 256 Hz tone was presented binaurally while they performed naming and reading tasks. However, Weinstein (1959) failed to confirm this finding; masking noise led to poorer performance in some patients; 10 of 18 patients did better in quiet than with noise. Schuell and co-workers (1964) also tried this procedure and found it not helpful. Finally, Wertz and Porch (1970) administered six tests from Eisenson's *Examining for Aphasia* to 15 aphasic patients while simultaneously presenting a sawtooth noise at a level 70 dB above the patients' threshold for a 500 Hz tone. The patients were correct on 68 per cent of the tasks in quiet, on 66 per cent during noise, a nonsignificant difference. Latency of response was significantly shorter in the noise condition. The performance of the patients was so variable on the various tests that the investigators were unable to generalize concerning the effect of masking noise.

Background Noise. Siegenthaler and Goldstein (1967) found that aphasic patients generally perform with reduced efficiency when there is background noise. They studied both auditory and visual figure-background perception in 30 aphasic patients. The auditory performance involved response to auditory signals buried in a noisy background (a continuous babble of a male voice recorded seven times on top of itself and played backward); visual perception was tested with a hidden figure test. On both tests the patients showed a generally lowered perceptual performance in comparison with normals. Whatever the modality, background noise apparently reduces the efficiency of aphasic patients' performance.

Regarding their efficiency of performance, aphasic patients tell us the same thing. Skelly (1975) reported interviews of 50 aphasic patients, and Rolnick and Hoops (1969) reported interviews of six other patients. The patients interviewed commented on the destructiveness of noise on their performance. Some patients said that they could not follow TV programs unless they were alone, nor could they do their homework if there were people around talking. Patients repeatedly report that competing signals interfere with auditory and visual reception and comprehension.

Directness of Wording. What else can be varied about the stimulus beside its loudness or its freedom from noise interference? Green and Boller (1974) varied the directness of the wording of test items, contrasting directly worded commands ("Point to the ceiling") with indirectly worded commands ("I would like you to point to the ceiling.") They also included a condition in which the directly worded item was preceded by an introductory alerting sentence ("Here's something: point to the ceiling"; "Tell me something: do you have any trouble walking?") Although the patients did not perform significantly differently on these three conditions when only correctness of response was measured, they did perform differently when another measure of response was used, namely, general appropriateness of their response to the stimulus: the more direct wording and the presentation of the stimulus with an introductory sentence enhanced response.

Position of Speaker. Albert and Bear (1976) reported that in intensive work with a single word-deaf patient, his performance on sentence comprehension and digit repetition improved when he could see the speaker's lips. Studying a group of severely impaired aphasic patients, Green and Boller (1974) found that patients' responses to questions were not significantly different whether the speaker was behind or in front of the patient, but their performance was somewhat better with the speaker in front. Another finding was that the voice channel has a significant influence: when stimuli were presented by a live speaker, patients made more correct and more appropriate responses than when the presentation was by tape recording. The difference was statistically significant and was found with regard to both in front and behind presentation and on all kinds of sentence stimuli. They reported that on tape-recorded presentation, patients often imitated the stimulus rather than responded meaningfully to it. Similarly, Boller and co-workers (1979) found in a study of the effect of emotional versus neutral content that their eight aphasic patients made significantly more responses to live than to recorded messages; in this case tape-recorded stimuli tended to result in a total lack of response rather than error responses.

Emotional Content. In this study of the effect of emotional content, Boller and associates (1979) used eight severely aphasic patients (two identified as having Wernicke's aphasia, six with global aphasia), who were presented 30 sentences with emotional content and 30 sentences judged to be emotionally neutral and matched to the emotional sentences in terms of number of syllables, syntactic transformations, and word frequency. The 30 sentences with emotional content consisted of 10 commands ("Say shit"), 10 yes-no questions ("Do you wet your bed?"), and 10 questions requiring information ("What would you do if you won a million dollars?"). Other sentences were of somewhat lower emotional value ("Show me how you drink beer," "Do you ever get hungry?"). Responses were scored in three ways: correct or incorrect, whether the response was appropriate even if technically incorrect, and by a judgment of change of the general behavior of the patient. Results indicated that the content significantly influenced the responses. Items of high emotional value elicited more correct responses and also higher scores by the judges concerning changes in the patient's behavior. The high emotional content of the input appeared to increase the responsiveness of the patients; emotional arousal was seen to have an impact on reception as well as expression of language.

Characteristic Sound. The potential of the characteristic sound of a stimulus to improve naming by aphasic patients was considered by Mills (1977). He presented stimulus materials to four subjects as follows: 32 words represented items having a characteristic sound such that the stimulus could be identified only by hearing its sound; 32 words were selected possessing no such characteristic sound. Mills then took 16 words from each of these two lists and composed Lists A and B in order to determine the effect of training with environmental sounds. The patients first had to demonstrate that they recognized the sounds; none demonstrated less than 91 per cent recognition. Then they were subjected to the naming training procedure as follows: (1) baseline testing was done on all 32 items of both Lists A and B without any accompanying characteristic sounds, the patients simply naming the pictures; (2) four training trials were given on either List A or List B; each picture was presented once, a "sound" word accompanied by its sound presented on tape by ear phones and a "no-sound" word presented by ear phones accompanied by white noise; if the patient named the picture correctly, his response was reinforced by a red lamp; if he responded incorrectly, there was no feedback; (3) a repeat baseline was obtained (P-4) where both lists were presented without accompanying sound; (4) the subjects received four more training trials of the kind described; and (5) a repeat baseline (P-8) without accompanying sound was obtained. Two measures were used, latency of response and error rate. Results showed that response latencies on the sound words were longer than the no-sound words at P-4, but there was no difference between the two lists at P-8. With regard to error rate, error rates on the sound words at P-4 were slightly smaller than for the no-sound words, but by P-8 the error rate on sound words that had been trained had decreased significantly. The second smallest error rate was on the sound words not drilled on. Mills concluded that the decrease of errors on the drilled sound words indicated that such practice resulted in a retrieval strategy that was internalized by the subject, eight training sessions being required for internalization. The strategy was generalized to a lesser extent to the nondrilled items. Mills believed that practice effect and feedback helped reduce errors but that a large part of the improvement was due to the use of sound cues. He suggested that the treatment of naming disorders might well involve use of environmental sounds as a basis for one retrieval strategy. Smithpeter (1976) has suggested a similar treatment procedure using olfaction.

It appears, then, that we should try to make the auditory stimuli we present to aphasic patients as salient, prominent, unambiguous, and clear as possible. Increased loudness will not help in all likelihood, but freedrom from background noise and distractions will. Direct rather than indirect wording and the use of an introductory alerter will help. Presentation of the auditory stimulus live is to be preferred to presentation by tape recording, and visibility of the clinician's mouth as he faces the patient may be helpful. Emotionally arousing content can improve responsiveness, as can utilization of supplementary sensory stimulation, such as characteristic sounds or smells.

Visual Input

Imagery. Our consideration of how visual stimuli can be selected in terms of their arousal power is especially important when we consider that recovery from aphasia may be related to increased activity of the nondominant hemisphere. Paivio (1971) has said, "Imagery is specialized for the symbolic representation of concrete situations and events, whereas the verbal system is characterized by its capacity to deal with more abstract stimulus information." It is well understood that verbal material is processed primarily by the left hemisphere, whereas visual imagery involves the right hemisphere. West (1977), drawing upon the theory and evidence presented by Paivio, points out that aphasic patients in most cases have intact right hemispheres, which may be tapped by using visual imagery in relationship to language performance. She has suggested that language is dually coded as it is learned, so an image of the word, event, or object may remain even though the verbal processes associated with the word, event, or object do not remain or are unavailable. The patient's seeing of the visual symbol may revive or evoke the verbal symbol. "Tapping the visual symbolic code may trigger retrieval of the verbal code." West thus suggests that visual imagery can serve as a facilitator to language performance. She suggests that material be chosen that effectively arouses nonverbal images. Words may do this, but pictures will do it better. Pictures of concrete ideas and pictures that relate to action will probably do it best (West, 1978). The use of color may further heighten the effect of the visual stimulus.

To illustrate her point, West quotes the results of a study by Altman (1977) with aphasic patients on a paired-associate learning task using picture to picture pairs, picture to printed noun, printed noun to picture, and printed noun to printed noun. The patients accomplished learning best in the picture to picture condition. West urges, then, that stimulation with aphasic patients should involve the use of pictures that involve color and action in order to heighten the visual imagery and involve the right hemisphere in language processing.

An increase in the responsiveness of aphasic patients through the use of visual imagery has been demonstrated by Faber and Aten (1979). They divided 20 one- and two-syllable nouns into two balanced lists and prepared bold black-and-white drawings of the objects represented by these nouns. One list was pictured by what might be called intact pictures whereas in the other list the objects were represented in a broken or damaged state (glasses with one broken lens, a torn coat sleeve, a broken pencil). Believing that the usual stimulus "What is it?" or "What is the name of this?" is calculated to lead to convergent language behavior, that is, naming only, they substituted the instruction "Tell me what you see" in the hope that it might facilitate divergent verbal behavior involving wide-ranging associations and more verbal output. The responses of 10 nonfluent aphasic patients with apraxia of speech and three fluent aphasic patients were rated on a five-point scale reflecting the number of uninterrupted grammatical word-strings produced; the mean length of these strings in words was calculated as well as the mean of the three longest strings. Results indicated no difference between the two lists when the measure used was accuracy of naming, but there was a marked difference between the amount of verbalization elicited by the two sets of pictures. (The behavior of the fluent aphasic patients was not different on the two conditions, so the rest of the analysis was devoted to the performance of the nonfluent patients only.) Subjects produced 90.5 verbalizations on the intact picture list, in contrast to 148 verbalizations on the list of "broken" pictures. They produced significantly more topically related words in response to the broken pictures than to the intact pictures. They also produced more uninterrupted grammatical word-strings, the length of these strings was greater, and the mean of the three longest strings was greater for the broken pictures than for the intact pictures. The subjects produced more simple active declarative sentences in response to the broken pictures (11.3) than in response to the intact pictures (5.7). The investigators thought that "broken pictures broke the verbal code as well!" The subjects appeared to respond in a genuine attempt to describe specific visual content; the broken pictures appeared to arouse multiple associations surrounding the concept of the object, associations related to fundamental sensory and motor experiences of the object in use. The instruction used probably facilitated greater output as well, the patients producing divergent language behavior that went beyond simple naming performance.

Color. Agreeing with West's notion of the usefulness of color in arousing visual imagery, Montgomery (1971), apparently herself an aphasic patient, has applauded the use of color with stimulus materials. She has suggested that in repetitious and often boring aphasia therapy, visual materials printed in a variety of colors rather than simply in black and white can heighten and maintain the attention of the patient. Apparently she herself found the use of color to be stimulating and attention-holding.

Realism. Another possible parameter for manipulation is the realism and the completeness of visual stimulus material. Data on this point are somewhat contradictory. Bisiach (1966) studied the naming performance of nine aphasic patients using three types of pictures: realistic pictures of objects, outline drawings of the same objects, and so-called mutilated drawings, which were outline drawings interrupted by superimposed jagged or curved lines. The patients were most successful in naming the realistic pictures. Bisiach reasoned that such pictures present the most information, outline drawings contain this information coded in a more economical manner, and mutilated drawings contain this economically coded information further altered by the superimposition of distracting foreign graphic elements, evidence again that a change in signal-to-noise ratio leads to increased trouble in naming.

Does it follow that objects are better visual stimuli than pictures or drawings? Benton and co-workers (1972) compared the naming performance of 18 aphasic patients in response to objects, large line drawings, and small line drawings. Although the patients recognized the drawings, the objects appeared to carry more information facilitating retrieval of the name, "possibly by arousing a larger number of associations." Even though they found a significant difference between naming of objects and naming of small line drawings, these investigators believed that the difference was too small to be important clinically.

Several other studies indicate that the difference is negligible or nonexistent. Stoler (1960) compared life-size and reduced-size photographs and found no difference in their effect on the ability of aphasic patients to name the items represented. He also compared the naming of objects with the naming of photographs of those objects and again found no difference. Christenson (1959) compared the naming and recognition performance of aphasic patients using an uncluttered stimulus (a photograph on a black background) with a cluttered stimulus (the same photograph with five to nine other photographs surrounding it); he found no difference between the two types of stimulus. Corlew and Nation (1975) studied the naming performance of 14 aphasic patients using the 10 items from the Porch Index of Communicative Ability (PICA) presented in one condition as objects and in a second condition as reduced-size uncolored line drawings; they reported no difference between the two conditions either on initial confrontation naming or on spontaneous self-correction by the subjects of their initial responses. (Bisiach [1976] criticized the study by Corlew and Nation: whereas he studied patients who met criteria for what Luria called "optico-amnesic" aphasia, Corlew and Nation apparently included "a wider variety of aphasic disorders." Whereas Bisiach controlled for visual recognition of the stimuli, he pointed out that Corlew and Nation apparently had not.) Hatfield and co-workers (1977) contrasted the ability of 21 aphasic subjects to name real objects versus photographs versus line drawings. They found no differences between the three stimulus conditions and concluded, "We have found no evidence to support the idea that realism . . . has any effect upon the finding of object names. Given that a patient recognizes the drawing of an object he is as likely to name it correctly as the object itself. . . . If there are any real advantages of realism in confrontation naming they are probably restricted to a very small group of patients."

Operativity. "Operativity" is a parameter which Gardner (1973) thought might influence naming by aphasic patients. He presented to 22 aphasic and 11 nonaphasic subjects four pictures, each containing 18 items to be named. Nine of each 18 items were "operative" (relatively discrete and separate from surrounding context, easy to manipulate, firm to the touch, easily available to several sensory modalities); the other nine were "figurative" (not meeting the criteria for operative words but picturable, elements continuous with surrounding context, not lending themselves readily to manipulation, difficult to grasp, not firm to the touch, known primarily by visual configuration). For example, in the picture of the interior of a room, operative and figurative words, respectively, were vase and ceiling; in the picture of a body, finger and hip; in the picture of a city, hydrant and curb; in the picture of the countryside, rock and cloud. Each set of nine words in each picture was divided into three levels of frequency of occurrence. The subjects named the pictures and were scored with regard to correctness of spontaneous naming and latency of response. When subjects could not name the picture spontaneously, they were given multiple choices and scored on correctness of choice. Results indicated that the aphasic patients differed from the normal subjects primarily in the ease with which they spontaneously named the pictures; both frequency and operativity made a substantial contribution to ease in naming objects, operativity making the larger contribution, particularly in the case of the aphasic patient.

In summary, activation of language function may be increased by making visual stimuli as salient, prominent, clear, and unambiguous as possible. Color may heighten interest, evoke more associations, and hold attention better than black and white. Visual stimulation is probably slightly enhanced by the use of real objects rather than abstractions of them, that is, drawings, especially small drawings. Operativity built into the visual representations may be facilitating. Novel representations, like "broken pictures," may evoke more associations and prompt more divergent, wider-ranging language behavior.

THE ROLE OF CUES, CONTEXT, AND REDUNDANCY

Cues

Can we help the aphasic patient understand better what we present to him aurally or visually by providing prestimulation or additional simultaneous stimulation together with the target stimulus? Can we "tune the patient into the task" or build a bridge to the new task? Can we help him by enriching the redundancy of the input, just as we help him by increasing its saliency and arousal power?

The usefulness of various cues was studied by Rochford and Williams (1962) in investigating the relationship between nominal aphasia and the acquisition of vocabulary in childhood. They compared the naming performance of 32 aphasic patients with that of 120 children, using cards picturing objects with component parts that might also be named. If a subject failed to name the pictured object, four cues were presented: (1) a description of its use; (2) an open-ended sentence calculated to evoke the word by association or by its use in context ("a brush and _____," "we bite with our _____"); (3) a rhyme ("not a chuckle but a [buckle]"); and (4) oral spelling of the word. They found that the order of difficulty of the test items accorded with the lateness of acquisition of the words by children, and the harder the item, the more cues necessary to elicit the correct response. The three latter types of cues were of about equal power, all three more useful than description of the object's use. It is of interest that subsequently Rochford and Williams (1963) studied 10 aphasic subjects from the earlier study who after a period of up to 3 months were almost completely recovered. They found a great decrease in the number of cues needed to elicit difficult names from the subjects, whereas easy names were evoked without the use of cues. They stated: "The results are taken to suggest that the act of naming an object depends on the threshold of the word and . . . thresholds are related to frequency of usage and are raised in dysphasia but may be lowered by a number of factors acting as cues."

The use of cues was also studied by Barton and colleagues (1969). They asked 48 aphasic patients to name 25 one-syllable nouns in different ways: (1) naming a picture spontaneously, (2) providing the name of a picture at the end of an open-ended sentence, or (3) naming a picture in response to a description of the item. They found that performance was facilitated most by the open-ended sentence cue. Naming a picture spontaneously was next easiest, and naming in response to a description of the item was hardest.

Context Plus Cues

The late Egon Weigl (1961, 1968) developed an approach in therapy called "deblocking," which is based on the provision of cues and context. He believed that the performance of a patient could be facilitated in a modality in which the patient was having trouble by earlier presenting a stimulus through a modality in which he was having less trouble. For example, if a patient were having trouble with auditory recognition, his recognition of a spoken word might be helped by prestimulation with the same stimulus through the visual channel; or, if the patient were having trouble naming words, he might be helped by prior hearing of the words. Weigl and Bierwisch (1973) even proposed that the patient need not hear the target word at a prior time; he might be helped by hearing some related word that would lead him toward the appropriate semantic field in his search of the lexicon. (It is in a development of Weigl's ideas that McDearmon and Potter [1975] have suggested the clinical use of prompting materials. They recommend the use of "symbolic prompts" (a written, printed, or spoken word) and "realistic prompts" (real objects, miniature objects, models, photographs, drawings, tactile sensations, odors, tastes, and demonstrations of the use of objects). They suggest the simultaneous presentation of stimuli in two modalities, gradually fading out the prompt. Thus, one might use printed words to help the patient name pictures or match pictures to objects; one might use writing by the clinician or by the patient to help the patient name pictures.)

Some of Weigl's ideas were tested by Podraza and Darley (1977), who studied the relative effectiveness of five conditions of picture naming with five aphasic patients: (1) presentation of the picture without prestimulation; (2) presentation of the picture together with prestimulation of the initial phoneme plus schwa; (3) prestimulation of the picture with an open-ended sentence such as "You cut with a _____"; (4) prestimulation with the target word together with two foils completely unrelated semantically or phonologically to the target word, for example, *fish*, shade, cheese); and (5) prestimulation with three words all semantically related to the target word represented by the picture, for example, *watch*, time, wrist, clock. Results showed that naming performance was facilitated to about an equal degree by prestimulation with the initial phoneme, the open-ended sentence, and the target word accompanied by two unrelated foils; no particular hierarchy of improvement emerged among these three conditions. Performance was not facilitated but rather was worsened by the prior hearing of three semantically related words. A common observation is that when aphasic patients misname pictures and objects, they often produce associated words; this condition seemed to foster just that sort of misnaming.

Pease and Goodglass (1978) also studied the effects of six types of cuing on picture naming by aphasic patients. Twenty aphasic patients, 17 moderately to severely impaired and three mildly impaired, were presented with 173 pictures representing words with a wide range of frequency of occurrence in the language. When a patient was unable to name a picture spontaneously, six different kinds of cues in random-ized order were presented: (1) the first syllable of the word (la- for ladder); (2) a superordinate (name of class), such as, "It's a kind of silverware; it's a _____" to elicit the word spoon; (3) location (environmental context), such as, "It's on the beach; it's a [shell]; (4) a rhyme, as in "It is not butter; it is [shutter]; (5) function (action or use normally associated with the object), such as, "You cut with it; it's a [knife]; and (6) an open-ended sentence, such as "She bought a new saddle for her [horse]." It was found that the degree of naming disorder was inversely related to the patient's responsiveness of cuing (−0.61); the more severe the patient's problem in naming, the less responsive he was to the various cues. The most effective cue, significantly more effective than all others, was the first syllable of the word. The open-ended sentence was significantly more effective than superordin-ate, function, or location. There were no significant differences be-tween superordinate, function, location, and rhyme. Only first syllables helped the most severely impaired patients; if the patient was less severely impaired in naming ability, other cues helped. The investiga-tors suggested that a minimum naming performance of 25 to 33 per cent indicates likely ability to benefit from cues other than first syllables. Finding that the same pattern of responses across cues was found with patients variously identified as having Broca's, Wernicke's, anomic, and other aphasias, Pease and Goodglass concluded that responsiveness to cuing is probably a reflection of differences in severity of naming impairment; the more accessible a word, regardless of "type" of aphasia, the more likely it is that it can be elicited by cues. It should be noted that the cues designed to mobilize semantic knowledge of the target word (for example, location, action, and superordinate) were least effective for all subjects.

The effect of plausibility of context of visual stimuli presented to aphasic subjects was studied by Hatfield and associates (1977). Thirty aphasic patients with naming problems were shown pictures repre-senting six different nouns, a sentence appearing under each picture with a missing last word for the patient to supply; the sentences represented three different levels of plausibility of context. It was found that level of plausibility of context did not affect the patient's naming ability. These investigators also studied the relative effects on naming of presenting pictures of objects in isolation in contrast to pictures of objects in context. They found that appropriate contextual information did not lead patients to correct responses more often than presentation of objects in isolation.

Similarly, Rochford and Williams (1965) contrasted the ability of 10 aphasic patients to name eight pictures of objects and eight parts of the experimenter's body in context as opposed to pictured representa-tions appearing in isolation. They found no differences in performance with the two types of input; the realism of the body parts in context, for example, did not help the patients evoke those words better than pictures of those body parts in isolation. Christenson (1959) also compared naming of objects presented in isolation on a neutral background with in-use presentation of the same objects being worn or manipulated meaningfully. He found no significant difference between the two methods of presentation.

Returning to a consideration of auditory input, it should be recalled that in their study, reviewed earlier in this chapter, Green and Boller (1974) found that aphasic patients comprehended and performed better when oral instructions were preceded by an introductory alerter, such as "Tell me something" or "Here's something."

Redundancy

The effect of redundancy in auditory stimulation was studied by Gardner and co-workers (1975). A group of 46 patients demonstrated their comprehension of words by pointing to pictures in response to each of five conditions of presentation: (1) presentation of the word alone at normal speed (for example, cat); (2) incorporation of the word into a neutral sentence spoken at normal speed (You see a cat that is nice); (3) incorporation of the word into such a neutral sentence spoken slowly; (4) incorporation of the word into a sentence containing a related word, a redundant element (You see a cat that is furry); and (5) incorporation of the word into a sentence containing a final unlikely or counterredundant word calculated to impede comprehension (You see a cat that is sour). The patients performed best when the word was spoken in isolation, when a redundant ("semantically supporting") word was included in the sentence, or when a neutral sentence was spoken slowly. The investigators suggested that in therapy one might adopt the following sequence: "Begin with the word alone, move next to the word in a slowly enunciated, semantically redundant utterance, then gradually eliminate redundant semantic cues and increase the rate of speaking."

In a related study, Wiig and Globus (1971) provided clue words to 11 aphasic patients who were asked to name 20 pictured nouns. The target words were accompanied by clue words of four different types: (1) a word of high association strength, based on Michigan Word Association norms, and logical semantic relationship (representing the name of the category to which the target belonged, that is, superordinate; a word representing a member of a category to which the target word belonged, that is, subordinate; or similar, as "car" is similar to the target word "automobile;" (2) a word of high association strength but of infralogical relationship based upon such factors as location, part of the whole, or some preceding response; (3) a word of low association strength and logical semantic relationship; (4) a word of low association strength and infralogical semantic relationship. Results indicated a pattern of progressive facilitation of naming by presenting clue words of low association value and logical semantic relationship, to words of low association value and infralogical semantic relationship, to words of high association value and infralogical semantic relationship, to words of high association value and logical semantic relationship. In brief, it was found that the retrieval and encoding of target words was best facilitated by accompanying clue words of high association strength which logically related to the target words.

Thus far in this section, all the investigations discussed have pertained to the retrieval of words (comprehension or naming) or the understanding of sentences. Data are also available concerning the facilitation of comprehension of paragraph-length material.

Stachowiak and co-workers (1977) asked 76 aphasic patients, 19 nonaphasic patients with right cerebral lesions, and 19 normal subjects to match a story text with a picture. Each subject was read a six-sentence story (in German), the story ending in an idiomatic metaphorical comment that summarized the theme and the outcome of the story, expressions such as "He is already following in his father's footsteps" or "There he feels as comfortable as a fish in water." After each story was presented, the subject selected the most appropriate picture from an array of five pictures, one representing the literal meaning of the idiom, one reflecting the true metaphorical meaning, the others being irrelevant or misleading. The investigators were surprised to find that the aphasic patients were not significantly poorer than the control subjects in selecting the appropriate pictures. The aphasic patients were not free of comprehension problems, for on the Token Test they performed significantly more poorly than the control subjects; but on the task of listening to the text and then finding the correct picture, they did as well as the control subjects. Why? It was concluded that the redundancy of the text, that is, the availability of more cues, enabled the aphasic patients to perform at normal levels. They performed much better on the paragraph task than they did in comprehending words and sentences; the difference appeared to lie in the greater redundancy of the paragraphs. If a patient missed a part of a paragraph, there were enough other cues in context that inference of the part missed was possible.

The comprehension of paragraph-length material was also studied by Waller and Darley (1978) in a group of 20 aphasic subjects. In one experiment, the patients were read a number of highly factual redundant paragraphs preceded by one of four conditions: (1) presentation of a picture, (2) presentation of a verbal introduction, (3) simultaneous presentation of the picture and verbal introduction, or (4) a control condition with no antecedent presentation. The presentation of the picture alone proved detrimental to the patients' understanding of the paragraphs, perhaps because it introduced an extra encoding step;

however, simultaneous presentation of picture and verbal introduction significantly helped patient comprehension. In a second experiment, less cohesive paragraphs were presented and two conditions were contrasted, a control condition with no antecedent and a condition in which a verbal introduction was presented. Presentation of the prior verbal context significantly facilitated the comprehension of the paragraphs by the aphasic subjects. (Interestingly, Waller and Darley [1979] did not find that prestimulation [presenting antecedent verbal information] improved the comprehension of syntactically difficult *sentences* by these aphasic patients. Only accuracy of response was scored [selecting the correct picture from four foils after hearing each sentence], not latency of response or extent of retention, so the investigators did not fully exhaust the possibility of favorable influence by antecedent information. But the syntactic structures built into the sentences were known to be difficult for aphasic patients, and it appeared that they required analysis to a degree that the context did not help.)

The application of pragmatic principles of language usage to the auditory comprehension abilities of aphasic patients was undertaken by Wilcox and co-workers (1978a,b). Their intent was to maximize extralinguistic context in natural communication settings, to convey as much information as possible to their aphasic listeners by way of information about the perceived environment, nonverbal cues typically provided by speakers and listeners in interaction, suprasegmental aspects of speech, and information about the specific situation in which speech occurred. In each of two experiments, they studied the performance of 18 aphasic patients (nine high-level, nine low-level in terms of performance on aphasia tests) and seven control patients. In the first experiment, patients were shown 40 videotaped interactions between two participants in four different settings — kitchen, office, living room, and hallway. In 20 interactions the situation ended with one participant making an appropriate response to a statement by the other participant, whereas in the other 20 interactions an inappropriate response was made. In all of these situations the indirect requests to which the actors were responding contained a positive intent, as in "Can you open the door?" or "Can't you answer the phone?" After seeing the videotaped sample each subject was supposed to respond "Yes" when the response was appropriate, or "No" when the response was not appropriate. The aphasic patients as a group did just as well as the control subjects in responding to these situations, the high-level subjects performing more accurately than the low-level patients. In a second experiment the idea was conveyed by an indirect statement sometimes of negative and sometimes of positive intent; for example, negative intent: "Must you take the chair?" and "Should you erase the board?" Positive intent: "Can you carry the books?" Again the aphasic patients did quite well, but less well on items involving negative intent. In this case "the availability of extralinguistic cues was not sufficient to compensate for the aphasics' processing difficulties with linguistic stimuli." The general conclusion of the two experiments was that except for some requests conveying negative intent, aphasic patients are able successfully to combine linguistic and contextual cues and demonstrate accurate comprehension of many indirect requests. The aphasic patients did better on these pragmatic tasks than they did on standard tests of auditory comprehension (high-level patients: 76 per cent correct scores on standard tests, 94 per cent correct scores on contextual tasks; low-level aphasic patients: 45 per cent correct scores on standard tests, 86 per cent correct scores on contextual tasks). The correlation between the two sets of performance was not significant, indicating that although standard tests may differentiate high-level from low-level comprehension, they do not adequately reflect the receptive abilities of aphasic patients in natural communicative settings. It would follow that in therapy we should provide not only auditory stimulation but also rich contextual stimuli resembling those available in natural conversation.

Real-Life Situations. Admitting that there is no research yet available on the subject, Brookshire (1978b) has speculated as to why aphasic patients seem to perform better in some real-life comprehension situations than they do in test situations. Perhaps these discrepancies are not due to the patients' ability to make use of nonverbal situational, gestural, and contextual cues to the meanings of the messages, as has often been suggested; perhaps the aphasic individual makes use of his "knowledge of the world" to decipher the meanings of messages delivered to him in real-life context. This knowledge of the world may include utilization of context and history (in terms of what usually happens in given real-life situations), but it probably also includes cognitive strategies specific to the task of decoding incoming messages. Brookshire considers the situation in which the individual is required to make judgments relative to the truth or falsity of spoken messages, based on information presented in pictures. For example, on one trial the subject sees a picture of a boy hitting a girl and hears a sentence, "The boy is hitting the girl" or "The girl is hitting the boy." The subject must verify by looking at the picture that a boy and a girl are present and that the boy is in fact hitting the girl, or vice versa. On another trial, a picture shows a man carrying a box along with the sentence "The man is carrying the box" or "The box is carrying the man." The two sentences are syntactically alike and resemble the two previous sentences, but the latter sentence is quite different from the previous ones in terms of the usefulness of one's knowledge of the real world in decoding it. In this sentence our knowledge of the world tells us that it is unlikely, or impossible, that the box is carrying the man. Consequently, a sentence containing the words "man," "carrying," and "box" can almost certainly be expected to be structured "The man is carrying the box." In the earlier pair of sentences, knowledge of the world gives us no help in decoding; if one heard the words "hitting," "boy," and "girl," one would not be able confidently to predict the structure of the sentence. Brookshire points out that we do not know for sure whether aphasic patients make use of the constraints placed on messages that might be delivered within the real-world context to help them decide their meaning. But it seems reasonable to expect that especially patients whose cognitive ability is relatively intact might well make use of such strategies. If they do, we may explain the discrepancies between their test performance and their real-life performance on the basis of such strategies used by the patient together with his knowledge of the world. It follows that the materials we use and the conversing we do with aphasic patients should not present illogical, absurd, contrary-to-fact material but rather sentences and structures that allow the patient to use his knowledge of the world and his cognitive abilities to respond appropriately.

In summary, alerting statements and cues of different kinds can facilitate the comprehension and response of aphasic patients. These cues may be representational prompts or highly related words that add redundancy to the message, open-ended sentences that bridge the gap to the target, or the initial phoneme or syllable of a target word; rhyme, description, and superordinate word cues are considerably less useful. We can foster absorption of even lengthy and complex materials by providing lead-in information and by making the materials richly redundant so that details missed can be inferred from other parts. Our materials should not be sterile and spare but lifelike, with rich contextual detail such as one encounters in the real world. We should avoid illogical, absurd content; rather we should use reasonable sentences, ideas, and structures that allow the patient to use his knowledge of the world to respond appropriately.

SYNTACTIC AND SEMANTIC COMPLEXITY

Research reports (Wepman et al., 1956; Howes, 1964; Schuell et al., 1969) indicate that in their expressive performance, aphasic patients use words of high frequency and reduce their use of less frequent words of the language. The sentences they produce tend to be simpler than those produced by nonaphasic patients. Similarly, with regard to input, we find that patients respond differentially to stimuli that vary in syntactic and semantic complexity.

Syntactic Complexity. We consider first the influence of the syntactic complexity of what is heard or read by aphasic patients on their performance. Studies by Baker and Holland (1971), Levy and Holland (1971), and Levy and Taylor (1968) have shown that as the syntax of stimulus sentences increases in complexity, performance in response to these sentences by aphasic patients is impaired in terms of both adequacy and speed of comprehension. The comprehension of visually presented sentences is faster and more accurate for active positive declarative sentences (I fed the cat) than for passive (The cat was fed by me), negative (I did not feed the cat), or passive negative sentences (The cat was not fed by me). Shewan and Canter (1971) confirmed this finding by presenting orally to 27 aphasic patients sentences representing various levels of length, vocabulary difficulty, and syntactic complexity. The effect of syntactic complexity was tested by using sentences with simple active declarative form; a single transformation, either negative or passive; and two transformations, both negative and passive. The patients, who indicated their comprehension by pointing to one of four pictures, performed significantly more poorly than a group of normal subjects. The investigators reported that syntactic complexity constituted the most difficult parameter; increments in syntactic complexity led to greater impairment of performance than increments in either length or vocabulary difficulty.

Lasky and co-workers (1976) reported that 15 aphasic patients demonstrated better auditory comprehension of active affirmative sentences than of negative constructions, and they better understood passive affirmative sentences than active negative sentences. In a related study, Weidner and Lasky (1976) found that when their 20 aphasic patients were asked to answer orally presented yes-no questions, follow spoken directions, or repeat sentences of increasing length, their errors increased as the sentences increased in grammatical complexity.

Goodglass and associates (1979) investigated whether the auditory comprehension of ideas by 22 aphasic patients would be better if the ideas were expressed as a series of syntactically simple propositions than if they were combined into a single syntactically complex sentence. They built a test involving three different types of linguistic structures (embedding one simple proposition in another, using compound verb and noun phrases, and using prepositions of directionality or with-of agency). Each sentence was read to the patient, who then pointed to his choice of four pictures as representing the sentence he heard. Regardless of type of aphasia (Broca's, Wernicke's, conduction), the patients demonstrated that expanded sentences were significantly easier to understand than sentences that were syntactically more complex. In all the constructions designed, the expanded forms yielded superior performances over the compact forms. The investigators concluded that expansion into two simple propositions did indeed facilitate comprehension in contrast to embedded sentences, and, further, that comprehension of syntactically complex sentences is not simply a function of the amount of information the patient has to process but relates in part to the structure of the sentences being processed.

With regard to language output, the complexity of the task, including syntactic complexity, helps to determine how well patients perform. We will consider just one example reported by several investigators: One can ask a patient a question about himself, a picture, or a paragraph read to him that requires only a yes-no response (Are you wearing a necktie? Can you light a fire with matches? Did Peary reach the North Pole?) or one can ask information questions that require the patient to formulate and express an idea (How is your eyesight? Where were you born? What happened to the Antarctic explorers?) All studies agree on the outcome of these two types of presentations: patients respond significantly better to yes-no than to information questions even though the two types of questions relate to the same content (Boller and Green, 1972; Green and Boller, 1974; Waller and Darley, 1978; Boller et al., 1979).

Semantic Complexity. Turning to word level and how the semantic complexity of stimuli affects responses by aphasic patients, we consider first the frequency of occurrence of words in the language. Schuell and co-workers (1961) studied the relationship between auditory comprehension and the frequency of test words in 48 aphasic patients. They twice administered the Ammons Full-Range Picture Vocabulary Test, Form A, once before treatment and once after treatment, the range of treatment extending from 1 to 12 months (mean, 3½ months). The words were divided into four lists according to frequency, and the subjects were divided into four quartiles according to the number of errors they made on the test. The results showed that for all quartiles of patients, as word frequency decreased (as words became more rare), comprehension difficulties increased. Regardless of the severity of their aphasia, the patients experienced less difficulty understanding words in common usage. Furthermore, the gains made during therapy by the groups were greatest on the more frequent words.

Croskey and Adams (1970) similarly used an auditory word comprehension test, a patient being required to point to one of four pictures to demonstrate his recognition of spoken words. They found an inverse relationship between the patient's reaction times in pointing to the pictures and the familiarity of the words. Reaction time in responding to words, then, depends at least in part upon the frequency of their occurrence.

Bricker and co-workers (1964) used a spelling task to derive further information about the effects of semantic variables. They administered to 64 aphasic patients the Wide Range Achievement Spelling Test, consisting of 100 test words which the patients wrote to dictation. The patients were then ranked in four quartiles according to the total number of errors made. Results showed a predictable and orderly breakdown in the spelling performance of aphasic subjects. Both word length and word frequency proved to be significant variables in determining spelling performance. Regardless of which quartile they were in, that is, regardless of their level of spelling ability, spelling became increasingly difficult for aphasic patients as the frequency of word usage decreased and as word length increased.

Thurston (1954) reported a similar finding. He asked 30 aphasic patients, 20 nonaphasic brain-damaged subjects, and 60 normal subjects to spell aloud words selected from the Iowa Spelling Scale and representing four levels of difficulty. Results showed that the aphasic patients performed more poorly than the normal subjects, this inferiority being particularly marked on the more difficult words. They were more inferior in oral spelling performance than either of two groups assumed to be poor spellers (older normal subjects and normal subjects with lesser degrees of education). The nonaphasic brain-damaged subjects resembled the aphasic patients in total score but did not show the marked decrease in performance on the more difficult words noted in the aphasic patients.

In his study of operativity as a parameter of word stimuli, Gardner (1973) also considered the influence of word frequency. He found that his 22 aphasic subjects differed from his normal subjects in the ease with which they evoked the names of 18 items. One of the determinants of their performance was word frequency, although frequency was a less potent influence than operativity.

Other parameters than the frequency of occurrence of words may help determine aphasic patients' comprehension of or response to them. Siegel (1959) found that 31 aphasic patients on a reading-aloud task made more errors on adjectives than on verbs or nouns, more errors on long than on short words, and more errors on words of high abstraction level than medium abstraction level as judged by raters. Words representing concepts that were not able to be pointed at gave the patients more trouble than words whose referents were more concrete. Although Siegel did not study word frequency thoroughly, he found more errors on the more infrequent than on the frequent words.

Noll and Hoops (1967) found that 25 patients with mild aphasia had more trouble spelling aloud nonpropositional morphemes (for example, but, for, and, until, anything, against, whether, themselves) than nouns, verbs, and descriptive modifiers.

In summary, in order to facilitate the patient's comprehension and to get his best performance in output, we should use familiar, frequently occurring words, not the hardest words for the patient, or words of high association strength, and we should avoid nonpropositional words and words of high abstraction level. The instructions we give and the stimulus sentences we use for practice should be syntactically simple, not involving multiple transformations, expressing their point directly and in an expanded, not too compact, form.

AVOIDING INFORMATION OVERLOAD

The amount of information presented to the patient at one time appears to influence his comprehension and his performance significantly. The Token Test is built upon this concept and reveals minimal degrees of aphasic impairment of auditory comprehension. As one progresses from Part I, requiring the processing of two bits of information, to Part IV, dealing with six bits of information, one typically sees increasing deterioration of performance. A number of studies present experimental verification of the fact that as stimuli increase in length, performance is increasingly impaired in aphasic patients.

Some of the studies alluded to in the section on syntactic and semantic complexity of stimuli have dealt with the matter of information load as well. Weidner and Lasky (1976) used four auditory subtests from the Minnesota Test for Differential Diagnosis of Aphasia (identifying two and three pictures in sequence, answering yes-no sentences read to them, following oral directions, and reading sentences of increasing length). Their 20 aphasic subjects demonstrated more errors as the sentences in the various subtests increased in length (as well as in grammatical complexity). Shewan and Canter (1971) included among their control parameters the factor of sentence length, defined in terms of number of critical items and number of syllables contained in each sentence. Length was found to be detrimental to the performance of their 27 aphasic subjects, although it was less detrimental than syntactic complexity.

These studies have pertained to the processing of sentences of increasing length. Other studies have considered the processing of multiple items in sequence. Swinney and Taylor (1971) visually presented to eight aphasic subjects and matched normal subjects two-, four-, and six-digit strings followed by a single digit; they recorded the latency of the subjects' reports as to whether the single digit was in or not in the original list. The aphasic patients had an error rate 20 times that of normal subjects, mainly because of two patients who performed extremely poorly; when data from these two subjects were eliminated, the remaining six patients still made three times as many errors as the normal subjects. The latencies were greater for the aphasic than for the normal subjects and, as in the case of the normals, greater for the longer series of digits. The investigators concluded that aphasic subjects conduct a slow search of memory, quantitatively different from that of normals. Warren and colleagues (1977) reported a similar finding in a study of 10 aphasic subjects and concluded that search time, the rate at which information is scanned in short-term memory, is slower in aphasic than in normal subjects.

Do aphasic patients have a general defect in auditory verbal short-term memory or a selective defect in short-term memory for sequences, or both? Albert (1976) did two experiments to answer this question, using 28 aphasic subjects, 29 nonaphasic subjects with unilateral cerebral damage, and 25 normal subjects. Eighteen objects were used, readily identifiable by all subjects. Subjects were asked to point to four items in sequence on several trials, the type of errors being recorded (omission of an item or alteration of the sequence of items). The normal and the nonaphasic brain-damaged subjects did not differ from each other with regard to the total number of items correct, but the aphasic patients did significantly less well than both of the other groups, in terms of both total items correct and recall of the order in which they should point to the items. (To illustrate the magnitude of the errors: aphasic patients pointed correctly to only 201 of 336 items, whereas nonaphasic brain-damaged patients pointed correctly to 318 of 348; with regard to sequencing, aphasic patients got 24 of 336 correct, whereas nonaphasic brain-damaged subjects got 248 of 336 correct.) The aphasic patients appeared most different from the others on sequence-type errors, 34 per cent of their total errors being of this type, whereas only 20 per cent of the errors made by normal and nonaphasic brain-damaged subjects were of the sequence type. Albert concluded that aphasic patients have significantly impaired short-term memory for both total item information and sequences: "The influence of the defective memory for sequences becomes more pronounced as information load increases."

In his second experiment, Albert had the patients point to only two objects in sequence, giving them five trials with two different objects to be pointed to on each trial. In this case, the aphasic subjects made significantly more total errors (24 per cent) than the normal (2 per cent) and the nonaphasic brain-damaged subjects (2.5 per cent). The difference in total errors was due to omissions rather than sequence-type errors. To summarize both studies, it appears that aphasic patients have both types of short-term memory problem: "At low information load levels, the major form of memory deficit in aphasics is an omission type. As information load increases, defective memory for sequences becomes a critical factor."

Even word length warrants our consideration as a contributor to information overload. Filby and co-workers (1963) studied the effect of word length, word frequency, and similarity between words in 10 aphasic patients and 10 normal subjects. The task was to discriminate between visually presented words, pressing a button to indicate which of two words matched a sample word shown above. Words were selected in terms of their frequency, their length (eight, six, and four letters), and their similarity (based on the number of letters that the words had in common). The two groups did not differ in terms of the number of errors made, even though some of the patients were severely aphasic, but the groups differed significantly on latency of response, the aphasic patients taking significantly longer on the task. As the words increased in length, so did the response time of the aphasic patients.

Cohen and Edwards (1964), in a follow-up of this study, asked a group of 10 aphasic subjects to match a stimulus word to one of two words appearing below it, one correct and one incorrect, pressing a button to indicate their choice of the match. There were three levels of what the investigators called perceptual noise, that is, length of word. They also studied the presence and absence of color cues, the configuration of the word (the incorrect comparison words sometimes being reversed, sometimes scrambled), the pronounceability of the words, and the presence or absence of word meaning. Errors were counted and latency of response was measured. Results indicated that length of word was the only variable that differentiated significantly between the aphasic and the normal subjects. The investigators concluded that "as the perceptual field becomes more crowded, the discrimination of individual components becomes more difficult. While perceptual noise makes it difficult for normals to distinguish information carrying units, it is even more difficult for aphasics."

Noll and Hoops (1967) in the study alluded to earlier, found that when they asked their 25 patients with mild aphasia to spell aloud 100 words of varying levels of difficulty and grammatical function, the patients' errors were significantly related to the length of the words (as well as to grammatical function). Bricker and co-workers (1964) reported a similar finding.

The aphasic patients interviewed by both Skelly (1975) and Rolnick and Hoops (1969) offered advice about the length of sentences people should use. Rolnick and Hoops' patients asked speakers to use short sentences: "If you say a long sentence, a lot of time I forget it from the beginning." Head (1926) reported a similar comment made by a patient: "I like that young man; he's clever. I notice that clever people say everything in a few words, so I can understand." Skelly's patients warned against speakers asking too many questions at once; a second question or a too-quick repetition of the first question may interfere with the patient's processing of a given question. Skelly's advice is to "reduce the barrage, and ask one question at a time." It is probably input overload that makes it impossible for aphasic patients to make good use of explanations of their errors, which we may offer in an attempt to help them avoid them. Holland and Sonderman (1974) reported that their subjects did not appear to benefit from analysis of incorrect responses made on tasks similar to those in the Token Test. Instead of listening to the explanations, they usually went ahead and made some other responses. "Since impaired comprehension prevented the correct response initially, a longer auditory chain, that is, the explanation of the error, probably confused rather than aided the subject in making the correct selection."

In summary, we should limit the number of units of information that we ask the aphasic patient to respond to by controlling length of word and length of sentence and reducing the number of units presented in sequence. We must limit the information load.

SELECTION OF INPUT MODALITY

Can we expect better comprehension or performance if we use an alternative modality to one that the patient is having trouble with? (We are not referring here to the effects of deblocking, using prestimulation in a second modality to deblock function in an impaired channel. We are referring to the advisability of shifting to a completely different modality.)

Two studies indicate that in general the modality used for stimulus presentation does not significantly affect performance. Goodglass and co-workers (1968) studied the performance of 27 aphasic patients on the visual naming of objects, tactile naming, auditory naming (naming objects when the patient only heard characteristic sounds), and olfactory naming (naming objects when the patient only smelled characteristic odors). The experimenters found no significant differences between naming performances in the various modalities. With few exceptions, the naming scores were less than one standard deviation apart in all the modalities, leading the investigators to conclude that a modality nonspecific process intervenes between stimulus presentation and naming.

Gardner and associates (1975) studied the relative ability of aphasic patients to discover errors in sentences presented to them in two ways, through reading and listening. To 31 aphasic subjects and 20 normal subjects they presented 100 pairs of sentences, one of which was right, one wrong. In half of these pairs, the wrong sentence was syntactically deviant in any of six ways, and in the other half, the wrong sentence was semantically anomalous in any of seven ways. In the reading task, the patient would read the sentences, determine which sentences were wrong and where, and cross out the error; in sentences presented aurally, patients heard both sentences read while the examiner raised one hand for each sentence; the patient then pointed to the hand corresponding to the error sentence. Results indicated that the aphasic and the normal subjects did not show a difference in performance attributable to stimulus modality. All of the patients did equally well under auditory and visual conditions.

By definition aphasia is a multimodality disorder, so it is not surprising that these two studies of groups of aphasic patients should have turned out as they did. That is not to say, however, that we should overlook intermodality differences in individual patients. In a given patient, testing may reveal that one receptive or one expressive channel is functionally more intact than the others. We should capitalize on its intactness.

The next question is whether simultaneously providing stimulation in more than one modality helps the patient more than using a single modality of input. Gardiner and Brookshire (1972) gave eight aphasic subjects two tasks, picture naming and word reading; in each task they used three conditions: auditory (imitating the clinician), visual (naming the picture), and combined auditory-visual (hearing the clinician and seeing the picture simultaneously). The results showed that the visual condition resulted in fewer correct responses than either of the other two. If the more difficult visual condition and the combined condition were presented alternately, whenever the visual preceded the combined condition, performance in the combined condition was worse than might have been expected, the visual condition apparently having a debilitating effect; but performance on the visual condition was improved when it followed the combined condition. The combined condition was slightly better than the auditory condition alone, but the difference was minimal. The investigators arrived at two main conclusions: subjects vary in the effects of various input conditions; single-subject analysis suggests that a multisensory approach will not necessarily best meet the needs of all aphasic patients, although it may help some. Second, it appears that alternating the presentation of stimuli in combined and unisensory conditions will improve performance in one or both unisensory modalities.

Smithpeter (1976) was motivated to study the effect of olfaction in stimulating aphasic patients' responses by an experience she had with a patient who had not produced speech in response to the usual stimulation. One day Smithpeter held some perfume under her nose and the patient responded, "Perfume, perfume, perfume!" Subsequently, in response to odors she was able to name other objects; once she said a correct name in response to an odor, she never needed to smell it again to name it. Smithpeter went on to study the effects of olfaction on a group of 30 aphasic patients using 14 different odorous substances. She used several modes of stimulation, both unimodality and multimodality: seeing a substance and naming it; reading a printed word and matching it to a substance; hearing a word, repeating it, and pointing to the substance; taking away all substances and asking the patient to name as many as possible from memory; smelling the substance and naming it; smelling it, then naming it, and finding the substance smelled; simultaneously smelling and seeing the substance, then naming it; and smelling several substances and telling when a given substance was smelled. The results indicated that olfaction alone did not result in correct naming as often as conditions in which olfaction was used together with visual presentation of the substance, or when the patient smelled it and heard the name. Smithpeter concluded that patients did better on modes of presentation that followed olfaction alone and those using olfaction along with another mode of presentation. She concluded that olfaction can be used effectively to stimulate language in some aphasic adults, the best responses seeming to be to the more prominent odors (peppermint candy, mothballs, lemon, onion, coffee, perfume).

The performance of aphasic patients on a task using auditory information alone versus a task involving auditory and visual information was studied by Yorkston and co-workers (1977). Two groups of 13 aphasic subjects each were used, the groups being equated with regard to overall score on the PICA. Both groups were given commands from Part I of the Revised Token Test. One group heard the command and simultaneously saw a card with figures representing squares and circles; the other group saw no visual stimuli during the spoken command. Both groups were subjected to three conditions: 0, 5-second, and 10-second delay. Results indicated that the performance scores were significantly higher in the group that received auditory and visual information simultaneously, and their performance improved significantly as the length of delay was increased. During the delay period, all information was available to these subjects; their auditory and visual processing began as soon as the command was given and continued throughout the delay period, when there was such a delay. But the group with auditory information only had to retain it without being able to associate it with visual input until the delay period was over.

Another comparison using other modalities was made by Beukelman and associates (1980). They compared the performance of severely aphasic patients in response to input presented in three ways: verbally, by pantomime, and in a combined verbal-pantomime mode. Nineteen severely aphasic patients (mean PICA percentile of 22) were asked to respond to 10 commands involving object manipulation (brush your teeth, blow your nose, cut with the scissors, drink from a cup) and 10 commands requiring bodily movement (open your mouth, lick your lips, lift up your leg, cough, make a fist). Two response modes were used: a motor response (doing what was asked) and a picture identification response (pointing to colored photographs of objects being manipulated or body parts being moved). Results showed that in the motor response mode, the combined stimulation was best, followed by pantomime, then by the verbal mode, and all differences were statistically significant. The highest proportion of *prompt* responses also resulted from the combined condition, whose results were significantly better than the other two conditions, which were not different from each other. The examination of individual profiles indicated that with some patients a combination of verbal and pantomime instructions clearly facilitated performance, whereas in others there was little difference between the combined and the single mode. The investigators concluded that the combined mode of stimulation does not interfere with performance and in many cases may facilitate accurate motor responses. With regard to the other response mode, picture identification, results again indicated that accuracy was greatest in the combined condition; the verbal and the pantomime conditions were not different from each other.

In summary, we can expect aphasic patients to experience problems with all modalities, such being the nature of aphasia, but examination may reveal that in a given patient one input or output channel is relatively more intact, and we should exploit its intactness. Combinations of two input channels — auditory plus visual, olfactory plus visual or auditory, auditory plus gestural — may facilitate comprehension and performance by some patients. It is worth our while to investigate an individual patient's responses to determine whether multimodality stimulation may be useful.

VARIATIONS IN THE TIME DIMENSION

Patients tell us that they need more processing time in order to grasp what is going on and to respond appropriately. Patients interviewed by Rolnick and Hoops (1969) urged that speakers talk more slowly; one complained, "It moved too fast for me to know what you meant." Skelly's (1975) patients thought that they would better understand if speakers spoke more slowly. They also indicated that they needed more time to prepare and produce responses; having to hurry was "like having sand thrown in their gears."

Time can be manipulated in several ways in stimulating aphasic patients:

1. We may vary the rate of presentation of spoken input or visual stimuli.

2. We may vary the location and the duration of pauses within the auditory stimulus unit.

3. We may impose a delay upon the patient's response, making him wait for a designated period between the completion of the input and the initiation of the response. A considerable body of data reveals what happens when these variables are experimentally manipulated.

Rate of Presentation. Ebbin and Edwards (1967) tested 24 aphasic subjects on a speech sound discrimination task. Subjects were presented 25 syllable pairs, members of each pair being separated by no time delay or by an interval of 200 msec, after which the patients indicated whether the two syllables were the same or different. Results showed that same-different judgments improved when the time interval between the members of the pairs was increased, more with some patients than with others. The investigators suggest that clinicians would do well to determine just how interval-sensitive their patients are.

Parkhurst (1970) compared the responses of aphasic and nonaphasic subjects to spoken commands of varied length and complexity where rate was manipulated by electronically compressing or expanding the speech signal by 35 per cent. The aphasic subjects performed significantly more poorly in the compressed speech condition for all types of sentences. Some subjects improved in the expanded condition on longer, more difficult sentences.

Earlier reviewed was the study by Gardner and co-workers (1975) regarding the auditory recognition by 46 aphasic patients of words and sentences varied with regard to rate and redundancy. Their subjects performed more poorly when neutral sentences were spoken at normal speed than when the same sentences were spoken slowly. Albert and Bear (1974), working with one word-deaf patient, found that sentence comprehension and digit trigram repetition improved markedly at rates reduced to one third or less of normal. The patient did better when digits were presented with 3-second rather than with 1-second intervals, and his understanding of sentences was better at a rate of 45 words per minute than at 150 words per minute. In the study previously referred to, Weidner and Lasky (1976) presented 20 aphasic patients with four auditory subtests from the Minnesota Test for Differential Diagnosis of Aphasia, originally recording the stimuli at a rate of 120 words per minute, then slowing them to 110 words per minute and accelerating them to 150 words per minute. Performances at these two rates (110 and 150 words per minute) were compared. Patients who scored below the 50th percentile on the PICA did somewhat better on all four tests at the slower rate, and patients who scored above the 50th percentile on the PICA improved even more.

Cermak and Moreines (1976) studied five groups of patients — aphasic patients, alcoholic Korsakoff patients, patients with lesions of the nondominant hemisphere, alcoholic patients, and control subjects — comparing their performance on tasks involving the detection of repeated letters, repeated words, rhyming words, and words from the same category during the reading of a word list. The number of intervening words between the repeated items had a greater effect on the aphasic patients than it did on the other four groups, but when rate of presentation was slowed, the aphasic patients showed considerable improvement while the other groups maintained the same level of performance.

Sheehan and co-workers (1973) studied the responses of 30 aphasic patients to questions on 14 different kinds of language tests in which the stimuli were presented in three conditions: (1) 150 msec were interpolated between each pair of phonemes in words; (2) the same amount of cumulative time was inserted between words, thus producing slower speech; and (3) normal speech rate. Results indicated that only the younger patients, those under the age of 50 years, showed improvement, and this improvement was only in the first condition

involving interpolated silences, where the spacing was between phonemes rather than between words. The investigators believed that the
interpolated-silences condition perhaps helped the patient perceive
the correct sequence of phonemes (a task that Efron [1963] found to be
difficult for aphasic patients) and thus led to their better understanding
of words.

The effect of proactive interference on short-term recall by aphasic
patients and others was studied by Flowers (1975). His question was
whether aphasic patients demonstrate an unusual degree of proactive
interference, which occurs during a recall task when some aspect of
recalling prior items interferes with the recalling of subsequent items.
He studied 18 normal subjects, 18 nonaphasic brain-damaged subjects,
and 18 aphasic patients whose problem was generally mild (mean
PICA overall score of about 13). The mean digit spans of the three
groups were 6.06, 5.72, and 4.28, respectively. The experimental task
was presentation of six triple-consonant trigrams, followed by six sets
of three animal names, followed by another set of six triple-consonant
trigrams. The patient heard each trigram presented orally; then he was
required to count backward for 15 seconds; then during a 10-second
recall period he reported what the trigram was. The aphasic patients
did significantly more poorly than the normal subjects, but not significantly more poorly than the brain-damaged nonaphasic subjects. All
three groups showed about the same amount of proactive interference,
declining in excellence of performance especially between trial one
and trials two and three within each set of six trials. Similarly, all three
groups demonstrated about the same degree of perseveration from trial
to trial, another measure of proactive interference. With regard to
release from proactive interference, shown by a shift between the first
set of consonant trigrams and the set of animal trigrams and then
between the set of animal trigrams and the final set of consonant
trigrams, all groups showed this shift, but the aphasic patients did not
show as great a shift as the normal subjects. Whereas the control and
the brain-damaged subjects showed both the primacy effect (good
recall of the initial item in a trigram) and the recency effect (good recall
of the final item in a trigram), the aphasic patients demonstrated only
the primacy, not the recency effect. They demonstrated poorer recall of
final than of medial and initial items in the trigrams. Flowers concluded that proactive interference does not account for the poor performance of aphasic subjects any more than it accounts for the performance by the normal or the brain-damaged subjects; their poorer level
of performance overall appeared to have operated largely within trials;
he felt that the rate of presentation of the elements of the trigrams was
probably too fast for efficient processing. The number of items presented to them closely approximated the maximum number that the
patients could recall immediately, that is, their digit span. He ration-
alized the results thus: "The aphasic subjects may have been (1)

presented the second items of trigrams before the first items had been processed, (2) presented the third items while both the first and second items were being processed, and (3) required to begin counting before the coding process for the trigrams was completed. Accordingly, the aphasic subjects should have had particular difficulty recalling those items that were processed to lesser extents (the second and third items of trigrams), as was found in this study." Flowers also believed that the aphasic patients may have experienced intratrial retroactive inter- ference to a greater degree than the normal subjects because of the distracting effect of having to count during the retention interval. Here are seen, then, the probable deleterious effects of presenting material too rapidly and also introducing a distractor that interferes with retention. We will further consider the deleterious effect of a distractor later in this chapter.

How important are the duration of the period during which visual stimuli are exposed to aphasic patients and the length of the interval between such exposures? Brookshire (1971b) undertook two experi- ments with six aphasic subjects who were asked to name pictures or read words projected on a screen. In one experiment, the stimuli were exposed for 3, 5, 10, or 30 seconds, or at a rate determined by the subjects themselves. He found improvement in naming as the exposure time increased, and the subject-paced condition resulted in the highest rate of correct responses per unit of time. Since he found a rapid gain in improvement between the 3- and the 5-second exposures and less of a gain between 5 and 30 seconds, he recommended a 5-second exposure as optimal. In a second experiment, the stimuli were all exposed for 3 seconds, but exposures were spaced by intervals of 0, 3, 5, 10, or 30 seconds. Results revealed little difference between the 0-, 3-, 5-, and 10-second intertrial intervals but a significant increment in correct responding at the 30-second interval. The effects of increasing inter- trial time were much less than the effects of increasing exposure time.

In two other experiments, Brookshire found that patients per- formed better in conditions of only 10- and 30-second exposures than they did when they also had exposures of 3 and 5 seconds. It was apparent that the short exposures introduced stress, which interfered with performance. This interference was not confined to the short- exposure condition but persisted into longer exposure conditions.

Effect of Internal Pauses in Sentence Stimuli. A second way in which we can manipulate time is to introduce pauses within sentences. The first study to be considered manipulated both rate and internal pauses. Lasky and co-workers (1976) presented sentences to 15 aphasic patients in four conditions: (1) at 150 words per minute with 1-second interphrase pause time, (2) at 150 words per minute without pauses, (3) at 120 words per minute with 1-second interphrase pauses, and (4) at 120 words per minute without pauses. The pauses were inserted between the boundaries of the major constituents of the sentences — for example, "The boy / is hitting / the girl" and "The dog / is chased / by the cat." Results indicated that patients understood the stimuli better (pointed to appropriate pictures) when the sentences were presented at the slower than normal rate. The insertion of interphrase pauses in the normal-rate sentences also aided comprehension. Combining slower rate of presentation and interphrase pauses produced the greatest improvement. The advice of these investigators to clinicians is to slow the input and insert pauses at critical points.

The location of the pauses may indeed be critical. Liles and Brookshire (1975) studied the performance of 20 aphasic patients on a modified version of the Token Test. They inserted 5-second pauses at various points within some of the spoken commands and compared presentation with pauses with a standard condition without pauses. On Parts II and III of the Token Test, in which patients must process three and four bits of information, respectively, differences between the pause and nonpause conditions were significant. The placement of the pauses in Part III turned out to be rather important: if the pause was presented early, it helped; if late, it didn't. Apparently the patients could retain only a couple of items in immediate memory; pauses were effective when they broke strings of three or more bits into strings of two or fewer; pauses which left strings of three or more bits intact did not help. On Part V of the Token Test, these investigators did not obtain a significant difference between the pause and nonpause conditions. This part of the Token Test is linguistically different from the other four parts and requires processing, as Liles and Brookshire say, of both referential and relational information. This study suggests that pauses help the patient deal with sequences of lexical items but not with the grammatical components of sentences. A later study by Fehst (1976) failed, however, to confirm this finding; the hypothesis that pause time helps aphasic patients comprehend sentences that stress length and information but not sentences that stress grammatical relations was not supported; provision of pause time had little effect on the comprehension of either kind of sentence. In a further study, Salvatore (1974) demonstrated that in the use of training procedures on material such as the Token Test 4-second and 2-second pauses placed at significant boundaries within the sentences resulted in better performance than either 1-second or 1/2-second pauses.

Imposed Response Delay. The effect of imposing a delay upon the patient's response for some period of time after the stimulus is presented varies, depending upon the task involved. Toppin and Brookshire (1978), studying the performance of 12 aphasic patients on the Token Test, found that when items get harder, forcing the patient to delay his response leads to deterioration of performance, an effect not found in three normal subjects. The effect was not great in Parts I and II, in which only two and three bits of information are processed; it was considerably greater in Part III, requiring the processing of four bits of information. (The hypothesis was not tested on Parts IV and V because the patients were unable to do these parts.) A similar finding was subsequently reported by Brookshire (1978a).

Yorkston and co-workers (1977), in a study referred to earlier, used items from Part I of the Revised Token Test in two modes of presentation (auditory alone with token display covered versus auditory-visual, commands spoken with token display in full view) in three conditions of response: 0, 5-second, and 10-second delay. Results indicated that the group given auditory and visual information simultaneously improved their performance linearly as a function of increased length of delay. "Extra processing time increases efficiency of response in aphasic patients." The investigators also believed that the imposed delay perhaps prevented anticipatory errors, providing a self-monitoring period, and that it removed the pressure of time. In contrast, the group that received only auditory information and had to wait before they received visual information did not improve performance with increase of delay. The delay interval acted only as a retention, not a processing, period; the process of associating auditory information with visual information could not begin until the imposed delay period ended. The performance of these subjects did not deteriorate as the delay period increased. Stable levels of performance in all three conditions indicated that auditory retention was not the limiting factor in this comprehension task. (Of course only two bits of information were processed on this task; data from other studies suggest that auditory retention is a limiting factor with input involving longer sequences.)

The combined effect of delayed response and a distractor on short-term memory was studied by Butters and colleagues (1970). A group of 15 aphasic patients, one nonaphasic left hemisphere–damaged patient, and 11 nonaphasic right hemisphere–damaged patients were given three visual memory tasks (memory for geometric patterns, single written consonants, and consonant trigrams) and two auditory memory tasks (single consonants, consonant trigrams), all tasks being presented under four conditions: 0, 3-second, 9-second, and 18-second delays. During the delays, the subjects had to count backward by threes. Four trials on each task were given in each condition. Results indicated that patients with right hemisphere damage had more severe memory deficits on visual than on auditory input. The patients with left hemisphere damage who had a lesion in the parietal area had deficits on both visual and auditory tasks, whereas those with lesions in the left frontal lobe only had problems in the no-delay condition but no special memory deficits on the delay conditions for either auditory or visual tasks. The interesting finding is that the truly aphasic patients (those with left parietal lesions) had a steeper gradient with increase of delay than did the normals, between the 0 delay and the 18-second delay for the consonant trigrams. The aphasic patients suffered greater deterioration of performance as they were forced to delay their responses and as they were distracted by the interposed task of counting.

Further data are supplied by DeRenzi and co-workers (1978), who studied the performance of 15 aphasic patients mild to moderate in severity, 15 nonaphasic brain-damaged subjects, and 15 normal subjects in carrying out three-word commands on Token Test items in three conditions: (1) no delay, (2) a 20-second unfilled delay during which the tokens were covered, and (3) a 20-second delay filled with a counting-backward task. Results showed that the aphasic patients were no different from the others in their performance in the no-delay condition. The 20-second unfilled delay brought no decrement in performance to any of the three groups, but the condition in which the 20-second delay was filled with counting backward brought a decrement in performance to all groups. The rate of forgetting was significantly greater in the aphasic patients than in the others, even when degree of impairment of auditory comprehension of the subjects was corrected for. In an added experiment with 15 aphasic patients, these investigators introduced a 4-second pause before the patients started counting in order to ensure that they had had time to complete the linguistic analysis of the task. However, the aphasic patients did not benefit from this pause. The findings of the main study indicate that the steeper decay of the memory function on the part of the aphasic patients was not due to defective processing of information nor to overload of auditory memory span; rather, apparently they encoded the memory trace in a weak form so that introduction of the distractor task caused their performance to suffer significantly.

We take note at this point of a comment from Wepman (1972); he suggests that we observe how long it takes a patient to integrate a given stimulus. The patient may be said to receive the stimulus with his "shutter" open. As he becomes preoccupied with dealing with it, his "shutter" is closed to other stimuli. Wepman advised the presentation of stimulation according to the patient's rate of "shutter openings."

In summary, we maximize auditory comprehension and language performance by slowing overall rate of presentation, reducing the rate of phoneme production by prolonging words, and pausing at critical intervals to reduce the number of units of information that the patient must retain at one time. In presenting visual stimuli, we should extend exposure time to at least 5 seconds and also extend the intervals between exposures. Making the patient delay his responses may disrupt his performance, and introducing any intervening kind of distraction surely worsens his performances. But on some kinds of tasks — not those primarily taxing short-term memory — the opportunity for more processing time will likely be helpful. In general, we must allow more than average time for both auditory and visual processing and response.

SCHEDULING OF STIMULI PRESENTATION

A number of studies suggest how to set up a program of therapy and how stimuli within therapy sessions might best be scheduled. Many clinicians have concluded from their experience that the more intensive the therapy, the better. Pizzamiglio and Roberts (1967) present data derived from teaching 20 aphasic patients certain writing tasks. The patients had to supply the final word in sentences or name pictures, using an automated language retrieval unit and typing in the answers. One group was worked with daily, the second group on alternate days. The group having daily sessions made faster progress than the one having less frequent sessions. Massed therapy appears to be more efficacious than distributed therapy.

Repetition. Schuell and co-workers (1964) sanctioned the use of repetitive sensory stimulation. "Over and over, aphasic patients who looked perplexed and bewildered when a word, for example, was spoken once, showed instantaneous recognition when they heard it the fourth or fifth time. . . . The patient who could name five or six out of 20 pictures after 24 hours when he had received 10 successive auditory stimulations for each word, was able to recall from 15 to 20 words the next day, when he received 20 successive stimulations on each word." A study by Weigel-Crump and Koenigsknecht (1973) constitutes an experimental verification of the efficacy of the type of program suggested by Schuell and associates. Each of 150 words was presented to four aphasic patients 10 times in isolation, then in five simple sentences, and then 10 more times in isolation. The words were frequently occurring words in the language; the sentences were short and presented at a slow rate. Following such stimulation the patients were asked to say the words and supplementary techniques were used to elicit them (gestures, associated words, synonyms, carrier phrases, prompting initial phonemes). Eighteen 1-hour therapy sessions were carried out, two or three a week. After six such sessions the patients' scores rose from 0 correct to 61 per cent correct responses, after six more sessions to 74 per cent, and after all 18 sessions to 84 per cent. Response latencies were also decreased. The investigators reported progress not only on the words and categories worked on but on words and categories not worked on. Such generalization demonstrated to them that therapy is a mechanism for improving the general retrieval process and not a setting for teaching vocabulary via rote memorization.

As a further test of this procedure, Helmick and Wipplinger (1975) went about stimulus repetition therapy with a single patient in a somewhat different way. On odd-numbered days they stimulated the patient with 15 words in a maximum stimulation condition using 24 consecutive stimulations; on even-numbered days they stimulated the patient with 15 other words in a minimum stimulation condition using only six consecutive stimulations. Results indicated no difference between the minimum and the maximum conditions, both conditions resulting in improvement in naming. These investigators also reported generalization to words not worked on. They concluded that large amounts of stimulus repetition do not enhance naming skills more than small amounts but that the application of a systematic stimulation program does enhance naming skills.

Sequence of Tasks. Some information is available about the planning of the sequence of tasks in therapy. In a study not directly related to the language stimulation of aphasic patients, Engmann and Brookshire (1970) taught visual discriminations to 10 aphasic patients and concluded that the method of presenting stimuli to aphasic patients should proceed from simple to complex. The results of their study suggested that the use of single stimuli presented successively was wise at the beginning stages of training. Following the successful completion of this stage, one might move to simultaneous presentation of two or more stimuli and subsequently proceed to successive presentation of two or more stimuli. They believed that this sequence would lead the aphasic patient from a simple to a more complex task and thus minimize the number of trials needed to learn a given task.

Brookshire (1972) presents further information about the order of difficulty in which stimulus materials should be presented. He asked nine aphasic subjects to name pictures representing nouns three syllables or fewer in length, all falling within the first 4000 words in the Thorndike-Lorge list. In a pretest he determined for each subject which pictures were easy and which were more difficult to name. Then, in the experiment, he alternated easy-to-name with difficult-to-name pictures. Results indicated that exposures to difficult items interfered with the patient's subsequent ability to name what had been demonstrated to be easy items on the pretest, and exposure to easy items facilitated the patient's naming of difficult items that followed. In both situations the performances of the patients were better or worse than would have been expected on the basis of the pretest measures. Brookshire concluded that a task that causes a patient to experience a high proportion of failures may generate emotional responses capable of disrupting performance. These effects decay slowly over time, with gradual recovery of ability to respond. The clinical implications are clear: therapy programs should be designed to keep error rates low.

The preceding study involved an output naming task. Brookshire (1976) designed an analogous study of sentence comprehension by 20 aphasic patients using hard and easy items. Subjects pointed to pictures as instructed by sentence commands; in a pretest, it was determined which commands were easy and which were difficult; each patient's basal level (the sentence level at which no errors were made) and ceiling level (the sentence level at which all responses were in error) were determined. He then exposed the subjects to two conditions, a low-error condition using 40 basal items interspersed with 10 ceiling items, and a high-error condition using 40 ceiling items interspersed with 10 basal items. Results indicated that exposure to hard items degraded the subject's performance on easy items; errors in following spoken directions tended to generate additional errors on subsequent items. The conclusion follows that stimulation should be planned to keep error rates low and that when errors do occur, time should be provided for the effects of the errors to dissipate. (It is interesting to note that in this experiment Brookshire did not find that easy items facilitated performance on subsequent difficult items, unlike his finding in the naming task. Two of the subjects responded in this way, but the group as a whole did not.)

In still another study, this one dealing with nonlanguage stimuli, Brookshire and Lommel (1974) made a related finding: brain-damaged patients (both aphasic and right hemisphere–damaged patients) usually progressed through the task without incident until they failed a level. Following failure, their performance often was disrupted so that it was necessary to revert to what should have been extremely easy levels of the task before their performance recovered.

Selecting Vocabulary. Croskey and Adams (1969) have presented a rationale and clinical methodology for selecting vocabulary stimulus items for individual aphasic patients. They suggest administration of a 100-item picture-naming test twice in different orders to aphasic patients. One can assign a score of 1 if the patient passes the items both times, 2 if he fails the item both times, and 3 if he passes once and fails once. They suggest that a type 1 word need not be used for vocabulary building (using questions such as "What do you sleep in?"), since the patient readily retrieves it; such a word can be attached to other stimuli that are not so available. Type 2 words, which invite failure, should be postponed and worked on last. Type 3 words are appropriately used in vocabulary building work in order to get the patient to speak as soon as possible; stimulation with these next most available words improves chances of early progress and leads to generalization in improvement to items earlier found to be type 2 words.

Lack of Progress. What should one do if a patient's progress seems to be stalled on a given task? Brookshire (1968) developed an answer in a study of the performance of nine aphasic patients on a visual discrimination task: "If an aphasic patient fails to respond appropriately in early trials of clinical tasks, continued drill without change in the task is likely to have little value. In this study, performance of nonlearners improved only when the conditions were changed by manipulating the discriminative stimuli or by changing the consequences for certain kinds of responses. Consequently, in clinical activities, when a patient fails to respond correctly in early trials on a task, clinicians should not continue with extended drill of the same task but should change the task by changing discriminative stimuli, response consequences, or both." Brookshire further warns that patients' behavior is much influenced by initial experiences, so it is important not to start at too high a level on more complex speech and language tasks. Toubbeh (1969) offers similar advice. Having observed how aphasic patients perform on learning paired associates, a difficult task for them, he warns that increased practice when the patient has failed is detrimental. As his errors increase, there appears to be a conscious inhibition of all incoming stimuli pertaining to that particular task.

Timing of Reinforcement.   With regard to the timing of reinforcement, Brookshire (1971a) also has advice. Having worked with nine aphasic patients on a nonlanguage task, he concluded that "the performance of sizable numbers of aphasic patients is likely to be adversely affected by even relatively short delays between responses and their consequences, delays which do not affect the performance of nonaphasic individuals."

In summary, massed therapy is to be preferred to less intensive, distributed therapy. Therapy should provide much repetition of stimulus material, although perhaps the amount of repetition originally recommended by Schuell and co-workers is not more effective than lesser amounts. Therapy should be started at a level that is not difficult for the patient. Materials should be graduated in difficulty and their presentation planned to maximize successes and minimize failures, as failure tends to disrupt subsequent performance. Reinforcement should not be delayed.

SITUATIONAL FACTORS

Some data show that there are certain environmental or situational factors that warrant control if we are to maximize patient performance. The effect of fatigue on the communication performance of a group of 16 aphasic patients was studied by Marshall and King (1973). The PICA was administered twice under two conditions: (1) following isokinetic exercise in which the patient engaged in maximal exertion involving knee flexion-extension exercises, judged to be comparable to a normal physical therapy session, and (2) following a rest period. Results indicated a statistically significant difference between the exercise and the control conditions, indicating that fatigue has an adverse effect on test performance overall. Fourteen of the 16 subjects showed a performance decrement following exercise. Verbal and graphic subtests of the PICA proved most likely to be affected, apparently because they are more complex linguistically. Subtests involving matching were not affected by fatigue. The investigators concluded that it would be wise to schedule language therapy during morning hours, before patients have exerted themselves physically, and they should not have language therapy following strenuous activities, such as physical therapy.

If therapy must be scheduled following fatiguing exercise, the tasks engaged in should be those that are linguistically less taxing for the patient to avoid asking for performance beyond his processing capabilities, thus inviting failure.

Another facet of the same problem, the optimum time to schedule therapy for aphasic patients, was studied by Tompkins and co-workers (1980). To a group of 14 aphasic patients in a rehabilitation program, they administered 11 subtests of the PICA twice, once between 8:30 and 9:00 A.M. and once between 2:00 and 2:30 P.M.; at least 30 minutes had elapsed between administration of the PICA and activity in some other part of the rehabilitation program. Results showed morning mean PICA scores to be higher than afternoon mean scores in all cases. The overall communicative efficiency of the patients was significantly reduced in the afternoon, as measured by overall PICA scores, as well as by gestural, verbal, and graphic subtest scores. Examination of the individual subtests that proved most vulnerable indicated that afternoon scheduling affected the more difficult communicative tasks in particular. Buck (1968) also suggested the advisability of scheduling aphasia therapy in the morning, before a patient becomes fatigued.

In summary, data indicate that patients perform best on all kinds of language tasks — receptive and expressive — earlier in the day, when they are not fatigued by the rigors of other therapies or by physical exertion.

THE CONTENT OF THERAPY

We have already alluded to the advice that Schuell and co-workers gave about the value of working on words using abundantly repetitious stimulation. The studies by Weigel-Crump and Koenigsknecht (1973) and Helmick and Wipplinger (1975) demonstrated that such stimulation, using single words and words in sentences, leads to improvement in patient performance. But it appears that naming practice and prompting without the drill and stimulation that were built into these studies does not lead to improvement in performance, as shown by Brookshire (1975). To 10 aphasic patients, he made many presentations of pictures; every time they failed to name a picture, he said the name and the subjects repeated it. Results of this procedure indicated that spontaneous naming of the training pictures was slightly but not significantly improved by such prompting. Prompting did not move the patients from poor performance in early sessions to errorless or nearly errorless performance in the final session, and performance on probe words that were never prompted was often as good as or better than performance on training pictures, which were prompted. Brookshire concluded that prompting has a slight facilitating effect on the spontaneous naming of items prompted, but that these effects do not generalize to unprompted items. Prompting procedures appear not to constitute an efficient way to ameliorate naming deficits.

Some have advocated that the word level is not the correct level at which to provide stimulation. Beyn and Shokhor-Trotskaya (1966) provided repetitious stimulation to a group of 25 aphasic patients but excluded from the materials substantive words (nouns), working instead with words having a predicative character and expressing complete ideas such as "no," "there," "good," "tomorrow," "thanks," and "hello." They progressed as soon as possible to the use of complete sentences for stimulation. These investigators reported that they were able to prevent in their patients the development of a telegraphic style of response characteristic of most of the aphasic patients they had worked with previously.

Bloom (1962), reporting on work at the New York University Institute of Physical Medicine and Rehabilitation in group therapy with aphasic patients, contended that verbal behavior should occur in an environment where speaker and listener are involved in a functional situation, with appropriate reinforcement growing out of the relationship. She set up a number of everyday situations in group work categorized into four levels of severity: greeting situations, yes-no response situations, menu-ordering situations, and money-handling situations. These situations were constantly repeated, and appropriate responses were reinforced. She avoided teaching nouns, preferring to work on functional words like "sit down," which were of apparently greater operant strength; verbalization was encouraged in the situation rather than simply having the patient produce specific words. She felt that working on a stimulus word like "watch" might be meaningless alone, whereas stimuli like "Look at your watch" and "Where is your watch?" might be understood; the word "hello" might be meaningless as a word to be learned through reading, writing, or imitation, but it could become useful in conversation. Bloom reported that this type of work resulted in best progress in low-level aphasic patients who had the least residual of language function when they began their treatment. Higher level aphasic patients did better with more intensive and specific individual therapy sessions.

A similar experience is reported by Hatfield (1964), who used sentences in language stimulation with a single patient. As her patient emitted sentences and phrases, she took them down and "tailored them into a simple, concise, and correct form to serve as a model for him to read back, copy, or answer questions on." Whereas she found it hard to evoke single words from the patient, she elicited considerable contextual speech by concentrating on other than the word level. Relating speech work to occupational therapy and other real-life activities also seemed useful: "His speech is much more fluent than usual because he is engaged in creative activity (basketmaking) and is therefore mentally relaxed. . . . One could contrast this with the lack of motivation in a situation where the patient is merely asked to name two-dimensional pictures of objects for which he has no immediate need." With other patients, Hatfield incorporated speech into real-life activities, such as home redecorating, discussing samples of fabrics and wallpaper choices, and keeping a diary. She stressed "speech in action" and suggested working with sentences rather than words, paragraphs rather than sentences, situations rather than paragraphs, wholes rather than parts. (The application of pragmatic aspects of language discussed earlier in the section on redundancy and context should be recalled [Wilcox et al., 1978a,b].) Wepman (1976) similarly has urged that therapy should not be concentrated on names or other sterile drill but should deal with content and ideas. Because patients display a paucity of ideas, concreteness, and limited associations, Wepman suggests that they be stimulated with and encouraged to talk about things they are interested in. In contrast to his earlier advice (Wepman, 1951), he now counsels indirect rather than direct therapy.

What should be done when the patient makes errors? Should we correct them? Schuell and co-workers (1964) reported that in their experience, correction of errors does not reduce them. Brookshire's data (1975) on prompting in the case of error responses are in agreement. However, there are situations in which pointing out a patient's errors might be useful. Tikofsky and Reynolds (1963) suggest that if a patient is making many perseverative errors, these should be called to his attention. In a study of nonverbal learning, they discovered that unless perseveration errors were specifically pointed out to aphasic patients, they tended to persist. Pizzamiglio and Black (1968), using the language retrieval unit (a typewriter on which aphasic patients completed sentences and words), found that a frequent error was perseveration. But perseveration decreased as performance continued because the correct response was supplied to the subject each time an error was made. These investigators believed that that way of correcting perseveration, or at least pointing out what the correct response should have been, would allow the aphasic patient to reduce both perseverations and anticipations as quickly as any other type of mistake.

As mentioned earlier, Holland and Sonderman (1974) have shown that patients do not benefit from analyses presented to them of their incorrect responses. They appear not to listen to them; in fact, the message given in such an explanation probably only further confuses them because it is too long, too complex, and too much of an information load for them to handle.

In summary, stimulation therapy may profitably be planned at the word level, but one would perhaps do better to work with larger units. With at least some patients, we should move away from language-centered drills, fostering language use by concentrating instead on ideas and real-life activities out of which language grows. We should not spend much therapy time in prompting the patient when he misses an item, and correction and explanation of errors should ordinarily not occupy therapy time, except that it may be useful to point out perseveration errors to the patient.

OTHER FACILITATORS OF OUTPUT

Data presented in the foregoing sections suggest a number of parameters that can be manipulated in order to facilitate performance by aphasic patients on both input (comprehension) and output (expression) tasks of various kinds. Data that follow pertain specifically to maximizing output.

Berman and Peele (1967) have suggested a useful technique for improving the output of aphasic patients. They have observed that a patient who cannot evoke a desired response may produce parts of it or associated responses: synonyms, antonyms, definitions, gestures, part of a written word in substitution for an oral response, or part of a oral word substituted for a written response. They suggest that a clinician select from these various cues those that are especially efficient in leading the patient to produce the desired responses. Among the techniques they suggest are getting the patient to write a word that he wants to say, then sound out the word and say it; he can be led through these steps repeatedly until he follows the procedure spontaneously. If the patient uses associated words in word finding, the clinician can get the patient to listen to these words and make use of them rather than become angry and stop. If the patient unreliably produces "yes" or "no," one might discover a response produced consistently correctly to some obvious question ("Are you married?" "Are you dead?"), then teach the patient to ask himself that question when he wants to produce that response in other situations. Essentially these procedures encourage the patient to continue his search and use whatever association he comes up with to trigger an appropriate response. Rather than require stopping and concentrating on a single convergent response, the patient is encouraged to persist and produce divergent responses. The communication that results may not be exactly correct, but it may be fairly acceptable. The patient is helped to free himself from the inhibiting effect of responding negatively to his errors and ceasing the search for an appropriate response.

Pursuing this notion, Marshall (1976) recorded the conversations of 18 aphasic patients in nondirective therapy and noted examples of word retrieval behavior, defined as "a situation whereby the aphasic, unprompted by the clinician, illustrates that he is unable to retrieve a word and initiates some effort to do so without assistance from the clinician." He recorded 740 instances of five types of word retrieval behavior, ranked in the following order of frequency: (1) semantic association (producing one or more words related semantically to the target word), (2) description of what he was talking about, (3) general-ization (producing general words or empty words such as "whachama-callit" and "stuff"), (4) delay, and (5) phonetic association (producing a word phonetically similar to the target word). Semantic association led to the patient's evoking the desired word the highest percentage of time. It was used by all subjects but most effectively by higher-level aphasic subjects. Description, successful 57 per cent of the time, was used by all subjects, best by higher-level aphasic subjects. Generaliza-tion, successful 57 per cent of the time, was used mainly by lowest-level aphasic subjects but successfully only by higher-level subjects. Delay, successful 35 per cent of the time, was used only by higher-level subjects. Only one subject made much use of phonetic association, successful 17 per cent of the time. Marshall points out that these associations produced in searching for a word are not random but reflect how close the patient is to evoking the word. As suggested by Berman and Peele (1967), these observations help us become aware of the nature of the patient's searching behavior, the efficiency of which may be improved.

In a preceding section, it was pointed out that the differential response of patients to various types of questions provides another cue as to how best to maximize their performance. In Waller and Darley's study (1978), the aphasic patients always did better in answering yes-no questions than in answering information questions about the paragraphs. Boller and Green (1972) reported that jargon responses by patients were significantly more frequent in response to information questions than to yes-no questions. Green and Boller (1974) and Boller and co-workers (1979) also reported differential performance on yes-no and information-requiring questions. Patients may grasp many of the details presented to them orally, remember them, and respond appro-priately when given opportunities for yes-no answers to record their knowledge of them. They will not do that well when asked to retell a story or provide information, their capacities for verbal formulation and expression probably being overtaxed on this task.

Can a patient's writing be facilitated by the use of one or another writing method? Boone and Friedman (1976) studied the differential abilities of aphasic patients in reading and writing cursive and printed material. A group of 30 aphasic patients worked with four matched lists of 10 words each, reading aloud a list written in cursive, reading a printed list, writing in cursive words that were dictated orally, and printing words dictated orally. Scoring was in terms of the number of words written correctly and the number of consecutive letters written correctly. Results yielded no significant differences between the two styles on either reading or writing. Although there were no group differences, there were individual differences, with given patients doing better on cursive and poorer on printing. The investigators therefore suggest that in therapy "the writing style should be determined according to the individual patient's own preference and best performance."

Finally, we see how concentration upon input alone can facilitate output. Kushner and Winitz (1977) studied the effectiveness of what they call "comprehension training," differentiated from Schuell and colleagues' stimulation method in that they required a patient not only to listen but also to problem-solve as he listened, making a pairwise relationship between sound and meaning. They used a program for teaching foreign languages to nonaphasic patients, which requires no production of words but only repeated input following each time by pointing to pictures. Nineteen nouns were presented to a patient repeatedly in 106 frames, the patient being asked to point to the picture named. If he pointed incorrectly, the word was repeated and the clinician pointed to the correct picture. Training began during the second month post onset, 12 sessions being held during that month. No sessions were held during the third month, and nine sessions were held during the fourth month. During none of these sessions was the patient asked to say the words. Testing of naming was done after the second, third, fourth, fifth, and sixth months post onset. Results indicated that whereas the patient failed to name all of the 19 items prior to treatment, after 11 sessions he correctly produced 63 per cent of them. After a month of no treatment his percentage dropped to 42 per cent. After the third month, 100 per cent correct production was attained. Training on these lexical items generalized to comprehension of other words not treated, words selected from the Peabody Picture Vocabulary Test that were not included in the training program. These investigators view comprehension training as "a dynamic process as it involves a student in continuous discrimination and feedback activities." Regarding language production as the outcome of experience in language comprehension, they stated, "Linguistic information should be firmly established in memory storage prior to training and retrieval. . . . Controlled auditory stimulation, then, can be reinterpreted to mean the systematic teaching of language comprehension. Success in production should reflect success in comprehension."

In summary, the best way to improve an aphasic patient's output is to maximize input. Output will follow. Production of output may be facilitated by teaching the patient to recognize the value of the incorrect responses generated and to use those deliberately to get on target, rather than to reject and react to responses that are short of perfect. We should make use of more effective ways of tapping the patient's knowledge (such as yes-no questions) and individually preferred ways of performing in writing and speaking.

THE IMPORTANCE OF ATTITUDE

If we ask them, as Skelly (1975) and Toubbeh (1969) did, aphasic patients can tell us things clinicians do that are detrimental to patient performance. Skelly's interviewed patients stressed that clinicians should avoid presenting hints of impatience, such as sighs, tightened mouth muscles, shoulder or eye movements, or restless drumming of fingers. Some patients are highly aware of such nonverbal communication. The patients also acknowledged that they are readily daunted by a bellicose or indifferent manner on the part of a clinician. Toubbeh warns us that inattention on the part of the listener can be devastating to the patient.

Some experimental data on this subject are provided by Stoicheff (1960). Studying three matched groups of 14 aphasic patients each, she examined the differential effects of encouraging, discouraging, and neutral instructions on word-reading and picture-naming tasks. Whereas the three groups, each subjected to a different condition, performed equally well at the onset of the study, at the conclusion of 3 days of exposure those subjected to the discouraging condition performed significantly more poorly than those in the encouraging condition. The patients in the discouraging condition also rated their own performance more poorly than did those in the encouraging condition, and their motivation to participate had obviously been impaired by the condition to which they were subjected. It is interesting to note that the effect of these conditions was accomplished on a group of patients who had been aphasic on the average for 12½ months, and their exposure to the conditions was brief. Early post-onset experiences of patients may be even more critical than those explored in this study.

In summary, attitudes of acceptance, patience, encouragement, and optimism facilitate patient performance. Comprehension and performance are inhibited by expressions of impatience, hostility, indifference, inattention, and criticism.

From our foregoing review, it is evident that there are extant substantial data to guide us in our efforts to stimulate the patient's brain effectively and to improve the patient's language output. The data highlight certain activities that should be avoided. The data are not in complete agreement, but the agreement is substantial. They can serve as guides in our clinical approach to aphasic patients. They lead toward clinical work that is less intuitive, less the exercise of an art, more scientific, more defensible, and more effective in facilitating the recovery of aphasic patients.

References

Albert, M. L.: Short-term memory and aphasia. Brain Lang., 3:28–33, 1976.
Albert, M. L., and Bear, D.: Time to understand: a case study of word deafness with reference to the role of time in auditory comprehension. Brain, 97:373–384, 1974.

Altman, M. I.: Visual imagery as a facilitator of paired associate learning with aphasic adults. M.A. Thesis, Hunter College, University of New York, 1977.

Baker, N. E., and Holland, A. L.: Aphasic comprehension of related statements. In Holland, A. L.: Psycholinguistics and Behavioral Variables Underlying Recovery from Aphasia. Project report submitted to Social and Rehabilitative Service, DHEW, 1971.

Barton, M., Maruszewski, M., and Urrea, D.: Variation of stimulus context and its effect on word-finding ability in aphasics. Cortex, 5:351–365, 1969.

Benton, A. L., Smith, K. C., and Lang, M.: Stimulus characteristics and object naming in aphasic patients. J. Commun. Disord., 5:19–24, 1972.

Berman, M., and Peele, L.: Self-generated cues: a method for aiding aphasic and apractic patients. J. Speech Hearing Disord., 32:372–376, 1967.

Beukelman, D. R., Yorkston, K. M., and Waugh, P. F.: Communication in severe aphasia: effectiveness of three instruction modalities. Arch. Phys. Med. Rehabil., 61:248–252, 1980.

Beyn, E. S., and Shokhor-Trotskaya, M. K.: The preventive method of speech rehabilitation in aphasia. Cortex, 2:96–108, 1966.

Birch, H. G.: Experimental investigations in expressive aphasia. N.Y. State Med. J., 56:3849–3852, 1956.

Birch, H. G., and Lee, J.: Cortical inhibition in expressive aphasia. Arch. Neurol. Psychiatry, 74:514–517, 1955.

Bisiach, E.: Perceptual factors in the pathogenesis of anomia. Cortex, 2:90–95, 1966.

Bisiach, E.: Characteristics of visual stimuli and naming performance in aphasic adults: comments on the paper by Corlew and Nation. Cortex, 12:74–75, 1976.

Bloom, L. M.: A rationale for group treatment of aphasic patients. J. Speech Hearing Disord., 27:11–16, 1962.

Boller, F., and Green, E.: Comprehension in severe aphasics. Cortex, 8:382–394, 1972.

Boller, F., Cole, M., Vrtunski, P. B., Patterson, M., and Kim, Y.: Paralinguistic aspects of auditory comprehension in aphasia. Brain Lang., 7:164–174, 1979.

Boone, D. R., and Friedman, H. M.: Writing in aphasia rehabilitation: cursive vs. manuscript. J. Speech Hearing Disord., 41:523–529, 1976.

Bricker, A. L., Schuell, H., and Jenkins, J. J.: Effect of word frequency and word length on aphasic spelling errors. J. Speech Hearing Res., 7:183–192, 1964.

Brookshire, R. H.: A Token Test battery for testing auditory comprehension in brain-injured adults. Brain Lang., 6:149–157, 1978a.

Brookshire, R. H.: Auditory comprehension and aphasia. In Johns, D. F. (Ed.): Clinical Management of Neurogenic Communicative Disorders. Boston, Little, Brown, 1978b, pp. 103–128.

Brookshire, R. H.: Effects of delay of reinforcement on probability learning by aphasic subjects. J. Speech Hearing Res., 14:92–105, 1971a.

Brookshire, R. H.: Effects of trial time and inter-trial interval on naming by aphasic subjects. J. Commun. Disord., 3:289–301, 1971b.

Brookshire, R. H.: Effects of prompting on spontaneous naming of pictures by aphasic subjects. J. Can. Speech Hear. Assoc., pp. 63–71, Autumn 1975.

Brookshire, R. H.: Effects of task difficulty on sentence comprehension performance of aphasic subjects. J. Commun. Disord., 9:167–173, 1976.

Brookshire, R. H.: Effects of task difficulty on naming performance of aphasic subjects. J. Speech Hearing Res., 15:551–558, 1972.

Brookshire, R. H.: Visual discrimination and response reversal learning by aphasic subjects. J. Speech Hearing Res., 11:677–692, 1968.

Brookshire, R. H., and Lommel, M.: Perception of sequences of visual temporal and auditory spatial stimuli by aphasic, right hemisphere damaged, and nonbrain damaged subjects. J. Commun. Disord., 7:155–169, 1974.

Buck, McK.: Dysphasia: Professional Guidance for Family and Patient. Englewood Cliffs, New Jersey, Prentice-Hall, 1968.

Butters, N., Samuels, I., Goodglass, H., and Brody, B.: Short-term visual and auditory memory disorders after parietal and frontal lobe damage. Cortex, 6:440–459, 1970.

Cermak, L. S., and Moreines, J.: Verbal retention deficits in aphasic and amnesic patients. Brain Lang., 3:16–27, 1976.

Christenson, C. R.: The effect of photographic stimuli on responses in adult aphasics. M.A. thesis, University of Wisconsin, 1959.

Cohen, J. G., and Edwards, A. E.: Word length and discrimination behavior of aphasics. J. Speech Hearing Res., 7:343–348, 1964.

Corlew, M. M., and Nation, J. E.: Characteristics of visual stimuli and naming performance in aphasic adults. Cortex, 11:186–191, 1975.

Croskey, C. S., and Adams, M. R.: A rationale and clinical methodology for selecting vocabulary stimulus materials for individual aphasic patients. J. Commun. Disord., 2:340–343, 1969.

Croskey, C. S., and Adams, M. R.: The experimental analysis of certain aspects of an aphasic's recovery. J. Commun. Disord., 3:177–180, 1970.

De Renzi, E., Faglioni, P., and Previdi, P.: Increased susceptibility of aphasics to a distractor task in the recall of verbal commands. Brain Lang., 6:14–21, 1978.

Ebbin, J. B., and Edwards, A. E.: Speech sound discrimination of aphasics when intersound interval is varied. J. Speech Hearing Res., 10:120–125, 1967.

Efron, R.: Temporal perception, aphasia and déja vu. Brain, 86:403–423, 1963.

Engmann, D. L., and Brookshire, R. H.: Effects of simultaneous and successive stimulus presentation on visual discrimination by aphasic patients. J. Speech Hearing Res., 13:369–381, 1970.

Faber, M., and Aten, J. L.: Verbal performance in aphasic patients in response to intact and altered picture stimuli. Clinical Aphasiology Conference Proceedings, 1979. Minneapolis, BRK Publishers, 1979.

Fehst, C.: Effects of pause time on comprehension of comparative and enumerative sentences by aphasic subjects. M.A. thesis, University of Minnesota, 1976.

Filby, Y., Edwards, A. E., and Seacat, G. F.: Word length, frequency, and similarity in the discrimination behavior of aphasics. J. Speech Hearing Res., 6:255–261, 1963.

Flowers, C. R.: Proactive interference in short-term recall by aphasic, brain-damaged nonaphasic, and normal subjects. Neuropsychologia, 13:59–68, 1975.

Gardiner, B. J., and Brookshire, R. H.: Effects of unisensory and multisensory presentation of stimuli upon naming by aphasic subjects. Lang. Speech, 15:342–357, 1972.

Gardner, H.: The contribution of operativity to naming capacity in aphasic patients. Neuropsychologia, 11:213–220, 1973.

Gardner, H., Albert, M. L., and Weintraub, S.: Comprehending a word: the influence of speed and redundancy on auditory comprehension in aphasia. Cortex, 11:155–162, 1975.

Gardner, H., Denes, G., and Zurif, E.: Critical reading at the sentence level in aphasia. Cortex, 11:60–72, 1975.

Goodglass, H.: Studies on the grammar of aphasics. In Goodglass, H., and Blumstein, S.: Psycholinguistics and Aphasia. Baltimore, Johns Hopkins University Press, 1973, pp. 183–215.

Goodglass, H., Barton, M. I., and Kaplan, E. F.: Sensory modality and object-naming in aphasics. J. Speech Hearing Res., 11:488–496, 1968.

Goodglass, H., Blumstein, S. E., Gleason, J. B., Hyde, M. R., Green, E., and Statlender, S.: The effect of syntactic encoding on sentence comprehension in aphasia. Brain Lang., 7:201–209, 1979.

Green, E., and Boller, F.: Features of auditory comprehension in severely impaired aphasics. Cortex, 10:133–145, 1974.

Hatfield, F. M.: Rehabilitation of language. Sp. Path. Therapy, 7:68–77, 1964.

Hatfield, F. M., Howard, D., Barber, J., Jones, C., and Morton, J.: Object naming in aphasics — the lack of effect of context or realism. Neuropsychologia, 15:717–727, 1977.

Head, H.: Aphasia and Kindred Disorders. Vol. 2. New York, Macmillan, 1926.

Helmick, J. W., and Wipplinger, M.: Effects of stimulus repetition on the naming behavior of an aphasic adult: a clinical report. J. Commun. Disord., 8:23–29, 1975.

Holland, A. L., and Sonderman, J. C.: Effects of a program based on the Token Test for teaching comprehension skills to aphasics. J. Speech Hearing Res., 17:589–598, 1974.

Howes, D. H.: Application of the word-frequency concept to aphasia. In de Rueck, A. V. S., and O'Connor, M. (Eds.): Ciba Foundation Symposium: Disorders of Language. Boston, Little, Brown, 1964, pp. 47–75.

Kushner, D., and Winitz, H.: Extended comprehension practice applied to an aphasic patient. J. Speech Hearing Disord., 42:296–306, 1977.

Lasky, E. Z., Weidner, W. E., and Johnson, J. P.: Influence of linguistic complexity, rate of presentation, and interphrase pause time on auditory-verbal comprehension of adult aphasic patients. Brain Lang., 3:386–395, 1976.

Levy, C., and Holland, A. L.: Influence of grammatical complexity and sentence length on comprehension with adult aphasics. In Holland, A. L.: Psycholinguistics and Behavioral Variables Underlying Recovery from Aphasia. Project report submitted to Social and Rehabilitative Service, DHEW, 1971, pp. 1–26.

Levy, C. B., and Taylor, O. L.: Transformational complexity and comprehension in adult aphasics. Paper presented at ASHA Convention, Denver, Colorado, November 17, 1968.

Liles, B. Z., and Brookshire, R. H.: The effects of pause time on auditory comprehension of aphasic subjects. J. Commun. Disord., 8:221–235, 1975.

Marshall, R. C.: Word retrieval of aphasic adults. J. Speech Hearing Disord., 41:444–451, 1976.

Marshall, R. C., and King, P. S.: Effects of fatigue produced by isokinetic exercise on the communicative ability of aphasic adults. J. Speech Hearing Res., 16:222–230, 1973.

McDearmon, J. R., and Potter, R. E.: The use of representational prompts in aphasia therapy. J. Commun. Disord., 8:199–206, 1975.

McNeil, M. R.: Effects of diotic and selective binaural intensity variation on auditory processing in aphasia. Ph.D. dissertation, University of Denver, 1977.

Mills, R. H.: The effects of environmental sound on the naming performance of aphasic subjects: a pilot study. Clinical Aphasiology Conference Proceedings, 1977. Minneapolis, BRK Publishers, 1977, pp. 68–79.

Montgomery, J.: The importance of seeing red: self-teaching techniques for adult aphasia. J. Speech Hearing Disord., 36:250–251, 1971.

Noll, J. D., and Hoops, H. R.: Aphasic grammatical involvement as indicated by spelling ability. Cortex, 3:419–432, 1967.

Paivio, A.: Imagery and Verbal Processes. New York, Holt, Rinehart, and Winston, 1971.

Parkhurst, B. G.: The effect of time-altered speech stimuli on the performance of right hemiplegic adult aphasics. Paper presented at American Speech and Hearing Association Convention, November 22, 1970.

Pease, D. M., and Goodglass, H.: The effects of cuing on picture naming in aphasia. Cortex, 14:178–189, 1978.

Pizzamiglio, L., and Black, J. W.: Phonic trends in the writing of aphasic patients. J. Speech Hearing Res., 11:77–84, 1968.

Pizzamiglio, L., and Roberts, M.: Writing in aphasia: a learning study. Cortex, 3:250–257, 1967.

Podraza, B. L., and Darley, F. L.: Effect of auditory prestimulation on naming in aphasia. J. Speech Hearing Res., 20:669–683, 1977.

Rochford, G., and Williams, M.: Studies in the development and breakdown of the use of names. I. The relationship between nominal dysphasia and the acquisition of vocabulary in childhood. J. Neurol. Neurosurg. Psychiatry, 25:222–227, 1962.

Rochford, G., and Williams, M.: Studies in the development and breakdown of the use of names. III. Recovery from nominal aphasia. J. Neurol. Neurosurg. Psychiatry, 25:377–381, 1963.

Rochford, G., and Williams, M.: Studies in the development and breakdown of the use of names. IV. The effects of word frequency. J. Neurol. Neurosurg. Psychiatry, 28:407–413, 1965.

Rolnick, M., and Hoops, H. R.: Aphasia as seen by the aphasic. J. Speech Hearing Disord., 34:48–53, 1969.

Salvatore, A. P.: An investigation of the effects of pause duration on sentence comprehension by aphasic subjects. Ph.D. dissertation, University of Minnesota, 1974.

Schuell, H., Jenkins, J. J., and Jiménez-Pabón, E.: Aphasia in Adults: Diagnosis, Prognosis, and Treatment. New York, Hoeber, 1964.

Schuell, H., Jenkins, J., and Landis, L.: Relationship between auditory comprehension and word frequency in aphasia. J. Speech Hearing Res., 4:30–36, 1961.

Schuell, H., Shaw, R., and Brewer, W.: A psycholinguistic approach to study of the language deficit in aphasia. J. Speech Hearing Res., 12:794–806, 1969.

Sheehan, J. G., Aseltine, S., and Edwards, A. E.: Aphasic comprehension of time spacing. J. Speech Hearing Res., 16:650–657, 1973.

Shewan, C. M., and Canter, G. J.: Effects of vocabulary, syntax, and sentence length on auditory comprehension in aphasic patients. Cortex, 7:209–226, 1971.

Siegel, G. M.: Dysphasic speech responses to visual word stimuli. J. Speech Hearing Res., 2:152–160, 1959.

Siegenthaler, B. M., and Goldstein, J.: Auditory and visual figure-background perception by adult aphasics. J. Commun. Disord., 1:152–158, 1967.

Skelly, M.: Aphasic patients talk back. Am. J. Nursing, 75:1140–1142, 1975.

Smithpeter, J. V.: A clinical study of responses to olfactory stimuli in aphasic adults. Clinical Aphasiology Conference Proceedings, 1976. Minneapolis, BRK Publishers, 1976, pp. 303–314.

Stachowiak, F. J., Huber, W., Poeck, K., and Kerschensteiner, M.: Text comprehension in aphasia. Brain Lang., 4:177–195, 1977.

Stoicheff, M. L.: Motivating instructions and language performance of dysphasic subjects. J. Speech Hearing Res., 3:75–85, 1960.

Stoler, L. S.: A study of factors affecting visual recognition in adult aphasics. M.A. thesis, University of Wisconsin, 1960.

Swinney, D. A., and Taylor, O. L.: Short-term memory recognition search in aphasics. J. Speech Hearing Res., 14:578–588, 1971.

Thurston, J. R.: An empirical investigation of the loss of spelling ability in dysphasics. J. Speech Hearing Disord., 19:344–349, 1954.

Tikofsky, R. S., and Reynolds, G. L.: Further studies of nonverbal learning and aphasia. J. Speech Hearing Res., 6:329–337, 1963.

Tompkins, C. A., Marshall, R. C., and Phillips, D. S.: Aphasic patients in a rehabilitation program: scheduling speech and language services. Arch. Phys. Med. Rehabil., 61:252–254, 1980.

Toppin, C. J., and Brookshire, R. H.: Effects of response delay and token relocation on Token Test performance of aphasic subjects. J. Commun. Disord., 11:65–78, 1978.

Toubbeh, J. I.: Clinical observations on adult aphasia. J. Commun. Disord., 2:57–68, 1969.

Waller, M., and Darley, F. L.: The influence of context on the auditory comprehension of paragraphs by aphasic subjects. J. Speech Hearing Res., 21:732–745, 1978.

Waller, M., and Darley, F. L.: Effect of prestimulation on sentence comprehension by aphasic subjects. J. Commun. Disord., 12:461–479, 1979.

Warren, R. L., Hubbard, D. J., and Knox, A. W.: Short-term memory scan in normal individuals and individuals with aphasia. J. Speech Hearing Res., 20:497–509, 1977.

Weidner, W. E., and Lasky, E. Z.: The interaction of rate and complexity of stimulus on the performance of adult aphasic subjects. Brain Lang., 3:34–40, 1976.

Weigel-Crump, C., and Koenigsknecht, R. A.: Tapping the lexical store of the adult aphasic: analysis of the improvement made in word retrieval skills. Cortex, 9:411–418, 1973.

Weigl, E.: The phenomenon of temporary deblocking in aphasia. Zeitschr. Phonetic. Sprachwiss. Komm., 14:337–364, 1961.

Weigl, E.: On the problem of cortical syndromes: experimental studies. In Simmel, M. L., (Ed.): The Reach of Mind: Essays in Memory of Kurt Goldstein. New York, Springer, 1968, pp. 143–159.

Weigl, E., and Bierwisch, M.: Neuropsychology and linguistics: Topics of common research. In Goodglass, H., and Blumstein, S. (Eds.): Psycholinguistics and Aphasia. Baltimore, Johns Hopkins University Press, 1973, pp. 10–28.

Weinstein, S.: Experimental analysis of an attempt to improve speech in cases of expressive aphasia. Neurology, 9:632–635, 1959.

Wepman, J. M.: Aphasia therapy: a new look. J. Speech Hearing Disord., 37:203–214, 1972.

Wepman, J. M.: Aphasia: language without thought or thought without language? ASHA, 18:131–136, 1976.

Wepman, J. M.: Recovery from Aphasia. New York, Ronald Press, 1951.

Wepman, J. M., Bock, R. D., Jones, L. V., and Van Pelt, D.: Psycholinguistic study of aphasia: a revision of the concept of anomia. J. Speech Hearing Disord., 21:468–477, 1956.

Wertz, R. T., and Porch, B. E.: Effects of masking noise on the verbal performance of adult aphasics. Cortex, 6:399–409, 1970.

West, J. F.: Heightening the action imagery of materials used in aphasia treatment. Clinical Aphasiology Conference Proceedings, 1978. Minneapolis, BRK Publishers, 1978, pp. 201–211.

West, J. F.: Imaging and aphasia. Clinical Aphasiology Conference Proceedings, 1977. Minneapolis, BRK Publishers, 1977, pp. 239–247.

Wiig, E. H., and Globus, D.: Aphasic word identification as a function of logical relationship and association strength. J. Speech Hearing Res., 14:195–204, 1971.

Wilcox, M. J., Davis, G. A., and Leonard, L. B.: Aphasics' comprehension of contextually conveyed meaning. Brain Lang., 6:362–377, 1978a.

Wilcox, M. J., Davis, G. A., and Leonard, L. B.: Diagnostic and treatment implications of an analysis of aphasic adults' contextual language comprehension. Clinical Aphasiology Conference Proceedings, 1978. Minneapolis: BRK Publishers, 1978b, pp. 247–254.

Yorkston, K. M., Marshall, R. C., and Butler, M. R.: Imposed delay of response: effects on aphasics' auditory comprehension of visually and non-visually cued material. Percept. Mot. Skills, 44:647–655, 1977.

6 • THE TREATMENT PROGRAM

Introduction
Where to Begin: Improving Input Processing
    Selecting an Appropriate Auditory
        Comprehension Task
    Determining Baseline Performance
    Keeping Record of Change
    Establishing a Criterion for
        Acceptable Performance
    Selecting a Simple Response Mode.
    An Array of Auditory Comprehension
        Tasks
    Graduated Reading Tasks
Moving On; Expressive Tasks
    A Hierarchy of Speaking Tasks
    Graduated Writing Tasks
Working with High-Level Patients
General Principles in Treatment
    Multiple Tasks Per Session
    Stimulation Plus
    Adjusting the Rate of Presentation
    Progress Through the Hierarchy of
        Difficulty
    Avoidance of Correction of Errors
    Relevance to the Patient's Needs
    Encouragement and Reward
    Adequate Intensity of Therapy
    The Clinician's Attitude
    The Patient with Multiple
        Communication Problems
Special Management Procedures
    Group Therapy
    PACE Therapy
    Melodic Intonation Therapy
    Working with Globally Aphasic
        Patients
    Possible Adjuncts to Therapy
The Family: Patient/Clinician
    Clarification of the Nature of the
        Problem and What to Expect
    How to Communicate with the
        Patient
    Helping the Spouse Cope
    The Family Member as Clinician
References

The clinician's role is not that of a teacher. . . . Rather the clinician tries to communicate with the patient and to stimulate disrupted processes to function maximally.

HILDRED SCHUELL

The time comes to design a program of treatment for the aphasic patient. In accomplishing the evaluation procedures outlined in Chapter 2, we have discerned the extent of the patient's language dysfunction; we have an estimate of the length and complexity of the message

237

that he can grasp and the adequacy of his response to the message. When we know what he cannot do in language processing and what he somehow manages to do in coping with his aphasia, we will be ready to embark upon a program designed to activate his brain functions with the goal of improving language processing capability.

What is involved in designing and carrying out a management program has been conceptualized by Wepman (1953). He suggests three parameters along which patients differ: stimulation, facilitation, and motivation. These guide us in our remedial program and ultimately determine its outcome.

As discussed in Chapter 5, it is necessary through *stimulation* to activate the brain to improved function. We design the stimulation so as to ensure that the stimuli are perceived by the brain.

We capitalize upon the readiness of the brain to be stimulated; the external stimulation brought to bear upon the patient "cannot effect a change in the patient unless he is in a state or set or condition which permits the integration to be made. When such a state does exist, the stimulation has its effect and the patient's efforts are *facilitated*." We exploit the opportunities that seem to indicate that the patient's nervous system is physiologically ready to respond.

The patient's psychologic readiness is the third essential for development of new neural integrations. The word *motivation* encompasses the psychologic readiness, "the level of goal-directed behavior possessed by the patient" — his drive to communicate, his desire to work at it, his capability to participate actively in the activities planned.

These three elements interact inextricably: "Therapy is organized, goal-directed stimulation, based upon a recognition of the patient's needs, his drives, his motivation. As stimulation is provided at a time when the organism is capable of response, it tends to facilitate neural integrations. If the direction of the stimulation at the proper time is in keeping with the patient's psychological state of readiness, if the stimulation is within the modality of language which meets the patient's needs, if the stimulation provides the end reward by realizable and recognizable goals of achievement, then success in therapy is more likely to follow" (Wepman, 1953).

The clinician's responsibility, therefore, is to design a patient-specific regimen of language stimulation, cognizant of the dimensions that heighten the arousal power of stimuli and maximize input to the brain; to present it according to a schedule that takes into account awareness of obstacles to the patient's performance and that exploits his capabilities to respond; to focus it at that level where failure threatens but success is possible; and to graduate it to broaden the patient's capabilities of response and provide rewarding communicative experiences. The program must be individually patterned, uniquely presented, continuously tailored to signs of progress and signals of failure.

WHERE TO BEGIN: IMPROVING INPUT PROCESSING

Selecting an Appropriate Auditory Comprehension Task. Tempting though it is to try to get the patient to talk better right away, we are well advised to concentrate first on auditory comprehension. As von Stockert (1978) points out, the major disadvantage of many therapy programs is that "they start with having the patient *say* something — but precisely this, in our experience, is the hardest job for him to do." We remember the evidence offered by Kushner and Winitz (1977) showing that "linguistic information should be firmly established in memory storage prior to training and retrieval." We recall the dictum offered by Schuell and co-workers (1964) that "auditory stimulation is crucial in control of language processes." We recall the fundamental clinical observations made by Schuell concerning the efficacy of auditory stimulation and the evidence supplied by Weigel-Crump and Koenigsknecht (1973) and by Helmick and Wipplinger (1975) confirming the efficacy of such a therapeutic strategy. We have reason to expect that every aphasic patient will have some degree of impairment of auditory comprehension. On the basis of all of these considerations, we begin with activities that provide auditory input whose goal is the increase of the patient's ability to recognize, discriminate, retain, sequence, and recall language units of increasing length and complexity.

The task to be selected first is one that involves a message of a length and complexity which the patient is just able to process. Recalling data concerning the deleterious effect of failure on the performance of an aphasic patient (Brookshire, 1972, 1976), we select a task which the patient can perform correctly but inefficiently, our intent being to improve efficiency and help the patient move on to a harder task which at present he cannot perform correctly. Basso (1978) emphasizes this point: "The best exercise is one that pushes the patient a little beyond his capabilities. The gap between what he can do and what he is asked to do should be small enough to be bridged by the facilitating techniques used in rehabilitation." Wepman makes the same point: "We must . . . construct a training program which frustrates him just beyond his presenting ability, that he may be led or guided toward his goal of communication" (1973).

Our test data tell us what such a task would be. A convenient way to think of it is in terms of the PICA multidimensional scale and the advice that Porch has offered about how to use test data in planning a program of therapy. A range of six values in the multidimensional scale represents responses that are correct but in some way short of perfect. The scale value of 13 represents a correct but *delayed* response; 12 indicates an *incomplete* response; 11 indicates an *incomplete delayed* response; 10 indicates that the patient spontaneously *corrected* an initially wrong response; 9 indicates that he required a *repetition* of the stimulus before he could respond correctly; 8 indicates that he needed additional *cuing*, some information beyond just repetition in order to respond correctly.

Our task is to review the various auditory comprehension subtests used in the evaluation instrument and determine the highest level of performance at which the patient was just failing of being completely correct. We select a task involving the presentation of stimuli of that simplicity level from among the Tasks AC1 through AC8 presented later in this chapter.

Determining Baseline Performance. Whatever task is selected initially, one must determine the baseline performance of the patient on that specific task. One can select a number of items of the type to be used in the task and present them to the patient to determine what percentage of them he responds to correctly. In connection with his presentation of the programmed stimulation method called Base-10, LaPointe (1977, 1978) suggests the use of ten items representative of the task. These should be administered two or three times within a session, deriving a mean score for the several performances, for if we are to measure progress from the baseline, we want to be reasonably sure that the baseline measurement is fairly stable.

Keeping Record of Change. As we use the therapy task in a program of rich repetitive stimulation, we should from time to time, probably daily, objectively reassess the patient's performance on this task. For this purpose we may again use the Base-10 Response Form developed by LaPointe (see Fig. 6–1) and re-present the ten baseline items. Performance on each of the ten items may be scored right or wrong (plus or minus) and the percentage correct determined, or further quantitative refinement can be introduced by using the PICA multidimensional scale, then summating the ten numerical values assigned and dividing by 15 (since 15 represents an accurate, prompt, complete, and efficiently produced response). This percentage is entered on the graph.

The periodic presentation of these ten baseline items does not constitute the therapy itself but is rather a probe used following therapy to determine its effect. As the same task is presented from day to day, the patient's successive scores on the baseline items can be determined and plotted on the graph portion of the form.

In a given therapy session, a number of tasks at the level selected can be chosen employing different materials but making use of essentially the same type of stimulation. For example, if one is operating at the level of Task AC1 described later (recognizing spoken words), one may engage in a period of therapy devoted to presentation of a given noun and may design a second, then a third, and possibly a fourth similar activity, presenting an adjective, a verb, or a preposition, in which the patient engages in the same type of active listening and makes the same kind of response as he made in the initial activity involving a noun. Probes can be presented with regard to each task at

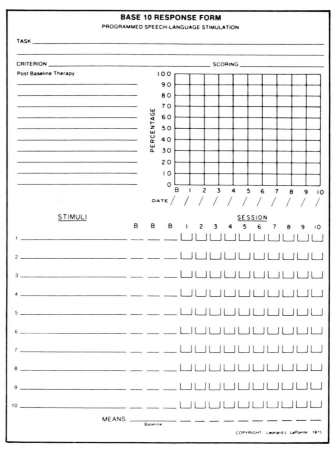

Figure 6–1. Base-10 Response Form designed by LaPointe (1977). Copyright 1975 by Leonard L. LaPointe.

the end of the session to determine the patient's level of performance.

Establishing a Criterion for Acceptable Performance. One continues the selected activity for as long as necessary to accomplish the desired gains. It is to be expected that as the task is presented repeatedly and the patient engages in a discriminative response to the items presented, his performance will gradually improve, and this improvement will be reflected on the Base-10 Response Form graph by a rising curve. To what level do we expect the curve to rise? A target of 100 per cent correct performance may be unrealistic, or it may be an unnecessary achievement, since the therapist would have done better to have moved on to a somewhat harder task. One may follow LaPointe's suggestion of a 90 per cent criterion, that is, the patient performing correctly on the baseline measure on 90 per cent of the items or better on three consecutive probes. However, the criterion to be established need not be inflexible. If a person achieves something less than 90 per cent correct performance — say, 75 or 80 per cent performance — and holds that level for several sessions, this plateau may be accepted and the decision made to move on to the next task despite the fact that the patient has not met the pre-established criterion. Thus we move on, graduating tasks in difficulty in such a manner that at each level the patient comes to experience success with a minimum amount of failure. If, however, the patient does not improve in his performance on the selected task over a number of sessions but continues to compile an impressive record of failures, the decision must be made to move back to the next simpler task and consolidate the patient's hold on that level of auditory processing.

Selecting a Simple Response Mode. After selecting a task at which the patient is just failing, we set the stage for him to succeed. In order to facilitate his performance, we must give him a way to respond that is not more difficult and threatening than the task itself. We do not measure the patient's ability to *recognize* single words by making him *say* those words; rather we select a response mode that is simpler — namely, having him point to an appropriate familiar picture or object. In all succeeding tasks we must remind ourselves to organize each task and select the response mode in such a way that when we measure patient performance, we are measuring ability to handle that task and not some *other* incidental task.

An Array of Auditory Comprehension Tasks. Following are eight tasks aimed at increasing the patient's ability to recognize, discriminate, retain, sequence, and recall what he hears and to process increasingly long and complex auditory linguistic units. The concepts and the words to be used in these tasks should relate to everyday activities and to the patient's needs and interests. A suggested lexicon of nouns, adjectives, verbs, and prepositions that might constitute the basic vocabulary for these activities is presented in Table 6–1. In the case of nouns, adjectives, and verbs, pairs of words are given that constitute opposites and from which the patient can select the word to be presented at a given time. The patient's discrimination between the contrasting words is tested, particularly in Task AC1, requiring the recognition of spoken words and forcing the patient to point to one or another picture in selective response to the verbal stimulus. This vocabulary can also be extended for use in the tasks that follow, so that repetition of the items in the basic lexicon constitutes a further reinforcement of the patient's recall.

Task AC1: Recognizing Spoken Words. Select a pair of words, for example, "box-book," and present one of the words in a series of phrases or sentences, accompanying the verbal stimulus with appropriate pairs of pictures or objects. Ask the patient to point to the appropriate picture or object in each case. If he fails to point appropri-

Table 6–1 A SUGGESTED LEXICON FOR INPUT STIMULATION

NOUNS	ADJECTIVES	VERBS	PREPOSITIONS
spoon-fork	big-little	sit up-lie down	on
knife-hammer	red-blue	sleep-wake	in
boy-girl	green-yellow	cut-sew	beside
cup-glass	black-white	find-lose	inside
bed-dresser	hot-cold	break-fix	under
mother-dad	early-late	cook-eat	near
milk-coffee	sick-well	walk-run	on top of
chair-table	old-new	read-write	after
bread-water	old-young	listen-talk	before
house-garage	clean-dirty	plant-pick	to right of
dog-cat	broken-good	wash-dry	to left of
coat-pants	soft-hard	take off-put on	up
dress-hat	wet-dry	sit-stand	down
shoes-stockings	sweet-sour	give-take	away from
hand-foot	tall-short	pick up-put down	through
tree-flower	fast-slow	pull-push	above
box-book	fat-skinny	love-hate	below
paper-wood	short-long	win-lose	off
man-woman	raw-cooked	fill-empty	behind
radio-TV	round-flat	build-tear down	in front of

ately, the clinician points, repeats the stimulus, and proceeds to the next stimulus. The patient must not listen passively to the stimulus but actively and discriminatively, and must respond every time by pointing.

For example, if one selected the pair "box-book" and the target word "box," one might present the following and other stimuli, asking the patient to point to a picture of the box or the box itself in each case:

a box of Kleenex   the box of firewood

a big box   a new box

a box of matches   a black box

a box of Wheaties   he broke the box

a yellow box   she found the box

the box is broken   a paper box

it's an old box   mail the box

this box is pretty   you can sit on this box

this is a wooden box   this box is cardboard

put the papers in the box   put the pencils in the box

Later one might use the word "book" as the target word and present stimuli such as the following:

read the book	this book has lots of pages
a little book	the book is torn
a red book	this book got wet
a book with a red cover	she lost her book
where's the book	read the children a book
the book is under the table	she tore up the book
a paperback book	the book got dirty
a hardcover book	fix the book
it's an old book	have you read this book?
find your book	Johnny sat on the book

Extend the work on recognition of spoken words beyond nouns to the other parts of speech shown. For example, one might select the adjective pair "big-little" and the target word "big," presenting stimuli such as the following:

This one is the big car.	The coat was too big.
This child is big.	This is a big house.
Use the big dish pan.	That is a very big tree.
Use the big box.	Take the big knife.
He is a big man.	This car is big.

In each case the patient points to the correct picture or object in the pair presented to him.

Or selecting the verb pair "read-write" and the target word "read," the following can be used:

We read books.	Read the newspaper.
Let's read the big book.	He must read the sign.
Mother will read to the baby.	He will read the letter.
He is going to read in bed.	They're going to read together.
The girl likes to read.	They're reading a story.

In working with prepositions, present pairs of pictures to the patient and ask him to point to the one that represents the correct preposition. Using the target "on":

The book is on the box.	The cup is on the shelf.
The cup is on the table.	The teakettle is on the stove.
The cat is on the bed.	The hamburger is on the plate.
The child is running on the sidewalk.	The cat is on the roof.
The car is on the street.	The pillow is on the bed.

Task AC2: Processing Series of Two and Three Words. Arrange a group of eight pictures or eight objects on the table in front of the patient. Name two of the items and ask the patient to point to them in the same order as they are named:

spoon and book	hammer and box
knife and fork	cup and spoon
cup and glass	knife and hammer
book and box	box and spoon
spoon and knife	fork and glass

Use the same procedure for a series of two adjectives, using pictures:

red and yellow	white and flat
black and white	green and red
round and flat	blue and yellow
flat and blue	round and red
yellow and round	green and black

For verbs:

walking and reading	cutting and sewing
pulling and sewing	pulling and pushing
cutting and writing	walking and running
running and pushing	writing and sewing
reading and writing	pushing and reading

When the patient passes the criterion level for processing two items, move on to stimuli requiring the processing of three items in succession, increasing the number of pictures or objects presented as foils.

Task AC3: Executing One-Step Commands. Place an array of eight objects or pictures in front of the patient and ask him to perform a series of single actions:

Point to the dress.	Touch the knife.
Show me the bed.	Point to the hat.
Pick up the radio.	Show me the TV.
Give me the spoon.	Tap the spoon.
Pick up the fork.	Turn over the dress.

Using the environment of the room and the patient's own person, ask him to perform a series of one-step tasks:

Point to the window.	Point to the light.
Look at the floor.	Look at the ceiling.
Make a fist.	Close your eyes.
Raise your hand.	Touch your chin.
Show me a button.	Show me the door.

Task AC4: Executing One-Step, Three-Unit Commands. Present an array of pictures or objects to the patient and ask him to perform a series of single activities each of which requires the manipulation of two objects in some manner indicated by the verb or the preposition:

Put the book in the box.	Put the flower in the vase.
Put the book on top of the box.	Put the stockings on top of the shoes.
Put the book under the box.	Put the bed beside the dresser.
Put the book to the right of the box.	Put the paper under the table.
Put the spoon in the cup.	Put the radio in front of the dresser.

Task AC5: Executing Two-Step Commands. Using objects, pictures, or the patient's person and the contents of the room, ask him to perform two activities in succession, in the same order as the instruction is given:

Give me the spoon and take the fork.

Point to the milk and give me the glass.

Give me the picture of the baby sleeping and turn over the picture of the child running.

Look at the ceiling and point to the floor.

Show me the light and give me the fork.

Point to the bed and shake hands with me.

Touch the knife and look at the window.

Take the cup and give me the spoon.

Tap the table and close your eyes.

Point to the door and give me the cup.

Task AC6: Executing Complex Commands. Using pictures, objects, and the contents of the room, present a series of commands that involve the understanding of subordinate clauses or modifying phrases or critical prepositions and conjunctions for their correct execution:

After pointing to the broken glass, show me the good glass.

Before you give me the red ball, point to the blue ball.

If the light is on, point to it.

Show me the lady cooking, but first show me the one sewing.

Touch your nose without using your right hand.

When I tap the table, point to the flowers.

If there is something round on the table, give it to me.

After raising your hand, look at the door.

When I point to you, give me the spoon.

Give me the fork after your give me the hammer.

Task AC7: Answering Yes/No Questions About Pictures. Show the patient a series of pictures, each illustrating people performing various activities such as those listed under verbs in Table 6–1, as well as objects represented by nouns on the list and possessing characteristics described by adjectives on the list. Ask the patient to answer each question that you ask by "yes" or "no":

Is Dusty asleep?

Is the window broken?

Is the man tall?

Is the tree yellow?

Is the milk white?

Is there a cup on the table?

Is the little girl listening to Dad reading a book?

Is Jane taking off her shoes?

Is Emily under the table?

Is Edith cooking?

TASK AC8: Answering Questions about Oral Sentences and Paragraphs. Present the patient with a series of sentences. After each ask a relevant question to be answered "yes" or "no":

Claire dropped the vase on the floor and it smashed into a million pieces. Did the vase break?

Charles put on his underwear, shirt, and pants. Did Charles get undressed?

The Twins beat the White Sox. Did the White Sox win?

The doctor made mother stay in bed for several days. Did mother cook dinner during that time?

The center on our basketball team is seven feet tall. Is he a short man?

Mother cooked the cauliflower for 20 minutes. Did we eat it raw?

Sue put the car in the garage. Did the car stay in front of the house all night?

Their house was totally destroyed by fire. Did a flood wash away the house?

Brian drove to New York. Did he go by plane?

Jesse was hospitalized for a week. Did he require medical attention?

The senator won the election. Was the senator elected?

Similarly, read aloud a series of stories, each consisting of six to eight sentences. Then ask the patient to answer yes/no questions based upon the salient points of each story.

Graduated Reading Tasks. In the auditory comprehension tasks presented earlier, visual materials were used but no letters or words requiring reading. As we embark on reading tasks, we now use auditory stimuli coupled with visual linguistic stimuli. Again we have a hierarchy of difficulty beginning with something as simple as single letters progressing to comprehension of paragraphs.

Task R1: Recognizing Letters. Present an array of six large printed letters for the patient to examine. Ask the patient to point to the letters in succession. Similarly use a second array of six other letters, then a third.

Now present two arrays of the same six letters in different arrangements. Ask the patient to match the letters which are alike in the two arrays.

Present the patient with an individual printed letter and ask him to place it on top of the corresponding letter in one of the arrays used previously.

Task R2: Reading Single Words. Present the patient with two words printed in large letters separately on individual cards, using one-syllable words from the list in Table 6–1. Name one of the words and ask the patient to point to the corresponding printed word. Later, arrange arrays of six to eight words on cards, and ask the patient to point to given words named by the clinician.

Follow the same procedure with two-syllable words selected from Table 6–1.

Follow the same procedure in getting the patient to listen for and find the printed equivalent of three-syllable words chosen from what might be expected to be the patient's everyday vocabulary.

Task R3: Matching Words and Pictures. Select pictures from the activities used in auditory comprehension tasks and print corresponding words on separate cards. Present an array of pictures, four to begin with, six and eight subsequently, and ask the patient to match individual words to the pictures, saying each word as you present it.

Task R4: Pointing to Two Words in Sequence. Prepare an array of eight words selected from Table 6–1 and ask the patient to point in sequence to two words named by the clinician. Do the same for another array of words on a card, and move on to an arrangement of 12 to 15 individual words on the table; ask the patient to select a series of two named by the clinician.

Task R5: Arranging Words into a Phrase. Prepare cards containing words which when arranged in proper order constitute familiar phrases. Present these words randomly to the patient and ask him to arrange them in proper order, using words selected from Table 6–1:

cup of coffee	through the door
a black dog	a big box
a green tree	an old chair
a soft bed	a clean spoon
lie down in bed	a broken hammer
put on your pants	sit in the chair
a little boy	fill the box
under the table	build a house

Task R6: Executing Short Printed Commands. Print a series of short one-step commands for the patient to read and execute. The prepositions presented in Table 6–1, together with a number of objects or pictures, constitute good stimulus materials for this activity:

Point to the book.	Put the book inside the box.
Put the fork beside the spoon.	Point to the window.
Hold up your hand.	Look at the light.
Give me the hammer.	Ring the bell.
Put the cup beside the glass.	Give me the pencil.
Put the fork in the box.	Look under the table.
Put the spoon beside the box.	Make a fist.
Put the red square under the green square.	

Task R7: Reading Short Paragraphs. Prepare a series of three-sentence paragraphs, each containing factual material pertaining to a single subject. Ask the patient to answer questions about these paragraphs by responding orally "yes" or "no," nodding, or pointing to appropriate pictures related to the story:

Mother was in the kitchen fixing lunch. Peggy was playing on the floor with some pots and pans. Smoky the cat was begging to be fed, too. Questions: Was the family getting ready for breakfast? Was there more than one person in the kitchen? Did the family have a pet? Was Peggy doing the cooking?

Dad took the car down to the filling station. He wanted to fill it up with gasoline. Johnny went along for the ride. Questions: Was mother driving the car? Did Dad go to the filling station alone? Was the car being taken in for repairs?

In all of the previously described activities pertaining to auditory comprehension and reading, no demand has been made upon the patient to speak other than to respond "yes" or "no." We should not be in a hurry to work on or "force" spoken responses to any of the materials being used or any of the questions being asked. We should let these come as the patient is able to make such responses, and it is reasonable to expect that they will as the patient's comprehension is strengthened and his recall of basic vocabulary improves. At intervals during the carrying out of the auditory comprehension and reading activities, one might probe the patient's ability to name the pictures and to read the words. Ten-item probes can be built from among the vocabulary in Table 6–1. Ask the patient to name ten pictures, recording his performance on a Base-10 Response Form; ask him to read ten words aloud, and similarly record his score. This procedure can be repeated periodically to determine the patient's spontaneous gains in expressive ability despite the fact that oral expression has not been specifically worked on up to this point.

MOVING ON: EXPRESSIVE TASKS

Initial therapy endeavors have been directed toward establishing a firm base of comprehension on the part of the patient, first of auditory comprehension and then of comprehension of visual linguistic stimuli. In the usual course of events we would expect the patient's expressive performance to improve simultaneously without our concentrating on it. Now we are ready to proceed to tasks in which the primary focus is expression — first oral expression, then written. In trying to help the patient accomplish more efficient output, we have the opportunity to use multiple input channels; we ask the patient to listen as we read together words and sentences in preparation for the patient's making an oral response; he listens as he looks at a picture and then produces an oral response; he looks at a printed word, hears us say it, and then in response uses it alone or in a familiar expression or writes it; he may himself read it and say it and then follow with a written response. We use each modality to reinforce the other modalities and to move the patient toward more effective use of all modalities.

It may be necessary with given patients to begin expression work at a one-word level. The emphasis will not be on elicitation of the word as a single entity but rather on facilitation of his retrieval of the word for use in longer, more meaningful units. However, to do this we may need to determine what words are readily available to him, what words he is able to retrieve part of the time, and what words he seems unable to retrieve. It will be useful, then, to establish a kind of baseline for this expressive use of words — whether nouns, adjectives, verbs, prepositions, conjunctions, or other words. For this purpose, we may find it useful to follow the suggestions of Croskey and Adams (1969) for selection of words for practice in oral expression. We select a body of words, perhaps those in Table 6–1 and others, and present them to the patient for determination of which words he is able to evoke on two successive trials; we run through the entire list twice to determine which words he can produce correctly both times, which words he can produce once, and which words he cannot produce either time. It is easy to elicit nouns in this procedure by showing the patient pictures of things or objects; we will need to adopt a procedure for eliciting adjectives, verbs, prepositions, and other words such as showing him a picture, presenting a sentence, or asking the patient to complete a sentence by supplying the desired target word. ("This man is not short; he is _____"; "When you lose money, someone will surely _____ it.")

Having determined the hierarchy of knowledge of these words, we will probably elect not to work for the present on the words that the patient was unable to retrieve either time; we will probably concentrate our attention upon those words which he was able to produce once but not twice, and in order to facilitate his production of those words, we will make use of the words he produced twice, using them to build the stimulus sentences.

A Hierarchy of Speaking Tasks
Task S1: Completing Sentences with Single Words. Using appropriate pictures or objects for the words selected, present for each word an incomplete sentence, inviting the patient to supply the target word to complete the sentence. We can do this with nouns:

The dog chased the_____.

The fork ran away with
    the_____.

She put the book in the_____.

Mother is watching_____.

I'll have a glass of_____.

When you're thirsty, have a
    drink of_____.

On Easter, mother wore her
    nicest dress and a
    new_____.

You cut with a knife and pound
    with a_____.

When we're tired, we go
    to_____.

I'll have a cup of_____.

The flag is red, white,
    and_____.

I'd rather fly than take the train
    because the train is
    too_____.

We can cook the carrots or we
    can eat them_____.

That shirt isn't clean; it's
    really_____.

Put it in the washer so we can
    get it_____.

The world isn't flat; it's_____.

Grass is_____.

If she eats too much, she'll
    get_____.

It's two feet wide and three
    feet_____.

Do the same with adjectives:

In summer the leaves are green,
    and in fall they turn_____.

Do the same for verbs using pictures to illustrate the intended activity:

I'm going to_____.

I want to_____.

I can_____.

I must_____.

Or we can use other open-ended sentences:

I'll wash the dishes and you can_____ them.

At night you go to sleep and in the morning you_____.

It is easier to push than to_____.

This glass is very fragile so please don't_____it.

My glass is empty; please_____it.

For once our team didn't_____; it_____.

Don't walk to the store; please_____.

I'm going to write a letter with my_____.

When you are tired you should_____.

The lamp is broken; can you_____it?

Do the same with prepositions, referring to appropriate pictures:

The book is_____the box.

The lamp is_____the table.

The cat is asleep_____the bed.

They're going to climb_____the stairs.

She is not in front of him; she is_____him.

The car rolled_____the hill.

This box isn't underneath the sofa; it's_____the sofa.

The garage is_____the house.

The clothes are_____the drawer.

Put the dirty dishes_____the sink.

Task S2: Completing Sentences Using Adjective Plus Noun.
We explain to the patient that in response to a series of pictures a more complete expression is called for, the target noun plus an appropriate adjective:

They live in a *small house*.

This pet is a *fat cat*.

It's a *red car*.

This is a *little boy*.

It's a *tall tree*.

She carried a *little box*.

It's a *soft bed*.

He played with a *yellow ball*.

It's a *broken cup*.

He cut his meat with a *sharp knife*.

If the patient is unable to supply both words, the clinician can show the picture and say the appropriate sentence, then ask the patient to join in saying the whole sentence in unison, after which the clinician can show the picture, present the beginning of the sentence, and ask the patient to supply the two-word ending.

Task S3: Supplying Opposites.
Using the contrasting words suggested in Table 6–1 or others, present a word in a sentence and ask

the patient to supply its opposite in order to complete the second part of the sentence:

This tree isn't tall; it's_____.

This snowball isn't hot; it's_____.

It's not mother holding the baby; it's_____.

Mother isn't cutting up the material; she's_____it.

This child doesn't feel well; he feels_____.

They're not listening to the radio; they're watching_____.

This speaker doesn't want to listen; he wants to_____.

These dishes aren't dirty; they're_____.

She is not pulling the wagon, she's_____it.

This lemonade isn't sweet; it's_____.

As the patient develops skill in supplying the target words, ask him to go an extra step and produce the whole sentence after completing the target word: "This isn't tall; it's *short*. Now you say the whole thing."

Task S4: Completing Two Parts of a Sentence. Using appropriate pictures, present the patient with the opportunity to supply spontaneously both the noun and the adjective in a construction of the following type:

The *knife* is *sharp*.

The *coffee* is *hot*.

The *cup* is *broken*.

The *ice cream* is *cold*.

The *coat* is *torn*.

The *pants* are *dirty*.

The *house* is *red*.

The *man* is *old*.

The *fork* is *dirty*.

The *trees* are *green*.

The clinician can extend the procedure by then asking the patient in each case, "What thing are we talking about?" The patient responds, "The knife." Then the clinician asks, "Is the knife dull or sharp?" The patient answers, "Sharp." Clinician: "Tell me the whole thing again," and shows the picture to elicit "The knife is sharp."

Task S5: Answering Questions Using Sentences. Showing appropriate pictures, the clinician asks a series of questions, inviting the patient to answer the question by supplying the correct word but using it in a sentence:

"What barks?" Patient: "A dog barks."

"Who cooks dinner?" "My wife cooks dinner."

"Where do we sleep?" "We sleep in a bed."

What do we eat ice cream with?

What do you put in your coffee?

Where do we put the car?

What do we do with seeds?

Where do we keep the matches?

What do we sit on?

What kind of pet does she have?

What did she do to the glass?

What's he doing with his clothes?

What's he doing with that pencil?

Where did she put the towels?

Task S6: Using Prepositions.   Using pairs of objects which can be manipulated relative to each other, ask questions which require the patient to use an appropriate preposition: "Where is the book?" (The book is in the box. The book is under the box. The book is on top of the box. The book is to the right of the box. The book is to the left of the box. The book is beside the box.) "Where is the spoon?" (The spoon is in the cup. The spoon is beside the cup. The spoon is in front of the cup. The spoon is behind the cup. The spoon is on top of the cup.)

Task S7: Answering Questions About Pictures.   Use a series of pictures representing situations involving several people doing a variety of activities. Ask the patient to answer questions about the characters and the situation: Where are they? How many people are there in the picture? What's mother doing? Are there any animals around? What time of day is it? Which one is the oldest? What's going to happen? If the patient is unable to answer a question, supply the answer in a sentence and later repeat the question, endeavoring to elicit a similar formulation of the answer on the part of the patient.

Task S8: Answering Questions About Self, Family, and Everyday Information.   Ask the patient a series of questions involving almost "automatic" answers: Where you are now? What time is it? How old are you? How old is your spouse? How many children do you have? How old are they? What day is today? What month is this? What year is this? Who is the president of the United States? Where does the president live in Washington? What number comes after 13? What month follows June? In what month do we celebrate Christmas? In what month do we celebrate Thanksgiving Day? In what room do you eat your meals at home? What do we call the first meal of the day? What are the other meals called? What do you like to drink with your meals? What TV programs do you like to watch?

Task S9: Formulating Sentences in Response to Pictures.   Show the patient a series of pictures portraying people and animals doing things. Ask the patient to describe who or what is doing what task. If the patient is unable to formulate the response, ask a leading question; then ask the patient to restate the information about who is doing what.

Graduated Writing Tasks.

Task W1: Copying Words. Using a selection of words from all grammatical categories in Table 6–1, present the patient with a written word. Ask him to read it aloud, spell it, and then copy it three times.

Task W2: Finding Two Words Embedded in One. Present the patient with a series of written or printed words in which two words are joined:

gingerbread	brokenhearted
mailman	bluebonnet
snowman	washpans
newspaper	breakwater
breadstick	afterthought
football	downcast
flowerbed	stairway

Ask the patient to say the whole word, to say the two component words separately, and to write these words separately, saying them as he writes them.

Task W3: Writing Words Spontaneously in Response to Pictures. Using the stimulus pictures representing nouns, adjectives, and verbs that were used in earlier activities, ask the patient to say and to write each target word spontaneously. If the patient is unable to produce the word and write it, present an open-ended sentence, which should elicit the word, tell him the word, spell it for him, and then ask him to write it.

Task W4: Writing Sentences in Response to Pictures. Present a series of pictures showing persons and animals engaged in activities; ask the patient to write one or more sentences about each picture explaining who or what is doing what. By a series of questions, the clinician can elicit from the patient expressions of greater length and greater complexity of structure, and can build into this activity words of increasing length and unfamiliarity.

WORKING WITH HIGH-LEVEL PATIENTS

The kinds of procedures that have been outlined previously may not be difficult or challenging enough for patients who have recovered to a significant degree but who may still not be completely whole in language function; they may still have subtle comprehension deficits, experience some delays in word retrieval, or lack morphosyntactic finesse. They may benefit from activities calculated to stimulate thinking and keep the flow of ideas going (Wepman, 1972, 1976). Following are tasks that may help keep these patients moving ahead and content with trying to improve their language skills. Other suggestions have been presented by Darley and others (1980).

Task HL1: Divergent Language Behavior Tasks.   Encourage the patient to engage in a wide-ranging search of language storage by asking him to perform a series of tasks that elicit divergent language behavior. Table 6–2 lists tasks of this type.

Task HL2: Formulating a Précis of Heard Information.   Read to the patient a paragraph consisting of three or four sentences organized into a coherent essay, such as the following:

> In A.D. 64 the city of Rome was almost completely destroyed by fire. The emperor Nero blamed the Christians for it. Many of them were executed as arsonists.

Ask the patient to present a summary of this paragraph incorporating in his own words as many of the salient facts as he can recall. When he has finished, review the paragraph with him to find out what omissions he made. Use a series of such paragraphs to improve the patient's retention and recall and capacity to abstract from material he has heard.

Task HL3: Formulating a Précis of Read Paragraph-Length Material.   Have the patient read a three- or four-sentence paragraph to himself, after which he is to give a précis incorporating as many as possible of the salient points in the paragraph. Review each paragraph with the patient to indicate his omissions.

Task HL4: Describing a Situation Picture.   Present a series of pictures to the patient representing people or animals doing things. Ask the patient while viewing each picture to describe it fully, including all possible details.

Task HL5: Scrambled Sentences.   Present to the patient a series of sentences, in each of which the words have been randomized. Ask him to arrange the words in the proper order in order to constitute the proverb: "a flock of feather together birds" becomes "birds of a feather flock together;" "saves a time in nine stitch" becomes "a stitch in time saves nine." After the patient has arranged the words in the proper order, ask him to explain the proverb, to abstract the meaning of each.

Task HL6: Building Sentences from Three Words.   Present to the patient three words and ask him to build from them a meaningful, coherent, complete sentence:

photograph, identify, murder   bluejays, birdseed, feeder

color blind, signal light, railroad   predator, victim, tiger
    crossing
                                  dust, vacuum cleaner, wind

bus, passengers, baggage

Table 6–2 ACTIVITIES TO FACILITATE
DIVERGENT LANGUAGE BEHAVIOR

---

1. Think of all the words that rhyme with each of these words:

cat	man
dime	sick
paste	fire
chum	cane
ship	pile
sail	pill
child	door
stack	aim

2. Think of all the things you can possibly do with each of the following:

a book	a piece of string
a piece of chalk	an empty peanut butter jar
a can of spray paint	a battery
a screwdriver	Scotch tape
an ice pick	a piece of Kleenex
an empty coffee can	a nail
a gunny sack	a button
a match	a slice of bread
an old nylon stocking	poker chips

3. List all the items you can in each of these categories:

ways we can use leather	things we see in the water
furniture in your home	spherical objects
things we sit on	holidays (and reasons for celebrating them)
items in your bathroom cabinet	foreign cities
things we use in cooking	presidents of the United States
ways to fix hamburger meat	comedy entertainers
spices and condiments	magazine titles
kinds of buildings	movie stars
beverages	TV programs
weapons used to murder someone	comic strips
card games	colors and tints
things with holes in them	big United States industries
things that come in cardboard boxes	compass points
writing materials	things that roll
things we buy in jars	kinds of balls
household things made of wood	items of hardware
parts of a car	types of containers
articles of clothing	sections of a large Sunday newspaper
things colored yellow; blue; black; white; red	materials used in making clothing
	ways to fix eggs
things we see in the sky	wh- words

4. As in item 3, first think of items that belong in the larger category, then of items that belong in the subcategories:

United States cities:	Airlines:
state capitals	domestic
port cities	foreign
Parts of the body:	Regions of the United States
external	New England
internal	Mid-Atlantic
Birds:	South
song birds	Midwest
game birds	Southeast
predators	Rocky Mountain
Sports:	Pacific Coast
spectator	Musical instruments:
contact	reed

Table 6–2 ACTIVITIES TO FACILITATE
DIVERGENT LANGUAGE BEHAVIOR *(Continued)*

Sports:	Musical instruments:
one-on-one	string
using balls	percussion
using implements	Authors and poets:
Countries:	American
North American	British
South American	other
Central American	Foods:
European	fruit
Asian	kinds of soup
African	beverages
Common brands:	canned juices
canned foods	meats
beer	Animals:
automobiles	wild
Baseball teams:	domesticated
American League	climbers
National League	animals with horns
Modes of transportation:	animals that supply us with
water	something useful
air propelled	Words that begin with given letters:
wheeled	m l
Trees:	b d
deciduous	k z
non–deciduous	

In each case, after the patient has created a sentence, ask him if he can rearrange the words to form a second sentence of equal validity.

Task HL7: Discourse on Selected Topics. Present the patient with a topic on which he can be expected to speak at some length:

Where would you like to go on vacation? Why?

How did you come to choose your vocation? Who was influential in your choice?

What is your favorite recreational activity? How did you happen to get into this hobby and what does it mean to you?

Task HL8: Describing Activities. Ask the patient to describe systematically and completely how certain activities are performed:

starting a fire in a fireplace

fixing a leaky faucet

traveling from home to work

making baking powder biscuits

making popcorn

the sequence of the church service

making a cake

doing the laundry

scoring a bowling game

finding a city on a map

Task HL9: Playing Columnist. Select items from the "Dear Abby" or "Ann Landers" newspaper columns and read them to the patient. Ask the patient to state how he would answer each query.

Task HL10: Ascribing Ideas to People. Ask the patient to state what idea or ideas are associated with well-known public or historical figures: Franklin D. Roosevelt, Woodrow Wilson, Pablo Picasso, Adolph Hitler, Jesus Christ, Henry Thoreau, Thomas Jefferson, Karl Marx, Mahatma Ghandi.

Task HL11: Listing Similes and Metaphors. Ask the patient to think of as many similes or metaphorical expressions as possible concerning each of a number of categories:

animals: fat as a pig, wise as an owl, quick as a fox
colors: red as a beet, a brown study, a yellow streak, white as snow
body parts: stiff-necked, tight-fisted, a bare-faced lie, sharp-eyed

Task HL12: Making Grammatical Transformations. Present the patient with sentences and ask him to transform them in designated ways.

A. Convert declarative statements into questions and questions into declarative statements.
B. Convert a series of three simple sentences into a single complex sentence.
C. Change a present affirmative sentence to past negative; an active affirmative sentence to passive negative; a present active affirmative sentence to past passive negative (The bakery makes good cakes → Good cakes were not made by the bakery).

GENERAL PRINCIPLES IN TREATMENT

Multiple Tasks Per Session. It is usually possible in the course of a single session (30 to 60 minutes long) to plan several tasks of the types outlined above. Depending upon the patient's level of performance, one may use several tasks within a given modality or may present tasks from different modalities, in each case at a level appropriate for that particular modality performance. One will usually want to arrange the tasks so that the patient experiences considerable success at the beginning of the session and to plan a task at the end of the session which reassures the patient that he is able to perform and allows him to leave in a glow of achievement. Time should be allotted for accomplishing the Base-10 probes applicable to each task incorporated in a day's session — if not daily, then at frequent enough intervals to keep detailed track of progress.

Stimulation Plus. The activities already outlined all constitute a form of stimulation, programmed so as to challenge the patient at the level he is now and help him move on to tasks that are harder and harder. But there is more to it than simply providing something for the patient to listen to or look at. In every case the patient is asked to respond to each stimulus. He is not asked only to listen but to listen and choose a response, if nothing more complicated than simply pointing to the picture matching the auditory stimulus or nodding. He is asked not only to recognize a spoken or a written word but to discriminate between it and another word; this is the reason for the contrasting words suggested in Table 6–1. The patient, then, is an active participant in therapy, not a passive observer of it. If the patient cannot respond or does not respond appropriately, the clinician indicates what the response should be and moves on to the next stimulus.

Adjusting the Rate of Presentation. In every task the stimuli are presented in sequence at a rate appropriate to the patient's ability to respond. Give the patient plenty of time to listen, read, select, ponder, and respond. By definition the aphasic patient requires more processing time, so we patiently allow it and avoid rushing on to the next stimulus or too quickly prompting with the same stimulus. A leisurely pace helps the patient gain confidence in his responses; a feeling of haste to cover more ground may "throw sand in his gears."

Progress Through the Hierarchy of Difficulty. The clinician keeps track of the patient's progress on each task. He has established a criterion level of performance so he knows when the patient is doing as well as might reasonably be expected on that task. The patient's performance provides the cue to moving on to a more difficult task in the hierarchy. The clinician may want to backtrack intermittently to probe the patient's performance on a simpler task to see whether he is maintaining his earlier gains. Records allow the clinician to know exactly what the patient can do and how well. If the patient fails to make gains on a given task, indicating that he is stalled at a low level of performance on it, it is appropriate to step backward and resume work on a task of lesser difficulty for the time being. Records of the patient's day-to-day performance provide documentation of why he is doing what he is doing; thus, the clinician can provide accountability for his therapy plan with quantitative data far superior to a subjective impression that the patient "seems" to be doing better and "perhaps" is ready to try something harder.

Avoidance of Correction of Errors. The patient inevitably makes errors when introduced to a new task. Little purpose is served by pointing out what his errors were and explaining what he should have done. A better procedure is simply to supply the correct answer and move on to the next stimulus. The goal is to elicit more and more responses to language input without regard to the correctness of individual responses. In general, patients are unable to use explanations of their errors and are made uncomfortable when stress is on correctness (witness the experience of Holland and Sonderman [1974]).

So the clinician presents 15, 20, 25, or 30 stimuli on a given task, asking for a response every time, supplying the correct response if the patient cannot, but not making a big production of a failure.

Relevance to the Patient's Needs. We will probably help a patient most if we plan therapy activities so as to relate to his interests and everyday needs. The language we stimulate with and the language we try to elicit should be functional language, and the therapy activities should be functionally related to everyday life. If a patient has not written a letter for the last 30 years, it will probably not be useful to devote much therapy time to writing. If the patient almost never reads, activities might better be planned to focus on listening and speaking activities, on which the patient depends.

It follows that we should probably avoid certain activities, such as those that have almost no bearing on what we do linguistically in daily life. We almost never go about naming things, and we almost never repeat what somebody else says. Therapy activities that focus on naming and those that require repetition may impress the patient as artificial and irrelevant. We do relatively little reading aloud, nor do we write much to dictation; our reading is usually silent reading for ourselves and our writing is usually to convey a message spontaneously to someone else. It is probably advisable, then, to avoid naming, repetition, reading aloud, or writing to dictation activities, what Basso (1978) has called "transposition tasks" involving translation of a message from one modality to another. These activities have little communicative value and are not likely to impress patients with their usefulness.

Encouragement and Reward. Whatever the therapy activity, the clinician should see to it that the patient knows how he is doing and that he feels good about his performance. Each time the patient performs correctly, the clinician may nod and smile or say "yes" or in some other way indicate that the response was appropriate. If the response was in error, the clinician supplies the correct response without announcing a patient failure. Feedback about the patient's performance should be continuous and immediate. (Brookshire [1971] has shown that even relatively short delays in providing reinforcement can adversely affect the performance of aphasic patients.) At first reinforcement should be provided after every response. Later it may be possible for the clinician to provide it less frequently. The clinician can share with the patient knowledge of his progress from day to day by showing him curves on the Base-10 Record Forms or by playing back to him tape-recorded samples of his past and present performance, giving him tangible evidence that he is improving.

Adequate Intensity of Therapy. Clearly the benefits that accrue from therapy depend upon scheduling treatment in a quantity and a concentration that provide significant impact upon the patient's nervous system. Homeopathic dosage — half an hour once a week or an occasional check on what the patient is doing on his own — will fail. Data reviewed in Chapter 4 show clearly that when degrees of improvement of treated and untreated patients are contrasted, the greatest contrasts have resulted from therapy regimens with sessions held daily or at least three times a week. We can use our Base-10 documentation to justify the expenditure of time and money required to achieve measurable gains in limited time spans.

The Clinician's Attitude. The clinician must perform as an interested, alert participant in each activity, revealing by facial expression, bodily posture, and words that he is sincerely interested in what the patient is doing and pleased with his participation in therapy. His tone should be encouraging, optimistic, and subtly indicative of the fact that he expects the very best to happen. He should be endlessly attentive, sensitive to the attitude of the patient as he responds. The clinician continually provides information to the patient, gives insight about his performance, and offers encouragement. He helps to assuage the patient's tendencies to self-criticism, self-punishment, anxiety, and despair. His manner should be supportive and nonprovocative. He schedules the language stimulation so as to convey to the patient that his problem is understood and can be dealt with constructively; he lets the patient know that it is being dealt with currently in the most appropriate way. These attitudes and activities on the part of the clinician constitute an essential ingredient of the clinical situation. They perhaps make as much difference as the activities themselves in bringing about improvement of the patient's performance.

The Patient with Multiple Communicative Problems. Some aphasic patients display an associated apraxia of speech, and others may be dysarthric. The question arises as to which problem the clinician should focus his attention on — the language disorder or the motor speech disorder. The decision is an individual one and depends upon the relative severity of the component communicative problems. If the patient is severely aphasic, with evident severe restriction of auditory and visual input, one will probably want to put emphasis first upon language processing, selecting tasks from the suggested receptive activities. If the input is less restricted and the patient's inability to generate an easy oral response is an extremely frustrating obstacle to him, one might concentrate early on reteaching motor patterns. It is often desirable to work on both kinds of problems in the course of a therapy session, devoting part of the period to relearning of motor patterns and part to increasing understanding of language input. The problems are separate problems and must be dealt with separately. It is not to be expected that by concentrating on his aphasia, the patient's apraxia will automatically improve or that by relearning motor patterns the patient will automatically be able to handle longer auditory messages. The distinctions emphasized in Chapter 1 are fundamental in this regard. Which problem is to be treated first or what relative amounts of time are to be devoted to each problem will be determined by an estimate of the patient's overall communication skills and his most pressing needs in functional communication.

SPECIAL MANAGEMENT PROCEDURES

Group Therapy. The language problems of the aphasic patient and his individual reactions to them are so idiosyncratic that one would ordinarily consider the best treatment to be individually planned and administered. In this way careful track can be kept of the patient's gains in language processing and production and timely decisions made about moving to next higher levels of function. However, there may be profit in group therapy, even though this may not be highly focused on the individual's language needs. Group therapy can also supplement individual therapy with benefit.

In the Veterans Administration Cooperative Study reported by Wertz and colleagues (1978), both the patients who had individual therapy and those who had small-group treatment of a different sort made substantial gains, although such significant differences as appeared between the groups favored those receiving individual therapy. Activities that proved stimulating and restoring for the patients exposed to the group program included various kinds of socializing experiences, listening to lectures, holding discussions, going on excursions, working puzzles, and the like. A similar program was earlier described by Aronson and co-workers (1956). Their group activities for aphasic patients included group singing, other musical rhythm activities, listening to stories, participating in speech games (word lotto, proverb games), manipulating puppets, preparing tape recordings, and group discussions. The patients reacted favorably to these activities, which overcame self-absorption, strangeness, and anxiety and led to a kind of group identification. The patients came to support and encourage each other in the various language activities attempted in the group, and the activities provided carryover from individual speech sessions to group discussions.

Group activity with severely aphasic patients demonstrating little residual language has been found to be helpful. Bloom (1962) set up functional situations involving patients and clinicians engaging in everyday interactions: situations involving greetings, yes or no responses, ordering from a menu, and money-handling. The same activities were repeated day after day and appropriate responses were reinforced. Words were not worked on as words but rather as parts of total situations; for example, the greeting "Hello," which might be of limited value as a practice word in reading, writing, or imitation activities, became functional in conversation.

Under trained leadership, other group therapy sessions might be more directly focused on the adjustment problems of the aphasic patients. Oradei and Waite (1974) have used daily psychotherapy sessions with hospitalized patients recovering from strokes, including some with disturbances of verbal communication. These sessions made it possible for the patients to express intense feelings of hopelessness, despair, anger, and depression. Hearing others express concerns that were similar to theirs proved encouraging to them and facilitated their own expression of feelings. A cohesive group identity developed, and patients expressed appreciation for the fact that this group activity helped them cope with feelings of depression and withdrawal.

PACE Therapy. An aphasia management plan quite different from what has been presented in this chapter has been designed by personnel of the Memphis State University Department of Speech Pathology. This plan is called Promoting Aphasics' Communicative Effectiveness (PACE). This approach to treatment incorporates components of face-to-face conversation and is based upon the pragmatic approach to language, pragmatics being the study of how language is used in context.

As outlined by its designers (Davis and Wilcox, 1981), PACE is based upon four principles:

1. There is an exchange of new information between the clinician and the patient. Messages are represented by pictures of familiar objects, actions, and stories. A stack of such pictures is available to the patient and the clinician, who alternately draw from them and engage in transmitting messages to each other. The listener is unaware of the nature of the message before it is conveyed by the speaker.

2. The speaker has a free choice of communicative channels to use in conveying new information. The aphasic patient may use whatever oral language is available to him, or he may write the message, use natural and conventional gesturing, pantomime, drawing, and pointing to pictures, printed words, or objects in the room. These channels can be used singly or in combination in any way the speaker desires so as to convey the message as best he can.

3. The clinician and the patient participate equally as senders and receivers of messages. They take turns in conversation, alternately selecting a message from the stack of pictures. When the clinician speaks, he presents a kind of model showing the patient how to use different channels as well as different types of communicative behavior within a particular channel. The clinician determines whether the patient has comprehended the message. Then the roles are reversed, and the patient conveys the message, determining whether the clinician has received his message.

4. Feedback is provided by the clinician in response to the patient's success in conveying a message. Emphasis is not on trying to improve the patient's nicety of verbalization, but rather on his accomplishing adequate conveyance of messages.

The developers of PACE indicate that it can be readily modified to deal with different degrees of severity of aphasia and different special problems in communication. How such adaptation can be accomplished has been described by Davis (1980). The most complete description of the rationale and the procedure used in PACE is presented by Davis and Wilcox (1981).

Melodic Intonation Therapy. Another unconventional approach to the treatment of aphasia, Melodic Intonation Therapy (MIT), has been developed by personnel of the Boston Veterans Administration Hospital (Sparks et al., 1974; Sparks and Holland, 1976). It is based upon the observation that some aphasic patients who are unable to produce meaningful words in speech are able to do so in singing. Melodic Intonation Therapy is a form of singing but with a difference. Whereas songs have melodies, melodic intonation is based on the spoken prosody of verbal utterances, using a vocal range limited to three or four whole notes. The prosodic patterns of spoken speech are converted into intonational patterns. A rather detailed hierarchy of procedures has been outlined, moving through four levels, with numerous steps at each level through which the patient progresses rather slowly, the clinician gradually withdrawing support and the patient increasingly demonstrating independent verbal initiation.

The designers of Melodic Intonation Therapy suggest that it is not ideal for all aphasic subjects. It is reportedly most appropriate for patients who have relatively good auditory comprehension but who are severely impaired in verbal expression, who have maintained such severe impairment of verbal expression for at least four months, and who have not benefited from prior conventional aphasia therapy. Helm (1978) has stated that "the best candidate for Melodic Intonation Therapy will display the syndrome known as 'severe phonemic articulatory disorder' " — the kind of patient we identify as predominantly apraxic in speech. In the experience of the Boston group, patients make language gains as well as speech gains in the course of MIT. The most recent description of the rationale and procedures of MIT is presented by Sparks (1981). Some special adaptations of MIT have been described by Marshall and Holtzapple (1976).

Working with Globally Aphasic Patients. The simplest tasks outlined in this chapter are suggested for use with patients who have a severe degree of aphasia in all language modalities. It is to be hoped that with intense, prolonged therapy they might begin to make gains in comprehension and output. For patients who fail to make significant gains, a number of other approaches have been suggested.

Helm and Benson (1978) have described a method called Visual Action Therapy (VAT), in which patients are taught to understand and produce symbolic gestures as a precursor to language treatment. A group of objects (razor, screwdriver, cup, etc.) readily manipulated with one hand and capable of being symbolized by a single gesture is selected. Large and small line drawings of these objects are also used, as well as line drawings of the objects being manipulated by a person. The patients are taught to match real objects with the large drawings, then with the small drawings. Then they are taught to manipulate the objects while looking at the action drawings. The patients become able to select the appropriate object from a group of objects and pretend to use it after being shown a selected action drawing. Then the patient is trained to recognize and produce a distinctive pantomime gesture in association with each object. By the time the program ends the patient can produce representational gestures to represent the small line drawings. The designers of this program have reported that globally aphasic patients exposed to this regimen have demonstrated an increase in auditory comprehension, in ability to communicate by gesture, and in the use of oral language as well.

Helm and Barresi (1980) have suggested another procedure for severely aphasic patients, which involves their developing voluntary control over involuntary utterances. The patient is shown printed words which he has been heard to say (even his stereotyped "no," "oh," "I don't know," or obscenities) and emotionally laden words likely to provoke some sort of response. If the patient is able to read a word aloud, it is printed on an index card, to be used in self-monitored drill. If, instead of uttering the printed word, the patient utters some other real word, the original word is discarded and the substituted word is printed on an index card instead. The patient's real word "errors" thus become correct responses. Subsequent practice in oral reading is done with these target words, using them in naming and other activities. Since only the patient's real word utterances are used, he seems to struggle less in processing them. He can practice his words with other patients or with family and gradually develop more verbal skills.

An approach suggested by Towey and Pettit (1980) emphasizes communication competence in nonlinguistic areas. It promotes a patient's ability to take in all available communicative behaviors, nonverbal as well as verbal, and to make appropriate selection from among the possible responses. They suggest nine important areas in improving communication competence in global aphasia. There are three important verbal behaviors: (1) The use of the patient's name or title in such a way as not to offend him but to establish a good relationship, avoiding first names if the use of titles would be more appropriate; (2) verbal responses: use by the clinician of expressions of understanding of and feeling for the patient's affect ("I know that you are very angry"); (3) avoiding interruptions of the speaker: allowing the patient to try to communicate and to avoid the rejection and frustration which result from interrupting his perhaps unintelligible message.

Four nonverbal behaviors are emphasized: (1) Eye contact, encouraged in patient and clinician, as lack of it might signify anxiety, poor self-image, or rejection; (2) head nodding, indicating participation, understanding, and desire to respond within an interaction; (3) pleasantness and appropriateness of facial expression, reflecting support, empathy, and concern; (4) reciprocity of affect displays: smiling, laughing, frowning, scowling, and other cues are responded to in a reflection of the patient's affect, indicating empathy and understanding of what the patient is feeling.

In addition, two proxemic factors are used: (1) Physical proximity during interaction, avoiding both being too close to the patient, which creates anxiety, and excessive distance, which causes discomfort and inhibits interaction; (2) general posture relaxation cues, making careful note of cues presented by the patient and in turn using postural cues that indicate comfort, participation, and attention. The designers of this approach indicate that patients (and clinicians) can be trained to be sensitive to nonlanguage means of communication and to use them increasingly; as they do, the patients reportedly also increase in language performance.

Some severely affected patients have to resort to communication boards, mechanical communication devices, sign language, or some method of communication other than conventional oral and written language. Some of the procedures that may be used have been described by DiSimoni (1981), and resource books for nonvocal communication have been published by Vanderheiden and Grilley (1975) and Vanderheiden (1978).

Possible Adjuncts to Therapy. Aphasiologists live in hope that new developments will come along that will facilitate the recovery of aphasic patients — some surgical procedure, some new medication or new regimen of an old medication, some psychologic manipulation that might somehow directly or indirectly improve aphasic behavior. So far no evidence exists that any technique other than language stimulation is clearly effective in facilitating recovery from aphasia.

The few reports available of the use of drugs as adjuncts to aphasia rehabilitation generally fail to support the notion that medication facilitates aphasic language performance. Several investigators have reported on the use of intravenous injections of sodium amytal (a sedative, hypnotic, and anticonvulsant). Linn and Stein (1946) reported a favorable result on a group of soldiers with post-traumatic aphasia, but Linn (1947) subsequently reported only transitory benefits with postsurgical (meningioma) aphasic patients and a patient with aphasia of vascular origin. Billow (1949) reported only temporary improvement in speech and mood in two aphasic patients. Bergman and Green (1951) used sodium amytal with 27 patients. They reported no significant improvement in any of them; in fact, larger amounts of the drug usually made the aphasia worse. In some cases there was an apparent increase in the patient's ability to speak or understand, but the increase was judged to be within the limits of the fluctuations that occurred spontaneously before administration of the drug. D'Asaro (1955) reported equivocal results with sodium amytal in 30 subjects; the only improvement in performance on various experimental tasks involved some automatic language.

West and Stockel (1965) reported the use of meprobamate (a tranquilizer, muscle relaxant, and anticonvulsant) and a placebo condition in a double-blind procedure with 29 aphasic patients. No significant differences were found that would indicate that language training was facilitated by the drug.

Sarno and associates (1972) administered hyperbaric oxygen to stroke patients; they reported a complete absence of effect on the course of aphasia. Altschuler (1974) studied the effect of supplemental oxygen inhalation (rather than hyperbaric oxygen administration) on the verbal, visual-motor, and oral neuromotor functioning of 12 subjects with aphasia of vascular origin. She concluded that the patients made slight but statistically significant improvement in the three skills measured while breathing supplemental oxygen for a period of 1 hour; a placebo had a slight but statistically significant effect in increasing overall communicative ability but did not affect oral neuromotor or manual visual-motor functions.

Darley and co-workers (1977) studied the effects of methylphenidate (Ritalin), a stimulant and antidepressant, and chlordiazepoxide (Librium), a tranquilizing drug used for the relief of anxiety and tension, on a group of 14 aphasic patients. Each subject served as his own control; intraoral administration of Ritalin, Librium, and a placebo constituted three treatment conditions, each treatment condition being given on three days for a total of nine administrations on consecutive days. Language behavior was measured with a battery consisting of 11 PICA subtests and the Word Fluency Test. No difference was found between treatment conditions; there was no suggestion of any difference between the effects of the two drugs or between the placebo and either of the other drugs.

The investigation of drug effects, whether indirect or direct, on language function in aphasic patients should probably continue. Other drugs should be studied, there are perhaps special kinds of patients whose management might well include a trial of some drug, and it would be worthwhile to know whether drug effects depend upon the stage of recovery from aphasia. But, so far, no drug has been shown to be a useful adjunct to language stimulation therapy.

Since aphasic behavior, although organic at base, presents functional components, the question arises as to whether language function might be improved in hypnotic trance or through posthypnotic suggestion. Kirkner and associates (1953) described the use of hypnosis, not in a bona fide case of aphasia but in a patient with "a complete ideokinetic apraxia of speech which is equivalent to motor aphasia." Usual speech retraining efforts had failed to produce vocalization by the patient, but with the aid of hypnosis he was induced to vocalize, after which traditional oral speech retraining proceeded with good results. Crasilneck and Hall (1970), discussing the use of hypnosis in rehabilitating patients with complicated neurologic problems, report its use in three patients with communication problems; one presented "expressive aphasia," one "the inability to communicate," and one "difficulty in following verbal commands." The authors conclude: "An increase in motivation for recovery seemed to be the major change elicited by hypnotherapy. . . . Hypnosis may be a useful way of approaching motivational problems in rehabilitating patients who manifest negativism toward conventional treatment." The general usefulness of hypnosis with aphasic patients has yet to be tested.

THE FAMILY: PATIENT/CLINICIAN

Aphasia constitutes a dramatic example of the fact that when a neurologic disaster strikes, the identity of the victim extends beyond the individual who had the stroke or tumor or suffered the trauma and includes the family — the spouse and the children as well. The family relationship and the roles played by all of the members of the family constellation are irrevocably changed. Everyone suddenly has to cope with the reality of a disabled loved one, and the coping is complicated by the fact that communication with the patient is impaired.

Everything is different. If the patient is breadwinner, for example, that role may be threatened. Because of his communication deficit, the patient gives up his dominant role and the spouse or one of the children assumes it, a role perhaps reluctantly relinquished later. There is great anxiety about the patient's health, how well he will recover, and whether there will be another episode of the kind that caused the aphasia. There may be uncertainty about the cause of the problem and possibly a naive attitude about the degree of recovery to be anticipated and how soon.

Family members wonder how best to communicate with the patient, how to fathom what he means but is unable to say, and how to comprehend and put up with his altered personality and his changing moods. As time passes, they begin to wonder how long the inconvenience, the worry, the irritation, and the anxiety are going to go on, and they worry about how they can continue to endure them and make the sacrifices in their own lives that have been occasioned by attention to the needs of the patient.

The patient's spouse, the children, and others important to the family need help of various kinds and in various forms at different stages of recovery and the rehabilitation program. Some of these needs have been documented in investigations (Malone, 1969; Malone et al., 1970; Kinsella and Duffy, 1978; Chwat et al., 1980) and are reviewed below.

Clarification of the Nature of the Problem and What to Expect.
From the onset, the family needs to be told the name of the patient's disorder. They need to become acquainted with aphasia, learn
that it is a common consequence of the medical crisis the patient has
gone through — whether stroke, surgery for brain tumor, a central
nervous system infection, or a traumatic event. They can be helped to
anticipate the kinds of behaviors associated with aphasia, which they
will have to live with. They must understand that the patient will
display reduced comprehension of spoken and written language and
reduced ability to convey information by speech and in writing. It is
not because the patient is stubborn, not because he has lost his mind,
not because he is now mentally defective, not because he has gone
crazy; rather it is because the circuitry in the brain responsible for
language processing is impaired as a result of a valid medical cause
that caused actual anatomic damage. They need to understand that the
patient's new language behavior may be inconsistent and quite puz-
zling. They can be helped to appreciate that the patient may not be able
to say something seemingly very simple while at times producing
unusual language behavior ("Why can't he say my name, even my
name? And why does he swear like that? He never used to do that!")

Those close to the patient need to understand that the experience
he has gone through is as devastating to his ego as it is to his language.
He is bewildered by the fact that apparently easy tasks are beyond his
reach, that people around him don't seem to be able to make any sense
out of what he says, and that part of the time they don't make much
sense to him. The patient's self-esteem has taken a beating, and
repeated failures to communicate leave him frustrated, impatient,
irritable, and sad. The family should be helped to understand that
sometimes the patient may *seem* to understand more than he really
does — as by a knowing look, a ready nod of the head, an automatic
"yes" he conveys complete understanding when in reality his understanding is quite incomplete. He may have responded to the accompanying gestures, the facial expressions, and the context of the situation and
have only fragmentary understanding of the language parts. It has been
demonstrated that spouses typically consider their aphasic husbands
or wives to be less handicapped than they really are, rating the patient's
communication performance as satisfactory in areas that objective
testing indicate are severely impaired (Helmick et al., 1976). This
misperception of the patient's handicap might on one hand seem to
lead to the family's providing emotional support for the patient, but it
may on the other hand lead to their building unrealistic expectations
concerning the language performance and to their using inappropriately complex language with the patient.

So, there is information about the causes and nature of aphasia that
the family needs and that the physician and speech pathologist can
convey soon after onset of the problem. This information-sharing task

can be aided by the use of printed materials such as those listed at the end of this chapter (see *Informational Booklets*).

How to Communicate with the Patient. Given some insight into the patient's language difficulties and their emotional tax on him, the family should then be helped to discover how best to communicate with the patient and what to do when he can't communicate with them. (This problem is not unique with family members but pertains also to the medical and paramedical personnel who work with the patient.) The family must be told that the aphasic patient has trouble processing all language input and output; they must assume that his comprehension is not efficient and complete. They can be given the following suggestions about how to speak to him and how to provide ample processing time before expecting a response:

- Secure the patient's attention before opening a conversation or offering instructions. Touch him on the shoulder if necessary, have him watch your face, and preface your remarks by calling his name.
- Speak somewhat more slowly than normal and insert pauses between the important parts of each sentence. If the patient does not respond or makes an inappropriate response, repeat the sentence, several times if necessary. Give him plenty of time to respond.
- When you repeat a question or an instruction, do not say it louder. The patient is probably not hard of hearing. Do not try to break the communication barrier by increasing the loudness level.
- Use short, simple sentences, slightly emphasizing a key word. For example, "It's *lunch* time"; "Do you want *coffee*?" When appropriate, accompany the sentences with gestures.
- In the attempt to simplify communication, do not talk down to the patient. Although his communication skills may be rudimentary, his social awareness and his sensitivities are not. An equal-to-equal approach is best in terms of tone of voice, facial expression, bodily posture, and general demeanor. Do not overpraise his attempts at communication or overshower him with kindness. Do not be oversolicitous.
- Whenever possible, questions should be simple, direct, and answerable by yes or no. If the patient can't understand, try writing the question.
- If the patient tries to express something that you cannot understand, ask him simple questions accompanied by pointing and gesturing until he indicates that you have found the correct subject area. If all fails, admit your difficulty and say "I'm sorry but I can't understand. Maybe we can try again later."
- Do not correct errors the patient may make. Encourage the patient to make more responses rather than make him struggle to correct erroneous ones.

- Communication is facilitated by establishing an encouraging, unhurried, uncomplicated atmosphere. Background music and the distraction of other people nearby conversing and making noise tend to disrupt the patient's ability to listen and respond.
- Do not exert pressure to elicit a response. A sense of urgency, an attitude of impatience, or squeezing a little harder in the hope that the answer will "pop out" will only inhibit the patient's response. Avoid frustrating remarks, such as "You said it yesterday; you can say it again."
- Avoid trying to talk for the patient unless it is absolutely necessary. Do not interrupt him when he tries to tell you something. Try to make him a real partner in conversation; do not put words into his mouth too quickly.
- Because the patient with aphasia has difficulty retrieving words and monitoring what he says, he may swear or produce jargon speech. Make no issue of it, downplay it by saying, "I know it's hard to say, but I think I know what you mean."
- Try to make every routine contact with the patient an opportunity for stimulating conversation. To make complex events happen in the brain, we must provide stimulation. Give the patient something to react to by telling him what you are doing, what forthcoming events will be, what happened yesterday, what came in the mail, what you're going to have for lunch, and so forth.
- Although the patient's understanding of language may be limited, he may enjoy watching television, listening to the radio, and looking through the newspaper and magazines. Person-to-person stimulation is best, but stimulation from the radio or television may be beneficial.
- Despite his limitations in comprehension, we should avoid discussing the patient's condition and prognosis in his presence as though he were not there or could not understand. Although severely aphasic, he may be able to grasp fragments of conversation and may be sensitive to the mood in which opinions are expressed.

Helping the Spouse Cope. In the early days after onset of the problem, spouses and other family members typically experience considerable support from medical and paramedical personnel working with the patient, from relatives and friends, and from each other. As times passes, the spouses may discover that there is a decrease in the amount of this support, and they ultimately find themselves seeming to cope alone. Increasingly, they may find that as they spend a great deal of time with the handicapped patient, they suffer a restriction of social contact with others; they develop the feeling that they are increasingly isolated, and indeed they may be. They find themselves essentially prisoners in their own homes, and they tire of unremitting contact with the patient.

They are bothered by their enforced neglect of other responsibilities. They lose sleep, are often fatigued, worry inevitably about finances, and wonder how things are going to turn out. Their loneliness is unrelieved by the usual kinds of communication with the loved one; because of the difficulty in communication, they are often unable to talk about even everyday things, much less about stressful situations that beset the family and worry the spouse. Difficulty in communication may lead to growing misunderstanding and tension.

Spouses come to find in some cases that there is a complete disruption of the marital relationship and a genuine loss of sexual partnership. The spouse experiences diminished sexual satisfaction and indeed may no longer consider the patient to be the kind of person to whom one would look for sexual satisfaction, being more like a (backward) child or a boarder than an intimate companion. With increased awareness of these feelings, there may be a growing feeling of guilt; and guilt feelings may in turn lead to even more dedication to and protection of the patient, which may keep him in a subordinate and helpless condition.

Spouses need an opportunity to express their feelings to people who can accept them insightfully, perhaps a professional counselor, perhaps a group of empathic patients' spouses who are in a similar situation and with whom common experiences can be shared. Certainly spouses need to be listened to, and they may need counseling and even psychotherapy (Newhoff et al., 1980).

The Family Member as Clinician.   This book has been addressed to clinicians whose professional activity includes the treatment of aphasic patients. The kind of professional treatment they can provide is probably optimal. However, the realities of everyday life — limitations of available professional care, geographic constraints, financial exigencies — make it likely that a member of the family will have to step in and attempt to help the patient if anyone is going to. Although some clinicians deplore the thought of asking a family member to assume the role of clinician and language stimulator, assuming that it involves a gulf too wide to bridge, the experience of many clinicians and even some research data (Goodkin et al., 1973) indicate that family members may indeed become improved communicators and effective "clinicians" with their aphasic spouses or parents.

The family member who is a candidate for the "clinician" role must be helped to understand the rationale of language rehabilitation and the role of stimulation in language recovery. He must demonstrate that he has the patience and the good will to engage with the patient in repetitious activities that may become boring; that he can create a psychologic set that facilitates participation by the patient in language rehabilitation; that he can keep the patient trying, provide needed reinforcement, and assuage rather than provoke feelings of disappointment, frustration, and panic.

It is helpful if the family member can observe a professional clinician at work in a series of sessions during the early days of therapy so as to catch a glimpse of how the work is done and the attitudes that must pervade the clinical situation. With the guidance of the clinician, he can understand where to start and how to know when to move on to other activities.

Fortunately, professionally prepared materials, which clinicians often use for language rehabilitation, are available commercially; these are often readily usable by family members as well. These compilations provide instructions and a variety of stimulus materials for improving input — auditory comprehension and reading — and they permit a variety of spoken and written responses. Several currently available workbooks which clinicians use and which family members can learn to use are listed at the end of this chapter. Not listed are a catalogue of other useful materials: word cards, picture cards, left-handed writing manuals, tape-recorded stimulus materials, and other materials and equipment available commercially. The clinician can share information with the family "clinician" about the uses of these and help secure them.

Informational Booklets for the Family

An Adult Has Aphasia by D. Boone. Danville, IL, Interstate Printers and Publishers, 1965.
Aphasia and the Family. New York, American Heart Association, 1965.
Communication Problems after a Stroke by L. K. Cohen. Minneapolis, Kenny Rehabilitation Institute, 1971.
Help the Stroke Patient to Talk by M. C. Crickmay. Springfield, IL, Charles C Thomas, 1977.
Stroke: The Condition and the Patient by J. E. Sarno and M. T. Sarno. New York, McGraw-Hill, 1969.

Workbooks

Aphasia Rehabilitation: A Speech and Language Workbook
    Cheryl A. Traendly
    C. C. Publications
    Tigard, OR 97223 (1974)
Aphasia Therapy Manual
    Joseph C. Aurelia
    Interstate Printers and Publishers, Inc.
    Danville, IL 61832 (1974)
The Aphasic Patient: A Program for Auditory Comprehension and Language Training
    William P. Baer
    Charles C Thomas
    Springfield, IL 62717 (1976)
The Bulloch-McLoughlin Adult Aphasia Program
    Kathleen L. Bulloch, Judy L. McLoughlin
    Word Making Productions
    Salt Lake City, UT 84115 (1977)

Clinician Controlled Auditory Stimulation for Aphasic Adults
    Robert C. Marshall
    C. C. Publications
    Tigard, OR 97223 (1978)
Graduated Language Training for Patients with Aphasia and Children with Language Deficiencies
    Robert L. Keith
    College-Hill Press
    Houston, TX 77035 (1980)
Photo Language Stimulation for Aphasic Patients
    Robert Canetta
    Interstate Printers and Publishers, Inc.
    Danville, IL 61832 (1974)
A Practice Book for Aphasics
    Milfred R. McKeown, Aleen Agranowitz
    Charles C Thomas
    Springfield, IL 62717 (1976)
Speech After Stroke: A Manual for the Speech Pathologist and the Family Member
    Stephanie Stryker
    Charles C Thomas
    Springfield, IL 62717 (1975)
Speech and Language Rehabilitation: A Workbook for the Neurologically Impaired and the Language Delayed
    Volume 1, Revised Edition
    Robert L. Keith
    Interstate Printers and Publishers, Inc.
    Danville, IL 61832 (1980)
Speech and Language Rehabilitation: A Workbook for the Neurologically Impaired
    Volume 2
    Robert L. Keith
    Interstate Printers and Publishers, Inc.
    Danville, IL 61832 (1977)
Workbook for Aphasia
    Susan H. Brubaker
    Wayne State University Press
    Detroit, MI 48202 (1978)

References

Altschuler, S. L.: The effects of supplemental oxygen respiration on aphasic hemiplegic adults. Clinical Aphasiology Conference Proceedings, 1974, pp. 21–26.
Aronson, M., Shatin, L., and Cook, J. C.: Sociotherapeutic approach to the treatment of aphasic patients. J. Speech Hearing Disord., 21:352–364, 1956.
Basso, A.: Aphasia rehabilitation: a note on methods and three examples. In Lebrun, Y., and Hoops, R. (Eds.): The Management of Aphasia. Atlantic Highlands, New Jersey, Humanities Press, 1978, pp. 9–21.
Bergman, P. S., and Green, M.: Aphasia: effect of intravenous sodium amytal. Neurology, 1:471–475, 1951.
Billow, B. W.: Observation of the use of sodium amytal in the treatment of aphasia. Med. Rec., 162:12–13, 1949.
Bloom, L. M.: A rationale for group treatment of aphasic patients. J. Speech Hearing Disord., 27:11–16, 1962.
Brookshire, R. H.: Effects of delay of reinforcement on probability learning by aphasic subjects. J. Speech Hearing Res., 14:92–105, 1971.
Brookshire, R. H.: Effects of task difficulty on naming performance of aphasic subjects. J. Speech Hearing Res., 15:551–558, 1972.
Brookshire, R. H.: Effects of task difficulty on sentence comprehension performance of aphasic subjects. J. Commun. Disord., 9:167–173, 1976.

Chwat, S., Chapey, R., Gurland, G., and Pieras, G.: Environmental impact of aphasia: the child's perspective. Clinical Aphasiology Conference Proceedings, 1980. Minneapolis, BRK Publishers, 1980, pp. 127–134.

Crasilneck, H. B., and Hall, J. A.: The use of hypnosis in the rehabilitation of complicated vascular and post-traumatic neurological patients. Int. J. Clin. Exp. Hypn., 18:145–149, 1970.

Croskey, C. S., and Adams, M. R.: A rationale and clinical methodology for selecting vocabulary stimulus materials for individual aphasic patients. J. Commun. Disord., 2:340–343, 1969.

Darley, F. L., Keith, R. L., and Sasanuma, S.: The effect of alerting and tranquilizing drugs upon the performance of aphasic patients. Clinical Aphasiology Conference Proceedings, 1977. Minneapolis, BRK Publishers, 1977, pp. 91–96.

Darley, F. L., Helm, N. A., Holland, A., and Linebaugh, C.: Techniques in treating mild or high-level aphasic impairment: panel discussion. Clinical Aphasiology Conference, 1980. Minneapolis, BRK Publishers, 1980, pp. 338–345.

D'Asaro, M. J.: An experimental investigation of effects of sodium amytal on communication of aphasic patients. Ph.D. Dissertation, University of Southern California, 1955.

Davis, G. A.: A critical look at PACE therapy. Clinical Aphasiology Conference Proceedings, 1980. Minneapolis, BRK Publishers, 1980, pp. 248–257.

Davis, G. A., and Wilcox, M. J.: Incorporating parameters of natural conversation in aphasia treatment. In Chapey, R. (Ed.): Language Intervention Strategies in Adult Aphasia. Baltimore, Williams & Wilkins, 1981, pp. 169–193.

DiSimoni, F. G.: Therapies which utilize alternative or augmentative communication systems. In Chapey, R. (Ed.): Language Intervention Strategies in Adult Aphasia. Baltimore, Williams & Wilkins, 1981, pp. 329–346.

Goodkin, R., Detler, L., and Shah, N.: Training spouses to improve the functional speech of aphasic patients. In Lahey, B. (Ed.): The Modification of Language Behavior. Springfield, IL, Charles C Thomas, 1973, pp. 218–269.

Helm, N. A.: Criteria for selecting aphasia patients for Melodic Intonation Therapy. 54th Annual Convention, American Speech and Hearing Association, San Francisco, 1978.

Helm, N., and Barresi, B.: Voluntary control of involuntary utterances: a treatment approach for severe aphasia. Clinical Aphasiology Conference Proceedings, 1980. Minneapolis, BRK Publishers, 1980, pp. 308–315.

Helm, N. A., and Benson, D. F.: Visual Action Therapy for global aphasia. Academy of Aphasia Annual Meeting, Chicago, 1978.

Helmick, J. W., and Wipplinger, M.: Effects of stimulus repetition on the naming behavior of an aphasic adult: a clinical report. J. Commun. Disord., 8:23–29, 1975.

Helmick, J. W., Watamori, T. S., and Palmer, J. M.: Spouses' understanding of the communication abilities of aphasic patients. J. Speech Hearing Disord., 41:238–243, 1976.

Holland, A. L., and Sonderman, J. C.: Effects of a program based on the Token Test for teaching comprehension skills to aphasics. J. Speech Hearing Res., 17:589–598, 1974.

Kinsella, G., and Duffy, F.: The spouse of the aphasic patient. In Lebrun, Y., and Hoops, R. (Eds.): The Management of Aphasia. Atlantic Highlands, New Jersery, Humanities Press, 1978, pp. 26–49.

Kirkner, F. J., Dorcus, R. M., and Seacat, G.: Hypnotic motivation of vocalization in an organic motor aphasia case. Int. J. Clin. Exp. Hypn., 1:47–49, 1953.

Kushner, D., and Winitz, H.: Extended comprehension practice applied to an aphasic patient. J. Speech Hearing Disord., 42:296–306, 1977.

LaPointe, L. L.: Base-10 programmed stimulation: task specification, scoring, and plotting performance in aphasia therapy. J. Speech Hearing Disord., 42:90–105, 1977.

LaPointe, L. L.: Aphasia therapy: some principles and strategies for treatment. In Johns, D. F. (Ed.): Clinical Management of Neurogenic Communicative Disorders. Boston, Little, Brown, 1978, pp. 129–190.

Linn, L.: Sodium amytal in treatment of aphasia. Arch. Neurol. Psychiatry, 58:357–358, 1947.

Linn, L., and Stein, M. H.: Sodium amytal in treatment of aphasia: preliminary report. Bull. U.S. Army Med. Dept., 5:705–708, 1946.

Malone, R. L.: Expressed attitudes of families of aphasics. J. Speech Hearing Disord., *34*:146–151, 1969.

Malone, R. L., Ptacek, P. H., and Malone, M. S.: Attitudes expressed by families of aphasics. Br. J. Disord. Commun., *5*:174–179, 1970.

Marshall, N., and Holtzapple, P.: Melodic Intonation Therapy: variations on a theme. Clinical Aphasiology Conference Proceedings, 1976. Minneapolis, BRK Publishers, 1976, pp. 115–139.

Newhoff, M., Florance, C., Malone, P., Ritter, G., and Webster, E. J.: Home and family: problems and payoffs. A panel presentation and discussion. Clinical Aphasiology Conference Proceedings, 1980. Minneapolis, BRK Publishers, 1980, pp. 346–351.

Oradei, D. M., and Waite, J. S.: Group psychotherapy with stroke patients during the immediate recovery phase. Am. J. Orthopsychiatry, *44*:386–395, 1974.

Sarno, M. T., Sarno, J. E., and Diller, L.: The effect of hyperbaric oxygen on communication function in adults with aphasia. J. Speech Hearing Res., *15*:42–48, 1972.

Schuell, H., Jenkins, J. J., and Jiménez-Pabón, E.: Aphasia in Adults: Diagnosis, Prognosis, and Treatment. New York, Hoeber, 1964.

Sparks, R. W.: Melodic Intonation Therapy. In Chapey, R. (Ed.): Language Intervention Strategies in Adult Aphasia. Baltimore, Williams & Wilkins, 1981, pp. 265–282.

Sparks, R. W., and Holland, A. L.: Method: Melodic Intonation Therapy for aphasia. J. Speech Hearing Disord., *41*:287–297, 1976.

Sparks, R., Helm, N., and Albert, M.: Aphasia rehabilitation resulting from Melodic Intonation Therapy. Cortex, *10*:303–316, 1974.

Towey, M. P., and Pettit, J. M.: Improving communication competence in global aphasia. Clinical Aphasiology Conference Proceedings, 1980. Minneapolis, BRK Publishers, 1980, pp. 139–146.

Vanderheiden, G. (Ed.): Non-Vocal Communication Resource Book. Baltimore, University Park Press, 1978.

Vanderheiden, G., and Grilley, K. (Eds.): Non-Vocal Communication Techniques and Aids for the Severely Physically Handicapped. Baltimore, University Park Press, 1975.

von Stockert, T. R.: A standardized program for aphasia therapy. In Lebrun, Y., and Hoops, R. (Eds.): The Management of Aphasia. Atlantic Highlands, New Jersey, Humanities Press, 1978, pp. 97–107.

Weigel-Crump, C., and Koenigsknecht, R. A.: Tapping the lexical store of the adult aphasic: analysis of the improvement made in word retrieval skills. Cortex, *9*:411–418, 1973.

Wepman, J. M.: A conceptual model for the processes involved in recovery from aphasia. J. Speech Hearing Disord., *18*:4–13, 1953.

Wepman, J. M.: Aphasia therapy: a new look. J. Speech Hearing Disord., *37*:203–214, 1972.

Wepman, J. M.: Aphasia: language without thought or thought without language? Asha, *18*:131–136, 1976.

Wertz, R. T., Collins, M., Weiss, D., Brookshire, R. H., Friden, T., Kurtzke, J. F., and Pierce, J.: Veterans Administration Cooperative Study on Aphasia: preliminary report on a comparison of individual and group treatment. 54th Annual Convention, American Speech and Hearing Association, San Francisco, 1978.

West, R., and Stockel, S.: The effect of meprobamate on recovery from aphasia. J. Speech Hearing Res., *8*:57–62, 1965.

INDEX

Page numbers in *italics* indicate figures; numbers followed by (t) indicate tables.

Accuracy, in testing, 71
ACTS, description of, 82
Adjectives, as stimuli, 243(t), 244
  sentence completion with, 253
Age, prognosis and, 137–138
  treatment results and, 179
Agnosia, prognosis for, 104
  verbal, auditory, and aphasia, 3
    models in, 40
Agrammatism, 42
  in Broca's aphasia, 38
Agraphia, alexia with, evolution of, 126
  alexia without, 41
Akinetic mutism, vs. aphasia, 27–28
Alexia, with agraphia, evolution of, 126
  without agraphia, 41
ALPS, description of, 80
Amnesia, verbal, 15
Amnesic aphasia, differentiation of, 125
Anarthria, 40. See also *Apraxia of speech.*
  prognosis for, 102
Anomia, 42
  in aphasia, 5
Anomic aphasia, evolution of, 126
Anticipatory errors, in apraxia, 11
Antonyms, use of, in treatment, 253
Aphasia, amnesic, differentiation of, 125
  anomic, evolution of, 126
  appraisal of, 61–79
  Broca's. See *Broca's aphasia.*
  central, 37
  definition of, 1, 42
  etiology of, prognosis and, 128–130
  evaluation for, 55–109
  evolution of, 126, 127(t)
  natural history of, 110–143
  patients having, performance of, 3–8
  treatment of, 237–278
Aphasia Language Performance Scales,
  description of, 80
Aphasia quotient, 114

Aphasia Severity Rating Scale, 69(t)
Aphemia, 15
Apraxia of speech, impaired auditory
    perception and, 18
  models in, 40
  prognosis for, 102
  vs. aphasia, 10–17
AQ, 114
  accuracy of, in apraxia, 13
  errors of, and aphasia, 17–18
  in apraxia, 10
  in contextual speech, evaluation of,
    67(t)
  in dysarthria, 9
  rating of, 68(t)
Articulated language, impairment of, 15
Associated speech problems, prognosis
  and, 102–103
Ataxic dysarthria, 9
Attitude, of clinician, treatment and, 231,
  263
Audiometric tests, for differential
  diagnosis, 75
Auditory comprehension, and aphasia, 3
  differential diagnosis and, 57
  improvement in, treatment and, 155
  in Token Test, 208
  presentation rate and, 214
  quantification of, 84(t)
  sentence pauses and, 217
  spontaneous recovery in, 116(t)
  summarization and, 257
  syntax and, 205
  tasks for, array of, 242
    selection of, 239–240
  treatment results for, 167–168
Auditory Comprehension Test for
  Sentences, description of, 82
Auditory imperception, and aphasia, 3
Auditory information, vs. visual
  information, comprehension and, 213
Auditory input, for language
  rehabilitation, 188–193

Auditory retention span, differential diagnosis and, 57
Auditory stimulation, redundancy and, 200
Auditory verbal agnosia, and aphasia, 3
prognosis for, 105

Background noise, in language rehabilitation, 190
Base-10 measurement, of treatment, 169–170
record of, 240, 241
Baseline performance, determination of, before therapy, 240
BDAE, description of, 80
Behavior, nonlanguage, evaluation of, 75–77
Bilingual patients, recovery in, 170–171
Binaural intensity variation, in auditory language rehabilitation, 189
Boston Diagnostic Aphasia Examination, 36, 39
and contextual speech, 66
description of, 80
for divergent language behavior, 65
Brain, anatomy of, language behavior and, 56
damage to, differential diagnosis of, 59
lesions of, localization of, 56
Broca's aphasia, 19, 20
agrammatism in, 38
differentiation of, 125
from diminished blood supply, prognosis for, 129
Brown model, of language function, 31–34

CADL test, description of, 81
Case studies, 163–175
Central aphasia, 37
Central language process, in Brown model, 31
Cerebrovascular accidents, aphasia from, prognosis for, 129
Characteristic sound, of auditory stimuli, in rehabilitation, 192
Classification, of severity, 86
Color, of visual stimuli, in language rehabilitation, 193
Commands, execution of, in treatment, 246–248
written, 250
Communication, disorders of, differentiation of, 2
functional, level of, determination of, 56
of family, with patient, 272

Communicative Abilities in Daily Living, description of, 81
development of, 163
Completeness, in testing, 71
Comprehension, auditory. See *Auditory comprehension.*
improvement in, measurement of, 124
information overload and, 208
training for, 230
Confabulation, in dementia, 24
Confrontation naming, in testing, 70
Confused language, vs. aphasia, 24–26
Consonants, articulation of, in apraxia, 10
Content unit, of speech, 69
Context, and cues, in language rehabilitation, 197–200
Contextual speech, 65–70
Convergent semantic behavior, and aphasia, 4
Cues, and context, in language rehabilitation, 197–200

Deblocking, as treatment, 197
Dementia, vs. aphasia, 23–24
vs. apraxia, vs. aphasia, 14
Depression, and nonlanguage behavior, 76
Differential diagnosis, language appraisal for, 55–56
of language disorders, 74–75
Divergent language behavior, assessment of, 62–64
facilitation of, activities for, 258(t)
Divergent semantic behavior, and aphasia, 4
Drugs, in treatment, 268
Dysarthria, ataxic, 9
prognosis for, 102
vs. aphasia, 8–9
Dysphasia, definition of, 2

Education, differential diagnosis of, 59
prognosis and, 138
Efficiency, in testing, 71
Electrophysiology, and brain lesions, 57
Emotional content, of language, in treatment, 191
Emotional disturbances, vs. aphasia, 26–27
Employment, prognosis and, 140
Environment, in language rehabilitation, 224–225
Errors, anticipatory, in apraxia, 11
correction of, 227
avoidance of, 261

Etiology, of aphasia, 2
  prognosis and, 128–130
  treatment results and, 182
Evaluation. See also *Test(s)*.
  examiner attitude and, 83
  family and, 78
  history in, 77
  home language practice in, 78
  language function in, premorbid level
    of, 77
  medical information for, 77
  of aphasia, 55–109
    principles of, 82–85
  of patient, 55–109
  personality in, 77–78
  predictions and, 85–106
  psychosocial information and, 77
  sampling in, 61
  social interaction and, 79
  testing for, 61–79
  tests for, description of, 79–82
    consistency and, 84
Evolution, of aphasia, 125–127
Expression, improvement of,
  measurement of, 124
Expressive tasks, treatment and, 251–256

Fair speech performance, definition of, 66
Family, communication with, in
    treatment, 272
  evaluation and, 78
  treatment and, 270–275
FCP, description of, 81
Feedback, in Wepman model, 30
  of performance, 262
Feigning, differential diagnosis and, 59
Flaccid dysarthria, 9
Fluency, of contextual speech, 67(t)
Functional communication, level of,
  determination of, 56
Functional Communication Profile,
  description of, 81
  language measure and, 112

Gesture, and aphasia, 6
Global aphasia, evolution of, 126
  prognosis for, 103
  therapy for, 266–268
Good speech performance, definition of,
  66
Grammar, differentiation of, 7
  evaluation of, 68(t)
  in Broca's aphasia, 38
  saliency from, 188
  transformations of, as therapy, 260
Group socialization, treatment and, 149
Group therapy, 264–265
Gunshot wounds, treatment in, 145

Hearing, aphasia and, 3
Hemiplegia, in stroke patients, prognosis
    for, 136
  nonlanguage behavior and, 76
Hemorrhage, aphasia from, prognosis for,
    129
High-Overall Prediction method, 98(t), 99
History, evaluation and, 77
  of aphasia, 110–143
HOAP slope, 98(t), 99
Home language practice, evaluation of,
    78
Hyperkinetic dysarthria, 9
Hypnosis, as treatment, 269
Hypokinetic dysarthria, 9

Illinois Test of Psycholinguistic Abilities,
  for divergent language behavior, 65
Imagery, of visual stimuli, in language
  rehabilitation, 193
Imitative responses, in apraxia, 12
Impaired auditory perception, errors not
  attributable to, 18
Impairment, of reauditorization, and
    aphasia, 3
  selective, and apraxia, 19
  severity of, prognosis and, 86
Imposed response delay, language
  rehabilitation and, 218–220
Infarction, of brain vessels, prognosis
  and, 134
Information, auditory, vs. visual,
  comprehension and, 213
Information capacity deficit, and aphasia,
  4
Information overload, 208–211
Input, auditory, for language
  rehabilitation, 188–193
Input modality, selection of, 211–214
Instrumental analysis, of speech, 20–22
Intelligence, prognosis and, 139
Intermittent auditory imperception, and
  aphasia, 4
IQ, and aphasia, 22, 23

Jargon, persistence of, prognosis for, 105
  responses in, 229

Language, appraisal of, 55–109
  shortcuts, in, 63
  brain anatomy and, 56
  Brown model of, 31–34
  change in, PICA measurement of, 120
    with treatment, 158, 159
  confused, vs. aphasia, 24–26
  evaluation of, factors in, 61(t)

Language (*Continued*)
  impairment of, differential patterns of, 56
  in dementia, 23
  models of, aphasia and, 28–41
  multiple, aphasia and, 6
  performance deviations in, rating of, 69
  premorbid level of, 77
  processing of, impairment of, 17
    comprehension and, 214–220
  testing of, self-correction in, 73
  Wepman model of, 29–31, *30*
Language behavior, convergent, assessment of, 62–64
    tasks for, for advanced patients, 257
  divergent, assessment of, 64–65
  facilitation of, activities for, 258(t)
  prognosis in, 103
  sampling of, 61
Language competence, residual, and aphasia, 6
Language dysfunction, differentiation of, 74
Language function, treatment and, 160
Language Modalities Test for Aphasia, 35
Language processing, visual, impaired, tests for, 62
Language rehabilitation. See also *Treatment.*
  auditory input for, 188–193
  context and, 197–200
  cues in, 197
  environment in, 224–225
  imposed response delay in, 218–220
  noise in, 190
  presentation rate and, 214
  processing time and, 214–220
  redundancy and, 200–204
  reinforcement timing in, 224
  repetition in, 221–222
  sentence stimuli in, internal pauses in, 217–218
  skills and, 160
  stimuli for, 186–236
  uses of, 144
  visual stimuli for, 193–196
  vocabulary selection in, 223
Language specificity, and aphasia, 22–28
Language therapy, intensive, efficacy of, 158
Lesion, location of, prognosis and, 130–235
Letters, recognition of, 248
Lip reading, rehabilitation and, 191
Literal paraphasia, 17
Loudness, in language rehabilitation, 188

Melodic Intonation Therapy, 157, 266
Memory, short-term, delayed response and, 219
Metaphors, as therapy, 260

Metathesis errors, in apraxia, 11
Milan Study, 171–173
Minnesota Test for Differential Diagnosis of Aphasia, and aphasic impairment, 35
  description of, 79–80
  for differential diagnosis, 57
Mixed dysarthria, 9
Modality, of speech, aphasia and, 28–41
  shifts of, in recovery, 116
Model(s), Brown, of language function, 31–34
  in apraxia, 40
  of language, 28–41
Monitoring, visual, and apraxia, 13
Morphosyntactic Comprehension Test, 122
Motor aphasia, 131
Motor disorders, and aphasia, differentiation of, 74
  and apraxia, 20
  prognosis and, 135–137
Motor speech programing, in Brown model, 33
MTDDA. See *Minnesota Test for Differential Diagnosis of Aphasia.*
Multidimensional scoring scale, for testing, 72(t)
Multilingualism, and aphasia, 6
Mutism, akinetic, vs. aphasia, 27–28

NCCEA, description of, 80–81
Neurological problems, in dysarthria, 8–9
Neuropathology, in akinetic mutism, 27
Neurosensory Center Comprehensive Examination for Aphasia, description of, 80–81
  for divergent language behavior, 65
Noise, buildup of, and aphasia, 4
  in language rehabilitation, 190
Nominal aphasia, 42
Non-aphasias, models in, vs. aphasia, 39–40
Nonlanguage behavior, evaluation of, 75–77
Nonstandardized tests, 85
No-treatment control groups, in treatment studies, 157–163
  lack of, in language rehabilitation studies, 145–157
Nouns, as stimuli, 243(t), 244
  sentence completion with, 253

Olfaction, as stimulus, 212
Operativity, of visual stimuli, in language rehabilitation, 196
Organic brain syndrome, nonlanguage behavior and, 76
  vs. aphasia, 23

PACE therapy, 265–266
Paragraph-length material,
 comprehension of, 201
Parallel tasks, in tests, 70
Paraphasias, 17
 in contextual speech, evaluation of,
  67(t)
 in running speech, evaluation of, 68(t)
Pauses, in sentence stimuli, language
 rehabilitation and, 217–218
Performance, testing for, 81
Personality, in evaluation, 77–78
 prognosis and, 139
Phonation, in dysarthria, 8
Phonemes, in apraxia, 11
Phonemic paraphasias, 17
Phonetic association, in aphasia, 5
Phonologic impairment, and aphasia, 17
Phrase-length ratio, changes in, 125
Physical condition in evaluation, 76, 77
 prognosis and, 135–137
PICA. See Porch Index of Communicative
 Ability.
PICA scale, therapy program and, 239
Playing columnist, as therapy, 260
Poor speech performance, definition of,
 66
Porch Index of Communicative Ability,
 36, 38
 description of, 79
 differential diagnosis and, 58
 recovery measurements and, 119–120
 scoring for, 72
Postpositioning errors, in apraxia, 11
Prediction, in aphasia, 55–109. See also
 Prognosis.
Premorbid level, of language function, 77
Prepositioning errors, in apraxia, 11
Prepositions, as stimuli, 243(t), 245
 in treatment, 255
Presenile dementia, vs. aphasia, 23
Presentation rate, adjustment of, 261
 auditory comprehension and, 214
Processing time, comprehension and,
 214–220
Prognosis, age and, 137–138
 evaluation and, 85–106
 factors in, 127–141
 for agnosia, 104
 initial severity and, 86
Programmed stimulation, therapy using,
 169–170
Promoting Aphasiacs' Communicative
 Effectiveness therapy, 265–266
Prompting, effects of, 225
Promptness, in tests, 71
Prosody, in apraxia, 13
 in contextual speech, evaluation of,
  67(t)
 in dysarthria, 9
 in schizophrenia, 27
Psychometric methods, for differential
 diagnosis, 59

Psychosocial factors, evaluation and, 77
 prognosis and, 138–141

Quantification, of auditory
 comprehension, 84(t)
Questions, types of, response and, 229

Radiology, and brain lesions, 57
Reading, and aphasia, 4
 comprehension in, differential
  diagnosis and, 57
 graduated tasks of, 248
 in apraxia, 11
 language evaluation with, 62
 oral, and apraxia, 12
 quantification of, 84(t)
 spontaneous recovery and, 116(t)
 summarization of, 257
 vs. listening, comprehension and, 211
Reading Comprehension Battery for
 Aphasia, description of, 82
Realism, of visual stimuli, in language
 rehabilitation, 195
 redundancy and, rehabilitation and,
  203
Reauditorization, impairment of, and
 aphasia, 3
Recovery, changes in, 116–127
 patterns of, prognosis and, 94, 96(t)
 prognostic factors in, 127–141
 spontaneous, period of, 110–116
Redundancy, in language rehabilitation,
 200–204
Reeducation, of patients, 110
 treatment results and, 146
Reinforcement, timing of, in language
 rehabilitation, 224
Reiterative errors, in apraxia, 11
Relevance, of treatment, 262
Repetition, in language rehabilitation,
 221–222
Residual language competence, and
 aphasia, 6–8
Resonance, in dysarthria, 9
Respiration, in dysarthria, 8
Response, to language stimuli, imposed
 delay in, 218–220
Responsiveness, in nonlanguage
 behavior, 76
 in tests, 71
Retention deficit, and aphasia, 4
Revan's Coloured Progressive Matrices,
 22

Saliency, in language rehabilitation, 188
Sampling, in evaluation, 61

Schizophrenia, Minnesota Test and, 58
vs. aphasia, 27
Scoring, of tests, 71, 72(t)
Scrambled sentences, rearrangement of,
in advanced patients, 257
Seizures, aphasia and, prognosis for, 132
Selective impairment, and apraxia, 19
Self-correction, in language behavior,
73–74, 73(t)
Self-correction scale, 73(t)
Semantic association, in aphasia, 5
Semantic complexity, language
rehabilitation and, 206–207
Senile dementia, differential diagnosis
and, 58
vs. aphasia, 23
Sensory deficits, prognosis and, 135–137
Sentence stimuli, internal pauses in,
effects of, on language rehabilitation,
217–218
Sex, prognosis and, 138
Short-Direct method, of prognosis, 99
Short-term memory, delayed response
and, 219
Similes, use of, in therapy, 260
Simple aphasia, classification of, 86
Simple response mode, in treatment, 242
Sklar Aphasia Scale, 38
description of, 81
Slow rise time, and aphasia, 4
Social interaction, and evaluation, 79
Sound, characteristic, of auditory stimuli,
in rehabilitation, 192
Spastic dysarthria, 9
Speaker, position of, in therapy, 191
Speech, and aphasia, 4–6
apraxia of. See *Apraxia.*
associated problems of, prognosis and,
102–103
characteristics of, rating of, 68(t)
content unit of, 69
contextual, 65–70
in dysarthria, 9
instrumental analysis of, 20–22
performance evaluation of, 66, 67(t)
problems of, prognosis for, 102–103
vs. aphasia, 8–21
productive defects of, differentiation
using, 125
quantification of, 84(t)
sound discrimination in, presentation
rate and, 214
spontaneous, improvements in,
measurement of, 121
spontaneous recovery and, 116(t)
tasks for, 252–255
territory of, in brain, 130
Speech effectors, in Brown model, 34
Speech in action, 227
Speech performance, poor, definition of,
66

Speech therapy, prognostic factors in,
152. See also *Treatment.*
Spontaneous recovery, period of,
110–116
Spontaneous speech, measurement of,
121
Spouse, treatment and, 273
Standardized tests, and aphasia, 22
Stimulus(i), for language rehabilitation,
186–236
presentation of, scheduling of, in
treatment, 221–224
Stimulus repetition therapy, 221
Stroke, and aphasia, prognosis for, 136
aphasia treatment with, 151
Substitution errors, in apraxia, 11
Summarizing, of heard information, 257
Symbolization, impairment of, and global
aphasia, 7
Symbols, in dysarthria, vs. aphasia, 8
Syntactic aphasia, 42
Syntax, and aphasia, 44, 45
complexity of language, rehabilitation
and, 204–206
in language confusion, 25
in schizophrenia, 27

Tasks, expressive, treatment and,
251–256
for auditory comprehension, array of,
242
selection of, 239–240
for input and output, in language tests,
62
parallel, in tests, 70
Tests. See also specific test names. See
also *Evaluation.*
accuracy in, 71
approach to, 63
audiometric, for differential diagnosis,
75
completeness in, 71
consistency in, evaluation and, 84
depth of, 82
differential diagnosis and, 57–60
efficiency of, 71
for aphasia evaluation, 79–82
for divergent language behavior, 65
for evaluation, 61–79
description of, 79–82
nonstandardized, 85
of input and output tasks, 62
open-ended, for divergent language
behavior, 65
performance patterns in, 93–102
prognosis and, 85–106
promptness in, 71
quantification in, 84(t), 85
responsiveness in, 71

Tests (*Continued*)
  scoring of, 71, 72(t)
  validity of, 63
Therapy. See *Treatment.*
Thinking disorder, differential diagnosis
  of, 56, 74
Thought process disorder, aphasia as, 65
Time, processing, comprehension and,
  214–220
Token Test, 43
  auditory comprehension and, 208
  description of, 81–82
  in language appraisal, 63
Trauma, aphasia from, prognosis for, 128,
  130
Treatment, 237–278. See also *Language
  rehabilitation.*
  action commands in, 246
  adjuncts to, 268–270
  antonyms in, 253
  assessment of, 144–185
  auditory comprehension improvement
    from, 155
  Base-10 approach to, 169–170
  clinician attitude in, 231, 263
  command execution in, 246–248, 250
  content of, 225–228
  effects of, 144–185
    without controls, 145–157
  efficacy of, 154, 176
  family in, 270–275
  graduated writing tasks in, 256
  group therapy as, 264–265
  intensity of, 179
    adequacy of, 262
  language changes with, 158, 159
  language function improvement and,
    177
  length of, 178
  letter recognition in, 248
  measurement of, syntactic complexity
    and, 206
  performance criterion for, 241
  preposition use in, 255
  principles of, 260–264
  relevance of, 262
  results of, aphasia type and, 180
    auditory comprehension and,
      167–168
    case studies of, 163–175
    in bilingual patients, 170–171
    in Milan Study, 171–173
    personal accounts of, 173–175
  simple response mode for, 242
  special procedures in, 264–270
  stimuli presentation in, scheduling of,
    221–224
  studies of, with controls, 157–163
    without controls, 145–157

Treatment (*Continued*)
  task sequence in, 222
  timing of, 177
  with multiple communicative
    problems, 263

Verbal agnosia, models in, 40
Verbal amnesia, 15
Verbs, as stimuli, 243(t)
Vision, testing of, and language
  dysfunctions, 75
Visual language processing, impaired,
  test for, 62
Visual monitoring, and apraxia, 13
Visual stimuli, answering questions
  about, 255
  in language rehabilitation, 193–196
Vocabulary, selection of, in
  rehabilitation, 223

WAB, description of, 80
Weigl Sorting Test, 22
Wepman model, of language function,
  29–31, *30*
Wernicke's aphasia, differentiation of,
  125
Western Aphasia Battery, description of,
  80
  for divergent language behavior, 65
Word blindness, 41
Word deafness, and aphasia, 3
  models in, 40
Word Fluency Measure, for divergent
  semantic behavior, 65
Word Fluency Test, description of, 82
Word length, and articulation, in apraxia,
  12
  as information overload, 209
Word recognition, and aphasia, 3
Word retrieval, 5, 228
Wording, directness of, in auditory
  rehabilitation, 191
Words, as phrases, 249
  copying of, as writing task, 256
  reading of, 249
  sentence building from, 257
  sentence completion with, 252
  series of, processing of, 245
  spoken, recognition of, 242–245
Writing, and aphasia, 6
  facilitation of, 229
  quantification of, 84(t)
  spontaneous recovery and, 116(t)
  tasks of, graduated, 256
  treatment effects on, 156